The Death and Life of Psycho Syd

Part One

Foxtrot Uniform Charlie Kilo

The Death and Life of Psycho Syd

By Syd Barnes

***

This is not medical advice. It is just my tale. I cannot and do not intend to advise anyone how to treat any disease including cancer.

This journey is my recollection of events that took place which other people named or unnamed may well have different memories and different accounts of. They are all fine and decent people. I merely describe my emotions, feelings and reactions.

The publication of this book was not intended to hurt or harm anyone. So, I ask you to respect everyone in the journey even if it appears that from my perspective they are in the wrong. Realise that they have their own pain and suffering and their own reasons for acting in such a manner. Through this journey we learn that love, compassion and forgiveness is always the answer. And I love every person in this tale and hold no anger or malice towards anyone.

***

Cover Design - Eugene Lewis Barnes
Image Photo - Peter Jeffereson

ISBN: 978.183002404

Published by: Psycho Syd Publishing

Revision Two

Contents

***

Foreword

My Name is Psycho

I ask you to envisage that you are my hearty shipmate as we embark on a reckless voyage across an unexplored ocean boldly going where no ship has gone before. On the stroke of midnight, we are both grinning at each other below deck on an age-old galleon. The cold wind is pelting rain against the tiny porthole, but we are safe and sound, clutching large glasses of dark rum. The timeworn beams creak as the flickering soft light from a brass lamp casts eerie, ghostly images of ancient mariners onto the warped wooden walls. The clink of our glasses echoes as the shadowy seadogs perform their "Dead Can Dance" show on this *Night of the Living Dead*. The generous gulp of red rum gives birth to a comforting warm glow inside as our very alive eyes sparkle and join this otherworldly dance. They jig with excitement while the lust for adventure races through our veins and we head valiantly into the unknown.

And shiver me timbers me old mate, what a mind-blowing adventure I have up my salty sleeve for you. So, get your sea legs pronto, because this turbulent voyage up until December 2014 will leave you dizzy and intoxicated as we sail from heaven to hell. A harrowing journey of terminal cancer, heartache and the unnerving struggle for survival.

My aim is to inspire you to fight and never give in, even when suffocating under the most dauntingly impossible circumstances. As well as to inform poor unfortunate souls who are diagnosed with cancer or have a loved one with the dreaded big C that there are ways to improve chances of survival or even defeat the evil monster. Also, to give an insight into a happier, healthier, more spiritual and compassionate life that is out there if you open your eyes.

After numerous changes, I finished up with the title, *The Life and Death of Psycho Syd*. The final change came by way of a lady online who had proposed that we unfuck together. To be honest, it was the opposite of what I was hoping for. I believe her implication was that the planet was totally fucked, and we should join forces to do our bit to unfuck it. Sounded good to me, but a leg-over, while we put the world to rights sounded even better. She went on to suggest the reversal of life and death and so even though my dreams of a passionate encounter in the flesh were never satisfied, hey presto, we had a title; as for the chapters...each one is named after a surreally relevant song title and the credit for that goes to my own unscrewed mind.

In the tale, my nemesis is known as the Wicked Witch of the East. After all, she started all this childish name-calling by nicknaming me 'Ghost-face,' but 'what's good for the gander is good for the goose', I have since smirked in immature satisfaction.

So, why am I Psycho Syd I hear you ask? First and foremost, let me get across that I am not some violent sociopath; in fact, this Psycho is a totally non-confrontational, compassionate, caring kind of bloke. I couldn't hurt a fly. So, without further ado, let me spill the beans.

Well, we must float back to about 1972 when I was the council estate hippy in bell-bottomed blue jeans, colourful tie-dyed t-shirts and long, flowing, blonde hair. I stuck out like a rainbow butterfly next to my hard, thorny mates who were either skinheads or 'suedeheads' and was nicknamed Psychedelic Syd. Cheeky young 'Manc' scallywags would scream and taunt "Weirdy, weirdo", but it didn't disturb my love and peace philosophy; in fact, I loved it as I proudly sauntered by dreaming of beach buggies and overland trips to India whilst humming Syd Barrett tunes. "Those Were the Days."

Next, we trip forward to the eighties when Psychedelic Syd spun the vinyl in the local nightclub; The Doors, Pink Floyd, Hendrix, The Stones and Hawkwind were played to the local hippies. The lights flashed while the colourful flower-power mob freaked-out as aromatic whiffs of patchouli and marijuana flavoured the smoky air.

A few years later I was the superstar DJ blasting out the latest alternative sounds. The Sisters of Mercy, Joy Division, The Pogues, The Smiths and Alien Sex Fiend were always on the playlist. Psychedelic was chopped to Psycho to suit the genre and the name has stuck like superglue ever since. My mother told me to her horror she sometimes heard people whisper, "There's Psycho's mum". I loved it. Norman Bates was alive and well and living in Chorlton-cum-Hardy, Manchester 21.

And another thing. It is a blooming miracle that you have this book in your hand. Some people thought that it would never happen. In a desperate effort to escape a hand-to-mouth existence on benefits I came up with the bright idea of writing a book. I was suffering with chronic fatigue because of my radiotherapy damaged thyroid and I was officially classified as unemployable. Scribbling my harrowing tale was the only option open to me. I dreamt that I could beat the cancer and have a best-selling book too, giving me and my kids a brand-new start. Only one problem; I had never written anything before.

Undeterred, I started in June 2015 expecting to finish within 12 months, but it took nearly four years. I hadn't considered the never-ending housework, taking care of my kids and how very sick I was. Revisiting that soul-destroying period played havoc with my shattered mind. The trauma of sifting through photographs and videos from both the torturous cancer battle as well as earlier happier times left me crushed and broken. I would stare at my laptop screen as rivers of tears ran down my face. Awakening in the dead of night in a cold sweat from a distressing nightmare, either about dying of cancer or being betrayed by the woman I loved was part and parcel of writing my tale of woe. It was an almighty slog, but I did it. And before the official publication was launched, I had sold almost 1,700 pre-publication copies that I had printed. Not half bad for an unknown nobody, hey?

But back to today. I'm a single dad raising a small son, (my elder lad is now at university) having lived through the most crushingly abusive relationship you could possibly imagine. I have two children living overseas too. I'm a plant-powered cancer survivor; I'm Psycho Syd. So, join me on an incredible journey to the centre of my mind, with so many out-of-the-blue shocks, twists and turns that it will leave you gobsmacked in disbelief. A little word of warning my loyal companion; the first seven chapters will be smooth sailing but once we reach 'chapter eight' wear your lifejacket and cling on for dear life because we will be battered by *The Perfect Storm*. Believe me, you're in for one hell of a trip.

I Hope You Die

(November 2012)

"Ghost-face, hurry up and die," screamed my wife.

What on earth was going on? Did she really say that, or had I lost the plot completely and just imagined it? After all, I had spent weeks living in chemical la-la land after a mind-bending concoction of chemotherapy drugs had been pumped into my dying frame. But that foggy nightmare of toxic madness had dissipated a few months back, awakening me to the brutal reality of terminal cancer. I was a death warmed-up bag of bones, sprawled half-comatose on a second-hand cream sofa in cold, rainy Blackpool, with stage four mouth cancer and a prognosis of just six months.

It was November 2012 and I was a burnt skeleton in complete agony after suffering the most unbelievably painful treatment, just to give me an outside chance of breathing in and out for a few months more. The skin around my neck was black and blistered, with scabs which oozed vile, foul-smelling pus. Yet that was nothing compared to my mouth's interior; red raw and swollen, it gave me the excruciating sensation of swallowing scalding water 24/7. The morphine hardly touched it.

The radiotherapy had destroyed my saliva glands and zapped most of my taste buds. No problem, because eating was out of the question. I had to keep myself alive to the fact that I was dying by pouring beige-coloured, sweet-smelling liquid into a peg tube in my stomach. I took sips of water, but each tiny droplet stung like acid, leading me to tightly grip the side of the sofa as I writhed in pain. The chunks of choked-up slimy blood-soaked phlegm that landed with a heavy splat in the bile-coloured, hospital bucket seemed infinite.

I was so weak and fragile and just gazed at my spouse in disbelief.

"You are so ugly, I am ashamed to be near you. I am not your wife; I am single," she spat. "You ugly Ghost-face, hurry up and die."

I stared at my spouse in horror as a white-hot dagger of pain stabbed the shiny scarlet flesh inside my burnt mouth. I looked down to a point on the floor where drops of pus had dripped from one of my open wounds. Finally, I gazed deep inside my mind to the ghastly realisation that as the cancer killed my body, my wife was murdering my soul.

Living in the Past

(1956 to 1988)

A red-faced baby screamed blue murder in a cot further down the maternity ward, crying out the bragging rights as the hellish Manchester United Red Devils defeated God's own team; the angelic sky-blue Manchester City. This was the day Psycho Syd drew his first breath and if that wasn't an omen of the forthcoming shit, I would have to undergo, then I don't know what was. It was 22nd September 1956 when I entered this life painfully, feet first. My tiny mind had already concluded that it wasn't too keen on yet another distressing ride on the Samsara merry-go-round of birth, ageing, sickness and death. The failure to reach Nirvana plus the bad karma from my previous life determined that I was born wailing at this breach of justice. I had no alternative but to endure yet another lifetime of suffering. I must reach enlightenment this time around to bypass a further unhappy spin on the big wheel of life, and instead live blissfully in seventh heaven as a larger-than-life spiritual being.

Well let's get down to brass tacks: I was brought up in Chorlton-cum-Hardy, South Manchester. It was a case of private house to council house then back to private house. My dad was a gardener and my mum a care worker. Two younger brothers followed in my footsteps. It was a warm, happy, loving family and holidays were spent in Blackpool and Rhyl, but I loathed those tacky holiday resorts, always preferring the wild mountains and moors. Two significant life-changing events occurred during my early years.

First there was my point-blank refusal, at the age of five, and as a member of a meat-scoffing family, to eat animals. I loved animals and just couldn't fathom how we could eat them if we loved them. Luckily, I was permitted to be a veggie in a meat-loving family in those 'vegetarian is unhealthy, weird and uncool' days. I have never eaten meat since and my parents became veggies too.

The second development was my dad taking a football-hating me to see a match when I was eight years old. I reluctantly went to watch Manchester City play Coventry City in a League Cup tie on 13th October 1965 and loved every minute of it. My team lost 3-2 but "The Sound of the Crowd", the energy, the noise and the floodlights mesmerised me. I was a fanatic from that moment.

School was always playtime, so I never tried, never completed any homework and was eventually expelled for having long hair. Next there was college for more fun and games, and it was a water into wine occasion when I managed to achieve two GCE 'O' levels. I had a list of jobs that would fit into an early Clash track - petrol pump attendant, factory worker, warehouseman, solicitor's clerk, transport manager, DJ, labourer and truck driver (but not a bus driver, ambulance man or ticket inspector).

Then I eventually opened my eyeballs and saw the folly of working to get pissed at weekends and clock-watching in a shit job, just to bring to life the vision of a three-week-long summer holiday away from Manchester. I knew there and then, that there had to be more to life than drowning in a 'dull as dishwater' office or factory; I had to break free.

Music was an essential ingredient in my "Lust for Life," changing direction, when I was 15 years old and I swapped my collection of top 10 singles for Island's double compilation sampler LP, interestingly named *El Pea*. As my feet terminated tapping to cheesy pop tunes, my skull began undulating to the strange new sounds of The Incredible String Band, Jethro Tull and Quintessence. The psychedelic phase of long hair and flower-power shirts quickly followed in a spaced-out dreamworld of Pink Floyd, Jimi Hendrix and The Doors. Next it was the raw energy of punk rock as I pogoed to The Sex Pistols, The Clash and The Buzzcocks. Up popped the alternative music scene which I embraced with open arms, turning on to bands like The Sisters of Mercy, The Cult and The Jesus and Mary Chain. Of course, it is only natural that I have a soft spot for *Madchester* [Manchester music scene] bands such as: The Smiths, The Stone Roses, Oasis, Joy Division, The Chemical Brothers and New Order. All in in all, my love of music has helped me dance, sing, laugh and cry through this insane roller-coaster of a life.

Another part of my lust for life was the opposite sex and I have been lucky enough to have had a love-life, many rock stars would be envious of. Now don't go getting the wrong end of my rhythm stick by presuming that I was a heartless "Wham Bam Thank You Ma'am" rotter; nothing could be further from the truth, because I was kind and loving. I confess to falling head over heels at the drop of a hat or a pair of scanty panties, eternally wearing my heart on my psychedelic shirtsleeve. Of course, I always ended up distraught to say the least, wishing one vital organ was no longer pumping and another less vital organ still was.

After two broken hearts, the initial caused by my first love who married my friend, and the second by a girl I was with for a year (who

6

dumped me for a woman), I decided that enough was enough and it was high time to travel the planet. So, in 1988 I hauled my heavy backpack and my even heavier crushed heart to sunny Singapore with the vague intention of returning overland to rainy Manchester.

The worldly pleasures of sex and drugs and pints of beer were left behind as my *Journey to the East* was a spiritual quest to seek the truth and heal my broken heart. On my first day in the orient I visited a small Chinese shrine. I sat as quiet as a temple mouse in this deserted place of worship as brilliant rays of sunlight from the half-open door reflected off an almighty golden Buddha illuminating the left side of this sacred building. *I was in the dark but maybe I was beginning to see the light,* I chuckled. I breathed in the potent twirls of sweet-scented smoke from the dozen burning incense sticks which were standing upright in a shiny brass pot. Concentrating on the buzzing and humming of nearby busy insects invoked a peaceful sensation of "Right Here Right Now". This otherworldly atmosphere awakened me to the sad realisation that most people sleep right through their whole lives; they never open their eyes. I left this holy structure with a gentle wise smile on my serene face. Then I asked myself, "Where is my Mind?"

Hello, I am "Right Here Waiting for You", it replied. *What about your true love who left you?,* it taunted. *You will never find another girl like her you know, and your broken heart will last forever,* it laughed.

I understood that my thoughts were unreal, and that they only created pain and suffering because I allowed them to. I must stop playing "Mind Games" with my very own spiteful mind. In fact, maybe it would be better if I lost my mind!

Each day was spent travelling by bus or train, locating a cheap guesthouse, buying some vegetarian food, with a spot of sightseeing thrown in for good measure. However, the highlight was taking refuge in a temple, a church or a mosque for thirty minutes to live in the moment. I would sit silently, focusing on my breath, the droplets of sweat on my skin and the whisper of the distant traffic. It did me the world of good leaving my crazy mind with its painful thoughts at the door of each sanctuary, but I always knew that it would return with a vengeance once I stepped outside. Nevertheless, I stuck firmly to my pursuit of inner wisdom for a full two weeks.

Then in the humid heat of the Cameron Highlands, Malaysia, recalling the tales old soldiers used to dreamily weave in my local back home, I gave into temptation and sampled my first Tiger beer. The soldiers would wax lyrical about this magical brew they'd supped during the war. The next blurry, painful recollection was the fully deserved, fallen angel hangover from hell, along with the piss-taking wisecracks bouncing around my banging skull from the trio of backpacking buddies I shared the cheap room with. They cried with laughter as they mimicked a Mancunian beer monster urinating in the corner of the hostel room during the night. At this point I mouthed those immortal words "never a-fucking-gain". No more insane drinking and no more literally pissing my travelling funds up against the wall.

After a tiring, humid, shirt-soaked third-class train journey my hot, frazzled body arrived in Georgetown, Penang. Upon eyeballing a massage parlour my jaded mind elected that my ready-to-drop-dead body warranted a refreshing treat. I was genuinely astonished when a scantily clad, slim young female appeared in the intimate air-conditioned room. I am telling the honest to God's truth, cross my heart and hope to die. I thought I was just going for a massage. I had, God forbid, never paid for or visited a lady of the night or even a lady of the hot tropical day in all my life.

Well, this seductively sensual Goddess of the East commenced to gently caress my trembling hairy chest before placing her perfect heavenly face so conveniently close to mine. Her inky black eyes gazed passionately into my mesmerised sky-blue peepers, which were also having a double-time eyeful of an advancing pair of bewitching eye magnets, inciting my council estate eyes to virtually explode out of my enraptured throbbing head. A jet-black tidal wave of long lustrous flowing hair cascaded, kissed and licked my scared-stiff face before her moist, blazing red. lips arousingly parted, whispering the enticing erotic pleasures up for grabs. Well blow me down! The universe had spoken, and I stood proudly to attention, ready to obey every command. I was spellbound and powerless to resist this out-of-this-world oriental Venus

"By Jupiter!" I chirped a short time later as I moonwalked out of the building with giant steps into the steamy, sticky hotness. I felt like a super-cool Englishman out in the midday sun as I grinned like a mad dog with my new-found knowledge: a coupling of spiritual and physical bliss is the method required to satisfy the conditions needed to attain enlightenment.

I spent the remainder of this four-month quest visiting temples, jungles, mountains and islands during the hot, tropical daytime and sultry, oriental girlfriends during the steamy passionate nights. I also got wasted on opium with a hill tribe in Northern Thailand and was spaced out for three days, thus successfully partaking in the three activities I had initially planned to avoid. The trip was a massive success because my realisation that spiritual and physical rapture was the way to Shangri-La had cured my broken heart.

Sugar Sugar

(1988-1994)

I returned to rainy old Manchester and instantly decided that my mind, spirit, body, soya meat and two veg firmly belonged in the Far East. Three months later I started teaching English as a foreign language to adults in Bangkok, Thailand and loved it. I was a fast learner and swiftly became a successful, popular instructor.

I recall one of my students, an extremely sweet lady named Honey, attending class one day wearing a very short, tight black mini-skirt and a tight black t-shirt, with the words 'A bob a job I'll suck your knob' screaming out their message in bright yellow letters across the front. I was speechless for once but didn't embarrass her by translating the X-rated phrase but do admit to crying into my coffee during the break because all my British coins were still in the UK! It will come as no surprise to learn that Honey became teacher's pet for the remainder of the term.

Life in the City of Angels was everything I had ever dreamt of. This densely populated city with its magnificent temples, towering skyscrapers and 'nudge, nudge, wink wink, say no more' nightlife captivated me. In all honesty I hardly ever bothered with the seedy sins of the flesh scene and would usually be found watching a live band or playing pool in my local, the Saxophone Pub. This vibrant trendy venue was just a 10-minute stagger away from my small studio apartment, which in turn was only a five-minute stroll from my workplace. No gridlocked rush hour madness for me!

I took to teaching like a pen to paper, meticulously planning each lesson before giving a powerful, entertaining and educational delivery. I looked forward to going to work, which made a welcome change. The happy-go-lucky Bangkokians seemed oblivious to the intense heat, insane traffic jams and never-ending chaos as they smiled with a good-natured '*Mai pen rai*' (never mind) acceptance. I pictured myself as an almost handsome devil in this heavenly city of angels and was having a hell of a time.

Well, this horny devil soon met and dated a horny angel, named Ladda after a species of flower. We met in the Saxophone Pub and she later revealed the bare-naked truth that it was my vegetarian lifestyle that had first attracted her; well that was an eye-opener coz I had always thought it was my good looks! She was an attractive, intelligent office worker in her mid-twenties who was fluent in English. However, we generally communicated in Thai because I was determined to learn the lingo, thus enabling me to interact with the locals without having to resort to a frustrating game of charades. After work, we would meet at a restaurant for a romantic dinner before dashing back to my pad for another climatic happy ending to one more mind-blowing day in Bangkok.

After just three months this blossoming relationship was sadly nipped in the bud with the tragic news that my father was dying of stomach cancer. Without delay I returned to Blackpool in the UK, where my parents had just relocated. This was a distressing, heartbreaking period of my life, as I crumbled inside while my poor old dad wasted away before finally passing on. A steady flow of letters from Ladda arrived pledging everlasting love. After heavy-hearted goodbyes to my poor mother and two brothers, I flew back to Bangkok with the pain buried deep inside. I hid my sorrow as invisible teardrops ran down my cheery face. Sometimes, the grief would bite with such ferocity that I would sit alone trembling as mournful tears blinded my eyes.

I recouped my old apartment, my old job and gave my not-so-old girlfriend a surprise call on the blower. The anticipated whoops of ecstatic hot glee never arrived, as I was brushed off with the cold shoulder. A flustered Ladda mumbled that she was extremely busy and couldn't meet me until next week. Not being as *Thick as a Brick*, I concluded that this unexpected snub undoubtedly implied that I had been dumped for a new partner. Elementary my dear Psycho!

This was not the time for beating around the bush, so my inner Sherlock Holmes responded with, "It is clearly obvious that you are not already on your way here because you have found a new lover."

Like a trapped Baskerville hound, she barked, "How dare you say that Peter. I never tell lies."

I slowly and very deliberately stressed each word out loud, "I-am-not-Peter - I-am-Syd."

The small mirror on my bedside cabinet reflected a self-satisfied smirk back to my triumphant eyes. I winked at my alter ego, imagining myself pacing the floor, dressed in a purple dressing gown whilst puffing on an old black pipe. The silence dragged on as I sat on the bed, praying that my halo wouldn't strangle me. Ladda apologised and confessed that Peter, who was her new boss in the golf shop where she was employed, was also her new boyfriend. I nonchalantly wished her good luck before carefully putting the phone down. I stared back into the mirror and grinned from ear to ear because I could already see the sensual beauty, smell the heady perfume, taste the intoxicating nectar, hear the lustful whispers and feel the stimulating touch of the next pretty petal that I would pick from this exotic flowerbed.

You don't have to be a supersleuth with a magnifying glass and a pair of binoculars to detect that another romantic flower arrangement was just around the corner. The fragrance of freshly baked bread and the scent of coffee floated in the air of the fashionable bakery a few doors down from my workplace. I sat at a small table by the window getting my caffeine kick from a latte and my nicotine fix from a cancer stick. The carefree chatter and spontaneous laughter from a cluster of university students filled this popular eatery with free-spirited optimism. They were immaculately dressed in their uniforms; the boys in white shirts and black trousers and the girls in white blouses and black skirts. Their youthful aspirations of love, lust and adventure were contagious, instantaneously infecting me with the very same fever. I didn't want to grow up.

I took one more deep drag on my cigarette and gazed outside, fixating on the bumper-to-bumper cars, buses and tuk-tuks making their stop-start progress along the busy main road. I pitied the perspiring motorcyclists struggling to make progress in the stifling heat and felt fortunate sitting in the air-conditioned atmosphere. I looked back towards the happy students and caught the eye of a slim young lady sitting at the adjacent table. We both smiled. She had long dark hair and was wearing a cream t-shirt and a shiny black satin skirt. I grabbed the opportunity to practice my smattering of Thai and I was glad that I had made the effort to learn it because she couldn't speak a word of English. From what I could gather she was unemployed and living with her elder sister in the north of the city.

My smidgeon of Thai must have been impressive because she agreed to a date the following evening. I danced home and transformed my one-room bombsite into a one-room love nest in the hope of attracting this pretty bird. A stylish vase of flowers, a pair of scented candles and a bloody good tidy up and hey, abracadabra, this wizard was ready to wave his magic wand and say the magic words; "open sesame!" However, I wasn't a heartless 'love em and leave em' lowlife merely after a conquest for a notch on my bedpost; I was seeking that elusive "Together Forever" true love partnership. Could she be the one? Possibly, because the first date was a cloud nine dream for this pair of high-flying love birds. Future

12

dates quickly followed with visits to the cinema, nights out in the pub, romantic walks in the park or just back to my place for a take-away dinner, a film and of course a fair bit of slap and tickle. So far so good.

A couple of weeks later Ladda waltzed into my apartment announcing that it was over with Mr Golf and that she was ready to walk hand in hand down the fairway with me again. With immense sorrow I let the cat out of the bag that there would be no future holes in one with me because I had met a new partner. This beautiful flower instantly mutated into a tree; a weeping willow! Karma can be a cruel bastard, but I didn't laugh loudest because I can never take pleasure in another's pain.

My new lady turned up at my flat looking flummoxed after having had an almighty row with her sister. She begged to move in with me until things were resolved, to which I readily agreed. After just a few weeks of living together I fell out of love with her. I knew there and then that we would never be compatible. The honeymoon was over, baby. Sharing a room 24/7 with a partner was a whole different ball game to having a candlelit dinner in the evening or visiting a temple on a Sunday afternoon before kissing goodbye until the next date. I couldn't quite put my finger on it, but the feeling of love had scarpered with its tail between its legs.

I decided to break the news as gently as possible by making it clear that I just wasn't ready to cohabit with anyone. Before I had the opportunity to deliver the painful words my lady greeted me with the happiest smile I had ever witnessed in my life, before declaring that she was pregnant. Oh my God, I was going to be a father, but the mother was a woman I hardly knew and even worse a woman I didn't love. I remained in this loveless relationship out of obligation, providing full support for the expectant mother and my unborn child. I felt imprisoned and reflected that my partner was indeed a flower; a Venus flytrap. Although I never blamed her because it takes two. I blamed my cocksure self for not bothering to use a condom, naively believing that it would never happen to me.

Nonetheless, I was excitedly looking forward to becoming a father for the very first time. Eight long months later my first child, a son, Eric Jay, released his introductory scream on planet Earth. And I guarantee that the jaw-dropping shock he delivers later in our adventure will leave you utterly gob-smacked. I was a loving father and a friendly partner during this challenging period, dutifully taking mother and son out for meals, shopping and sightseeing. It was tragic because she really loved me but sadly, I just didn't feel the same way.

***

Just under two years later the relationship was at long last "Dead and Buried" when I was offered the position of English teacher at a large sugar factory in north-eastern Thailand. It was like being handed the keys to my prison cell. The factory was right out in the sticks near the tiny village of Phu Khieo in Chaiyaphum province. I breathed a massive sigh of relief upon escaping the madness and pollution of Bangkok and a romance which had become as cold as a slaughterman's heart. I was as free as a released cage bird; eager to spread my wings and explore the mountains and forests of this wild landscape. I sprawled on my bed chirping with joy in my spiffy apartment.

The vegetarian breakfasts, lunches and dinners in the company canteen were supplemented with heaps of delicious fresh fruit scored from the local market. In the evenings I would either play tennis, football or snooker or just chill in my room listening to tunes. As well as teaching the factory staff I taught in the local primary school and gave tailor-made language lessons to the police and the medical staff at the nearby hospital. This newfound lifestyle was a breath of fresh air after two years of suffocating in my Bangkok jailhouse.

As an empathetic bloke I sympathised with my partner, understanding that she was suffering with a broken heart while I was jumping for joy. Sadly, this is usually the norm when a romance bites the dust; one partner is singing in heaven whilst the other is screaming in hell. Nothing is ever perfect in life, as the ache inside painfully confirmed... I was missing my son. I had no option other than to catch the overnight train to Bangkok each Friday evening to spend some quality 'dad and lad' time with Eric Jay. We had loads of fun as I spoilt him rotten with presents, afternoons of swimming, pizza and lots and lots of love. I treated my ex with compassion and kindness without giving her any false hope that the romance could ever be rekindled. On Sunday evening I would jump on the overnight train, ready for an "All Things Bright and Beautiful" Monday morning back at work.

After about six months my ex agreed to let Eric Jay live with me at the sugar factory. My first taste of life as a single dad was made easier with the help of a part-time nanny. I took good loving care of him in the evening as we watched cartoons together before I read him a bedtime story. Each weekend was an adventure as father and son bonded in nearby cities, towns and national parks. We ate in restaurants, walked up mountains, bathed in waterfalls and played hide and seek in forests. Our weekend breaks would always include a backpacker hangout for some western food and a welcome chinwag with intrepid travellers.

***

One of those mind-boggling events that sticks in your mind for the rest of your life occurred when we visited the quiet city of Loei. After a night in a cheap guest house we hit the road in search of a café. Sharing my wanderlust with Eric Jay was a great buzz and we were both ready for a filling breakfast before exploring the place. I wasn't optimistic about chancing upon any backpackers for my much-needed fix of Caucasian chitchat in this neck of the woods. It was well off the tourist trail; besides a couple of temples, a night market and a Chinese vegan café there was not an awful lot to do.

The blackboard outside a small shop which had coffee, tea, chocolate pancakes, muesli and ice-cold beer neatly written in yellow chalk was a sight for sore eyes, and hungry bellies too. We stepped inside this funky eatery and to my delight I spotted a smartly dressed young western man wearing a light-blue short-sleeved shirt and long cream trousers. We nodded to each other but there was something about him that was unnerving; he looked like he had just seen a ghost.

We made ourselves comfy on a timeworn green sofa before ordering vegetarian fried rice and a fresh orange juice for Eric Jay and beans on toast and a hot coffee for me. Large portraits of the King and Queen were prominent above the counter while Pornthip, the Thai girl who had won Miss Universe 1988, smiled at me from a colourful poster on the wall opposite. I scanned other posters of temples, waterfalls and Buddhist monks before browsing through some tired-looking guidebooks and novels on the shelf behind me.

"Hotel California" was playing in the background as I stole another peek at the young man; he really did look out of sorts. Curiosity eventually got the better of me as I chirped, "Hiya, mate, I am Syd and I live locally." Followed by the classic backpacker ice-breaker, "Where have you been and where are you going?"

He looked up with a shy smile and replied, "I have been to Bangkok and I am just here relaxing before deciding where to go next."

"Wow - Bangkok is something else; I bet you had a fabulous time," I responded enthusiastically.

"I didn't really see much of it to be honest," was his sombre reply.

I had my heart in my mouth as he recounted a shocking turn of events. He was a student from south-east England and had decided to spend a couple of months backpacking around Thailand. His very first night in Bangkok had been spent drinking with an Indian looking chap who had befriended him. His next hazy recollection was waking up in a hospital bed with drips in both arms. Obviously, his drink had been spiked because his passport, travellers' cheques and $100 had vanished. He endured two further days in a foggy blur drifting in and out of sleep, before being discharged from his sickbed. The British Embassy had provided an emergency passport and his travellers' cheques had been reimbursed. He'd made the gutsy resolution to resume his adventure but opted to sidestep the tourist hot spots, preferring to convalesce at a secluded location in the back of beyond.

Crikey! No wonder he appeared vacant and on edge. I sympathised with him and admired his stiff upper lip fortitude. What an appalling start to a dream holiday. Sometimes life can be a right bastard as our dreams are obliterated by a cruel twist of fate.

I ordered another coffee as a smiling south Asian bloke entered the café. A chair hit the floor with an almighty crash as my new friend leapt up and screamed, "That's the bastard." The newcomer's warm smile was instantly wiped off his face and replaced with an open-mouthed look of terror. He turned and fled for dear life with the English student hot on his heels. I sat frozen in astonishment. What the flipping heck had I just witnessed. Un-bloody-believable. Half an hour later two laid-back police officers, the enraged student and the now frantic south Asian man entered the eatery. Being the only person fluent in both languages, I was given the task of translating.

"To Cut a Long Story Short" the thief was from Bangladesh and had been financing his life on the road by drugging lone travellers before stealing their possessions. He was in tears pleading for mercy, explaining that as a poor Bangladeshi this was the only way he could see the world. The police eyed him with disgust prior to handcuffing him and carting him off. The student thanked me before heading to the cop-shop to give a statement. The likely outcome would be a lengthy spell in the monkey house for the villain and a feeling of retribution for the English bloke.

"Isn't Life Strange?" The probability of them meeting again in a tiny café in one of the least visited places in Thailand was next to nothing. On second thoughts, maybe the thief had come up with the clever idea of lying low in this out-of-the-way spot to ensure he didn't bump into his victim. Karma had other ideas.

There She Goes

(1994 to 2000)

Two years later the sweet gig at the sugar company was over, so I took up teaching at a language centre in the nearby city of Khon Kaen. This dynamic urban sprawl not only had cinemas, shopping centres and nightclubs but a sprinkling of ex-pats and western hangouts too. I instantly made friends with a group of Brits who I occasionally joined for a few beers. I was provided with a fully furnished detached house which I shared with two other teachers; a skinny Jewish lady from Manchester and her athletic Kenyan boyfriend. She confessed that she was a full-on rebel, only dating Arabs and Africans to piss-off her religiously devout mother. Her competitive nature meant that I faced an unholy tantrum whenever I beat her at scrabble, however we were single-minded teammates when tackling formidable cryptic crossword puzzles. Eric Jay joined me and was having a wonderful time in his new home and he had a new nanny to boot. Sometimes he would spend a week or two with his mother in Bangkok, which was fine by me because he needed us both.

Once again, I excelled at teaching and once again I fell libido over brain in love. This time I was smitten by a lady who had finished university and was studying English to boost her employment prospects. After just three months we relocated to a comfy apartment in Bangkok while Eric Jay moved back in with his mum. This was not an issue because her house was just a stone's throw away. I would visit him daily and once or twice a week take him to the cinema, a café or we'd go for a day out.

I kept the wolves from the door by teaching business English in nearby companies while my other half managed an upmarket beauty centre in a large shopping mall. This whirlwind romance ended up in wedlock just a couple of months later. Only Eric Jay joined us at the wedding ceremony because my missus' family were not "Dancing in the Street" at the thought of their daughter tying the knot with a foreigner.

The relationship had its fair share of ups and downs and ins and outs, nevertheless, we were still together one year later when we decided to relocate to England. The bright idea was to set up a travel company for Thai tourists visiting the UK. Alas, Eric Jay's mother would not permit him to join us, so I wished him goodbye and promised to keep in touch. It was comforting to know that in these modern times he was only a 12-

hour flight away if he ever needed me.

We stayed with my mother at the Wildlife Hotel in Blackpool. My parents had bought it with the vision of opening the very first vegetarian B&B in this popular seaside resort. I honestly assumed that a vegetarian hotel in this vulgar hotdog and beefburger daft destination would undoubtedly wind up as a sad lonely white elephant. As revealed in the previous chapter my father was diagnosed with advanced stomach cancer. This shocking event occurred just a few weeks after moving into the hotel and my poor father tragically died before he had time to live his dream. This unforeseen catastrophic slice of rotten luck had cruelly smashed his ambition to run a business with his lifelong partner.

Life can be so damn cruel at times, can't it? The Grim Reaper can snatch your breath away just when your dreams have come true. Started your perfect job, married your soul mate, relocated to your ideal location or had that baby you had been trying to conceive for so long? Well enjoy the moment, but never forget that the angel of death has a nasty habit of showing its morbid face when least expected. Nothing is permanent. After losing her husband my heartbroken mother picked up the pieces of her broken life and single-handedly created a successful business. There were guests most nights of the year and during the summer months it was often fully booked. I was so proud of her and I'm sure my dad was too as he beamed with pride in his heavenly abode.

The Wildlife Vegetarian Hotel stood out on this busy road with of over 100 hotels. You couldn't fail to spot the colourful front window mural with its dazzling array of foxes, sheep, pigs, cows, squirrels and owls. This eye-catching piece of artwork had been painstakingly completed by members of an animal rights group that held monthly meetings in the front lounge. The bedrooms were small but impeccably clean with modern showers. Once you stepped through the door of this little oasis you were greeted with an overwhelming sensation of calmness. The friendly ghost of compassion haunted this peace-loving haven as it uplifted your spirit to the higher realm of loving kindness. The breakfast was a massive serving of vegan sausages, tomatoes, mushrooms, baked beans and hash browns plus as much cereal, toast, fresh orange juice, coffee and tea as you could manage. Well done mum for proving me wrong; a shiny gold star for you.

My wife and I made the large room on the top floor home. This was where we would sleep, shower and watch TV. My other half became addicted to soaps such as *Coronation Street*, *EastEnders* and *Emmerdale*

Farm. I suppose they were easy to follow and had enough drama to keep her on tenterhooks until the next episode. The hotel kitchen was where we cooked and stored our food. We both helped mum serve the breakfasts and clean the rooms as well as designing tours for potential visitors.

The tour company began to take off and we led two groups of Thai visitors around the UK, visiting London, Nottingham, Blackpool, Chester, Conway and Bath. We excelled at supplying the Thais with a perfect holiday because, with my fluency in the language and deep understanding of the culture along with a Thai national as a partner, we knew just what they were looking for.

As fate would have it the economy in the Far East collapsed and suddenly the Thais no longer had any spare cash for holidays in the UK, leaving me with no alternative but to close the company. Shit happens. I became a telephone salesman but hated it, then a bread delivery van driver but my sleepy eyes weren't over the moon about the 4 am start. I finally settled for the freewheeling life of a cabbie. I loved driving and had always got on well with people, so it suited me down to the ground. Of course, I was homesick for my exotic life in the tropics, but I had to make the most of things in bloody Blackpool.

We not only slept, showered and watched TV in our room but there was a fair bit of monkey business too, so it should come as no surprise when you hear that Eugene Lewis, my second child, was born in 1997. I was there at his birth and what a magical moment that was. I was a doting dad with my little lad and carried on bringing the vegan bacon home as a taxi driver.

One Sunday afternoon, a lovely elderly couple riding in my taxi offered me a teaching position in China and without hesitation I pounced on this golden opportunity to fly across the sky away from my tedious routine in Blackpool. My other half wasn't champing at the bit for a new life in the land of the red dragon, but my wanderlusty feet were already itching for yet another intrepid adventure. We said farewell to mum who wished us luck. She joyfully continued living her dream; running the vegan hotel and fighting for the animals.

***

When Eugene was 10 months old, we arrived at Nanshan Foreign Language School in Shenzhen. Shenzhen was a ginormous modern city in mainland China about 30 minutes away from Hong Kong. This crowded metropolis of skyscrapers and shopping malls had an estimated population of 23 million. We rented a swanky fully furnished three-bedroomed ground floor apartment in the tranquil port of Shekou.

Shekou, which translates to mouth of the snake, acquired its name due to the shape of its harbour. This quaint seaside location on the southern tip of the city was something else. It gave off a kind of uncrowded holiday resort vibration. Dipping one's toes in the South China Sea whilst gazing at Hong Kong in the hazy distance was a must-do experience. Feeling the warm zephyrs brushing against your skin as you breathed in the salty seaside air was exhilarating. Upon turning around, you were left open-mouthed in awe as you beheld the green rolling hills gently hugging this charming settlement.

The cluster of western restaurants and bars included an Irish pub which surprisingly sold the cream of Manchester; *Boddingtons Bitter*. We bought many of our supplies from a tiny store which had a selection of western produce for the foreign devils who had made this gorgeous suburb home. I was chuffed to bits with the variety of vegan options that were up for grabs including my favourite; the yummy plant-based sausages. And finally, the modern high-speed ferry which departed from this port on its one-hour journey to Hong Kong was a huge plus. Indulging in a leisurely trip across the water for a day of British shopping in stores such as Woolworths and Marks and Sparks was a piece of vegan cake.

I buzzed as I taught English to large classes of primary school kids, who devoured nursery rhymes, new vocabulary, basic conversation and grammar with hungry enthusiasm. I recall dropping into the school canteen for lunch on the first day and ordering rice with steamed vegetables. I was aghast observing the Chinese staff matter-of-factly tearing and chewing the flesh off bones before flinging the meatless remains to the centre of the table. As a vegetarian, this corpse-munching knocked me for six. I somehow managed to finish my food without throwing up over the mountain of pig, cow and chicken bones that was steadily growing before my horror-stricken eyes.

As you can imagine I never visited the school canteen again, preferring to nip home for a fried tofu sandwich or a delicious vegan curry served up by my tasty better half. One memorable lunchtime I wasn't greeted by my wife holding a plate of vegan goodness but was met with a big smile of carnal badness and a seductive wink as she purred, "I want another baby."

I slowly began unzipping my neatly-pressed grey trousers before calmly oozing, "Your wish is my command."

Three weeks later she was pregnant and on August 7th, 1999, I was presented with a gorgeous baby daughter; Francesca Emma. By coincidence, it was my wife's birthday too, so I didn't need to fork out for a present because I had already splashed out nine months earlier, hadn't I? Ha-ha. I stopped teaching at the primary school to launch a language centre in equal partnership with a cool Taiwanese guy called Alex. The English courses were extremely popular, but they were merely the bread and dairy-free butter, because the serious spondulicks came from the generous commission received from British boarding schools for recruiting Chinese students.

***

My marital life wasn't a bed of red romantic roses though; more like a bed of painful sharp thorns. The relationship had broken down; we were civil with each other but were now sleeping in separate bedrooms. My sexy playmate would play no more. The only escape from the cold shoulder was the heart-warming joy of witnessing my kids playing happily together. I recollect an extraordinary evening when I decided to take my 'thorn in its side' body out for a few pints of *Boddingtons Bitter* at the local pub. As I was leaving my wife smiled prior to passing me two condoms.

With my usual laddish banter, I quipped, "Sorry love, I don't have time because I am off out for a beer."

She laughed, "Don't be silly, they are not for me. We are not sleeping together now so maybe you should find a Chinese girl and have a good time."

"Don't be bloody daft," I barked. "If you think I am going out to pull a woman after all the shit I have had with you then you need your flipping head testing." She laughed once more before insisting that I took the rubber johnnies with me. I rolled my eyes shrugging my shoulders before placing the contraceptives in a small compartment of my shabby wallet and strolled out into the warm tropical night without a second thought.

It was Friday night and the Irish boozer was full of its regular mishmash of Chinese and western party animals. I ordered a pint of *'Boddies'* and cheese on toast with chips and baked beans. I got chatting to an overweight Canadian man who was also standing at the bar. He had been here for a week searching for a teaching job. He left me flabbergasted when he drooled, "Jeez, have you seen that Thai bird who walks about town. The one with the long hair and legs up to her armpits. Man, she is so sexy. I have dirty dreams about her."

I smirked as I smugly replied, "I see her every day and every night because she is my wife."

He looked bewildered, instantly apologising before enviously expressing, "You lucky swine."

"Not as lucky as you think, mate," I laughed. "We have been married for six years and have two kids. However, it has been rocky and at present, we are sleeping in separate rooms. In all honesty, I don't think that she ever truly loved me and deep down believe that she only married me to visit the UK. If you think about it, there is no point in attempting to drive a sports car if it is broken; better to ride a bicycle, because at least you will get somewhere."

"I am sorry," he replied

"Don't be sorry mate. I have two beautiful kids and have had many hot passionate nights with my streamlined Ferrari wife but never forget that it hurts when you are in love with a beautiful woman. If I were you, I would be on the lookout for a reliable bike, my friend." We both laughed before I took out the two condoms from my wallet and placed them before his dumbstruck eyes." "My perfect wife gave me these in case I fancied a leg-over with a Chinese girl. You couldn't make it up, could you?" I returned the condoms to their secret compartment, grabbed my beer and plate of food and bade farewell to the startled Canadian.

I sat in a corner and leisurely scoffed my meal and sipped my beer as I looked around the small pub. The fifty-something-year-old-American owner who was of Irish descent and his young Chinese wife were busy behind the bar. The pool table was in full flow as The Human League's "Don't You Want Me?" played on the jukebox. The petite waitresses were serving dinner as noisy drunken laughter filled the hostelry.

I grabbed another pint and made my way through the cigarette smoke to the pool table. My turn next and without being cocky, I could normally remain on this 'winner-stays-on' table for as long as I liked. As an ex-snooker player, my deep screws were second to none, inevitably leaving the female onlookers open-mouthed and goo-goo eyed in admiration. My party piece was a massé shot: I would skilfully swerve the white ball around my opponent's ball before potting the object ball, which would have observers applauding as they shook their heads in astonishment. The more I drank the better I played.

After half a dozen games of showing off my pool table skills, I retired undefeated and went to sit with a couple of mates. Sam, a Scottish bloke who was teaching but hated it, and Kevin, a fellow Mancunian who was making a pretty penny from a book printing business he had set up. They both had Chinese partners. We were having a great laugh, which merited one last beer for the road.

I ordered my pint and when I put my hand in my jacket pocket my heart missed a beat. My fucking wallet was gone. Shit, I had been pickpocketed. What an effing downer. I was having such a good time too. There was about £200 in Renminbi and my debit card. It would be a pain in the arse cancelling it and waiting for a new one. I frantically searched my jacket pockets followed by my trouser pockets; bollocks, nothing there. Finally, I put my hand in my shirt pocket and pulled out my small blue Nokia mobile phone along with all my money and my debit card. I stared in frog-eyed confusion wondering what the hell was going on. I then recalled searching my wallet for a scrap of paper with a school's phone number on to hand to the Canadian bloke, on my last visit to the bar. I had taken all the money and my debit card out and popped them into my shirt pocket before locating the tiny bit of paper in the bottom corner of my moth-eaten wallet. In my drunken stupor, I had forgotten to return everything back to the wallet.

I smiled as I thought, *You jammy bastard.* I then burst out laughing as I visualised the thief greedily opening the wallet and to his disappointment, finding out that he hadn't come into money and all he had for his light-fingered dirty work were two flipping condoms. I held my sides and screamed with laughter as I mused, *I hope he comes into the condoms.* Everyone in the pub must have thought I had lost the plot and even the Canadian looked bemused as I placed a pint of beer before his eyes, slurring, "A pint from me."

I pissed myself laughing as I zig-zagged home and my wife laughed her pretty head off too as I recounted the strange unbelievable story. Imagine trying to explain to your partner that you still had your money and debit card, but your old dog-eared wallet and two condoms had been stolen. She would have been highly suspicious, and no doubt hit the bloody roof, accusing you of taking the piss because it was as plain as the lying nose on your face that you had been a no-good two-timing bastard. It was no problem with my missus because she didn't care, didn't love me and knew full well that goody-two-shoes Syd never told lies. Now, if it would have been a new possessive sweetheart who had heard this unfeasible tale, then that would have been a totally different kettle of fish, as a massive pile of shit would have hit the cheap night market fan.

***

After years of 'ins and outs' and 'ups and downs', this on-off relationship ultimately came to a non-stick end. We became unglued late September 2000, splitting up forever. I recall the bittersweet affair of observing my supposedly *'Till Death do us Part'* spouse step onto the Shekou ferry for the first leg of her return journey to Bangkok. Inevitably it was raining in my wishy-washy heart, but deep down I knew that every dark cloud had a silver lining and that the "Fat Old Sun" up above would soon be shining brightly because my tempestuous other half would be far away. However, my sorrowful eyes were not ogling at her athletic long legs or her lustrous dark hair blowing in the gentle breeze; they had zeroed in on one-year-old Francesca Emma who was in her mother's arms. My heart was not breaking for my wife but for my gorgeous little daughter. I held back the tears as I squeezed Eugene's hand.

Eugene was daddy's boy and had insisted on remaining with his old fella. I had pleaded with my missus to allow Francesca to stay with her father and brother, but she refused point blank, maintaining that Francesca needed her mum because she was just a baby. I cried inside while I focused on the ferry shrinking in size as it sailed across the South China Sea before it vanished into the far distance. When would I see my baby daughter again?

I hugged Eugene, then grasped his tiny hand as we started our soul-crushing death march back to the apartment. We passed the kids' playroom of the Nan Hai Hotel, where brother and sister had only last weekend spent a couple of hours, laughing and running wild. In fact, Francesca hadn't done much running since she had only just taken her first steps. A doting yours truly made endless frantic gallops past the plastic seesaw and around the bouncy castle each time his little angel toppled over. Once I was satisfied that she was okay I would set her on her feet again, giving her the go-ahead to chase after her elder brother.

Leaving the hotel and my memories behind we continued our mournful walk home via Shekou beach. Tear-jerking mind-movies of my two tiny tots building sandcastles and paddling in the sea flickered in my sorrowful skull. Without warning the unbearable pain, together with the grief-stricken shock, transported me straight into the present moment. The past and future had disappeared, as had the pain. I stood perfectly still with my feet on the warm golden sand listening to the squawking seabirds above my head. The pale blue sky with the white dinosaur shaped cloud above the green hills, the soothing waves lapping in perfect harmony with my gentle breath and the salty taste of the deep blue sea were perceived simultaneously for one split-second in time. Wow, this really was paradise.

Then in an almighty flash, I was back in hell. I had the enlightening realisation that paradise was a shithole dump of a town with my daughter in my arms, but this Shangri La was a living hell without her. Isn't it weird how on occasions when one is broken and in unbearable agony, some mysterious force floats us off to a peaceful pain-free land for a crystal clear glimpse of true reality? A pity our naughty monkey mind soon drags us back to the unhappy, unreal world of suffering.

Back home I turned on the *Cartoon Network* channel for Eugene and cooked his dinner. I looked on sympathetically, fully aware that he had lost his playmate too. No little sister to dance and run around with now. He was all alone just like me. I snuck off to my lonely bedroom and quietly wept. My shoulders heaved as my waterlogged eyes dripped with pearl shaped tears. The muffled sobs and the sorrowful atmosphere of despair stayed within the four forsaken walls. The last thing Eugene needed during this distressing period was to witness his destroyed father crying his heart and soul out.

What have I done with my life? "Alone Again, Naturally". But I wasn't alone, was I? I had Eugene and he had me. In an inspirational, eureka moment I fully understood what needed to be done. I dried my tears before returning to the living room and giving my son a warm hug and a tender kiss. I sat him on my knee and softly said, "Daddy loves you with all his heart so next week we are leaving and going on a very long exciting adventure. What do you think about that?" His little face lit up with excitement, he clapped his hands and gave me a massive loving hug. I went back to my bedroom and wept tears of joy.

15 Minutes of Fame

(2000 to 2003)

I was as busy as a blue-arsed fly buzzing about getting my shit together, so we could hit the "Road to Nowhere" for our "Once in a Lifetime" adventure. We donated all our possessions to friends except for a few clothes, a cheap video camera, the *Lonely Planet Guide to China* and Eugene's two favourite cuddly toys; a blue whale and a long green and yellow snake. Over the next few months whenever a girl made a fuss of Eugene, he would take out his snake and attack…stimulating the tickled pink female to scream and giggle. Like father like son! A future Hissing Syd in the making.

As luck would have it, now was the perfect moment to close down the language centre because, Alex, my business partner had foolishly invested all his money in a software company and had lost the bloody lot. Time to take my pennies and run. I was hoping that the dosh I had in the bank would support a shoestring journey of cheap guesthouses and low-cost street food for at least three months.

On 16th October 2000, with all our worldly belongings stuffed into a large rust-coloured holdall, we stepped onto the 7am VIP bus to Guangzhou. We were free, and I felt elated. We had no itinerary; we could do as we pleased and go wherever we liked. The world seemed very different today. It was marvellous being alive once more. I chuckled as my little lad attacked the Chinese ticket inspector with his snake. She laughed in glee and gave him a big hug. That's my boy. Two hours later we were at the crowded railway station ready to embark on a three-day train ride to Cheng Du in Western China. Psycho Syd was 44 and Eugene Lewis was just 2 years old.

The father and son wanderings didn't last for three months; our nomadic lifestyle continued for almost a year! And what an epic odyssey this pair of intrepid vagabonds undertook. Take our hand and accompany us on the pilgrimage to the centre of our minds. Sleep in a tiny blizzard covered temple at over two and a half miles above sea level. Feel the heat from the close at hand fire warm your frozen bones, as you absorb the unbelievable panorama before your awestruck eyeballs; an endless sea of snowy white fairy-tale mountain peaks. Slowly sip the revitalising hot noodle soup that has just been served up by a smiling red-robed Tibetan monk. Glow with new-born wisdom because at long last, you have discovered the meaning of life. And if you open your eyes, then you too will become aware that life is far too precious to waste away in a soul-destroying and meaningless job. When you are lying on your deathbed will you be content at having lived life to the full or will you be filled with remorse because you never really lived at all? There will be no point crying over spilt almond milk just before you meet your maker. However, the good news is that you can always change your life. And the time to do that is NOW.

Snatch a taste of life up in the sky as we horse-trek and wild camp above the clouds in the oxygen-starved thin air of the Himalayas.

Next, jump on board our tiny long-tailed boat for a two-day madcap voyage along a wild raging river. Sample full in-your-face fear as the adrenalin dashes around your bulging veins while your heart races like the clappers in your tight chest. Feel the knot in the stomach of your sopping wet body as the small boat struggles through countless sets of furious out-of-control rapids. Cling on for dear life and pray to the Lord above that we don't capsize, because there are no life jackets and we are at least a week's wilderness trek away from the nearest civilisation. We are living right at the razor-sharp edge of life and loving it. Proper hard-core, utterly insane and Eugene is just a tiny toddler!

If you are gagging for more then come on down, otherwise remain caged in your sad 9-5 existence, daydreaming that you too will taste freedom before you kick the bucket. Who are you kidding? Me or yourself? The sweat stings your eyes as humungous tropical insects buzz noisily around your head during an audacious week-long hike through scorching steamy jungles. Each evening we stay with an isolated minority tribe and leave the following morning for another exhausting wild trek beneath the rainforest trees arriving at the next remote village, an hour or two before sundown. No electricity and no roads in or out. Experience the strange sensation of being followed and watched by the whole village as they stare in astonishment at the peculiar foreigners; some had never seen a white man before! There were no showers and each evening we would wash the sweat and grime of our weary bodies in the river, to an audience of mesmerised onlookers.

Over 100 villagers sat on the soil outside the headman's wooden hut where we were staying in the hope of catching a glimpse of the mysterious strangers. Gorgeous little Eugene was the star attraction. I felt like a celebrity sampling the kind of life that John, Paul, George and Ringo had once experienced. Although sometimes I had the unsettling sensation of being a freakish curio, tasting the life the first African who had set foot on English soil must have undergone. It was weirdly enjoyable being the centre of attention for a while, but after a week of being followed, watched and pointed at, I thanked Almighty God when my "15 minutes of Fame", came to an end. There was no feeling of danger because these simple farmers were kind and welcoming, but understandably very curious. To them we were akin to aliens from a distant planet.

Each night we flaked out after being nourished with a bowl of rice and vegetables; not forgetting the large glass of potent homemade whisky which left a warm glow in my belly and a taste of paint stripper in my gob. The following morning the entire village turned out to wish their weird guests a safe journey. After another seven or eight hours of fighting through untamed jungle, we would reach the next Hmong or Akha village. I noticed how incredibly happy these isolated people were. Just a basic life of growing food, swimming in the river, falling in love and having children. No television or newfangled gadgets like in the wealthy west. It was plain to see that these simple commoners were far richer than us.

We managed to save money by spending a few months in a high school, and it really was a high school; 6000 feet above sea-level. We were provided with a comfortable room, free food and pocket money in exchange for two hours' English teaching a day. And luckily, I didn't have to witness piles of bones in the school canteen because the wealthy owner didn't eat meat. We had our very own VIP vegan dining room to scoff limitless dishes of cruelty-free meals.

To the front of the school was the dreamlike Daichi Lake and to the back the magnificent Western Hills, with ancient trails leading up to hidden temples with breathtaking views. At weekends and after lessons it was dad and lad playtime as we ran to the hills for a spot of outdoor fun. We sometimes caught the minibus to nearby Kunming to visit the supermarket and to gobble up western fayre such as beans on toast in a traveller's café.

Well, that is enough about this mind-bending trip for now, because the complete adventure will be scribbled in a future page-turning book; 'Careful with that Backpack Eugene.' The astute reader will recall that Psychedelic Syd was a fervent Pink Floyd aficionado, making it clear that Eugene was named after the spinetingling Floyd tune, "Careful with that Axe Eugene".' Far-out, man!

***

On 12th September 2001, I lifted my yawning head off the green pillow in a Vientiane guest house. We had spent 10 months tramping around western China and a month exploring Laos before arriving in Vientiane, the capital city. Eugene was still 'miles away' in the land of nod. I wiped the sleep out of my sky-blue eyes and focused on the large overworked fan lazily rotating on the faded yellow ceiling above my sluggish body. The gentle flow of warm humid air mopped my hot sticky skin. Out of the blue I remembered that my football team had played last night and was eager to discover the result. I left Eugene in dreamland and nipped downstairs for a 15-minute session on one of the computers available for guests.

The dark-skinned receptionist wearing a yellow 'Beer Lao' t-shirt and black jeans was also wearing a look of concern on her pretty face. She quizzed, "Have you heard about the terrible plane crash?" "No, I haven't, I have just woken up but will check online now," I answered. First things first. I opened the BBC football page and was over the blue moon at finding out that Manchester City had been victorious in a League Cup tie against Notts County. At the same time, my football mad ears pricked up upon reading that many people were up in arms because yesterday's matches hadn't been postponed considering the tragic air disaster. I lit a cigarette, glanced over to the receptionist who was busy on her laptop and mused, "Crikey, this must be mega serious." My initial theory was that an entire football squad had just been wiped out in an abominable aircraft catastrophe.

I sat stunned in open-mouthed horror as I fixated on the shocking videos of two jets smashing into the twin towers in New York. I read the full beyond-belief report and sat in silence before lighting another cancer stick. I gazed outside to the sunny street where a handful of backpackers were buying fresh baguettes from a smiling elderly lady at a wooden table shaded by a large blue parasol. At that very instant I decided to return to my mother in Blackpool. '*I want my mam!*'

We spent every minute of our final week in Bangkok, Thailand with my eldest son, Eric Jay. The two brothers bonded as we splashed about in a swimming pool, watched a family movie at the cinema and ate all our meals together as a joyful threesome. I loved my kids immensely, wishing my daughter was here to magically transform the joyful threesome into a perfect foursome. The scrap of news I had received regarding Francesca was that she was being raised by my wife's cousin somewhere in north-eastern Thailand, because her mother was in New Zealand with a new partner. I breathed a sigh of relief on hearing that my baby girl was happy and well but was quite rightly pissed-off that she wasn't with one of her parents; namely her loving dad. On the day of our flight back to England we said a heart-touching goodbye to Eric Jay. I hugged him closely, gushing how much I loved him before vowing, "I will be back."

***

We took to the skies with vivid memories of the wondrous adventure with my young boy playing in my head. Fortunately, I had shot over 20 hours of footage with my camcorder, meaning we could relive that remarkable trip any time we liked. When Eugene gets older, he will be agog when he views the outlandish expedition he undertook as a tiny tot. But before he is grown up, we will have at least one further journey to the east because I had a promise to keep, didn't I? Eric Jay was waiting.

My mother stared in overjoyed astonishment at the two unannounced guests standing at the front door of the Wildlife Vegan Hotel; her bedraggled son and grandson. She hadn't seen us in over three years. She ushered us indoors and the wildlife went wild. Scooby Doo, the black Labrador cross was howling and leaping in the air. Megan the brindled rescue whippet ran around in frantic circles and little Venus, the white Jack Russell with the cute brown patch on her face, sprang into my arms and yapped and yapped and yapped. I was jumping for joy too; feeling elated that the mutts had remembered us. They were so loyal, with pure love shining from their doggy eyes as their tails wagged in unrestrained euphoria, because we had returned to the pack. "Better than bloody women," I smiled; except for my dear old mum of course. I rolled around the floor in celebration with the hounds, before having a cuppa with mum while Eugene watched cartoons.

Mother was fit and healthy and in high spirits, taking good care of her baby; the vegan hotel. She had loads of animal rights mates and plenty of friends at her local church, which she visited twice a week. She had made a happy life for herself after tragically losing her partner. It always warms my heart when I hear of people who fight back and transform their lives after living through the most catastrophic losses that life can chuck at them. Well done mum. She led us to a small twin-bedded room and we were snoozing before our travel-weary heads hit the pillows. After all, just 15 hours ago we were sweating in the humid heat of Siam on the other side of planet Earth.

After 12 hours of deep slumber we finally awoke to a new life in

Blackpool. We made our way downstairs for a vegan sausage sandwich and a large glass of freshly squeezed orange juice. It was time for me to establish a motionless existence for the two footloose and fancy-free nomads. As a single bloke with a three-year-old son there wasn't a hope in hell of a career opportunity knocking on my door in this economically deprived area with sky-high unemployment. I had no option but to stand in line with the despairing people claiming benefits.

Eugene looked smart but strange with his tidy short hair, neat white shirt and red shorts on the day he started nursery. I stared in horror as he took his place with about 20 identical little humans. Each to be programmed into obeying robots that never questioned the shady elite who are running and destroying the world in their hidden quest for "Complete Control". *We don't want your thought control*, my Open Mind thought. I much preferred Eugene in his long straggly hair, scruffy jeans and crazy t-shirts, as he got a real education in the real world of look and see.

I made myself at home and helped mum with the hotel in return for food and board. We went shopping together and took the dogs for a run on the beach in the evenings. Sometimes mum would hire a cheap car and I would drive us to the Lancashire hills to give the dogs a long walk before grabbing a meal in a country pub. Mother really looked forward to these little family excursions and I was delighted that I had added these happy days to her life. Eugene was contented, and my mother adored him. She showered him with gifts for his birthdays and at Christmas. As a grandmother she glowed with pride, clapping her hands madly while watching her little grandson perform as a shepherd in the school's reception year nativity.

It was lovely spending time with my mother but as you can guess I didn't really belong in this dreary seaside town. One cold January evening I popped into the nearby pub for a pint. I was pondering what to do next with my life when I heard Coldplay's song "Yellow" in the background, while playing pool with a stranger. I suddenly had the answer; I was homesick for the orient, so it was time to shake a leg and escape unemployment in this "Dirty Old Town". My mother wasn't shocked and was in fact, surprised that we hadn't hit the road earlier; after all she had known me for 47 years. She wished us luck, gave us a bit of dosh to see us through the first period of our trip. We both hugged and kissed my mum before grabbing our backpacks and jumping into the taxi for the airport. Eugene was a big boy now. He was five!

I was glad that I had spent a couple of years with my mum and look back with fondness at the warm memories. Sometimes the universe sends us to a place where we don't wish to be for a reason which we only discover in the future.

Ever Fallen in Love

(With Someone you Shouldn't've)

(2003 to 2012)

I was alive once more, my body tingling with exhilaration while the fixed grin on my euphoric mush painted a showy picture of triumph. The jet plane roared through seventh heaven above cloud nine as it sped towards our next great adventure. The plan was to spend time with Eric Jay in Bangkok before backpacking overland through Thailand, Laos, Cambodia and Vietnam; eventually setting foot in China. Then I would find a job, get Eugene into school and employ a nanny. This wasn't a pie in the sky pipedream because as a multilingual native English speaker I would be able to pick and choose where I worked in that neck of the woods. A welcome change from the unwanted dosser thrown on the scrapheap back home, hey? The low cost of living would mean that an apartment, a school for my son and a nanny wouldn't burn a hole in my pocket, leaving a fistful of readies to live a comfortable life.

After touching down in the City of Angels we checked into our favourite guesthouse before contacting Eric Jay. He had grown into a tall and slender 12-year-old boy. He was rather shy and timid but seemed happy enough. We spent every moment with him because he stayed with us in the guesthouse too.

Each sunrise I floated all alone in the warm water of the large outdoor swimming pool. The early morning sun coloured the sky brilliant red while its rays splashed the clouds with gorgeous shades of pink. Gentle breezes stroked my skin as the water caressed my almost motionless body. I listened to my soft breathing while my hypnotised eyes gazed skywards at mother nature's exquisite work of art. In this meditative state my heart sang in harmony with the melodic dawn chorus of the wild tropical birds in the nearby coconut trees.

I smiled upon hearing my two boys laughing and splashing in the adjacent paddling pool. Then it was time for a hearty breakfast before spending the rest of the day doing whatever the kids' hearts' desired; an afternoon in the cinema, lunch at Pizza Hut, plane spotting at the airport or just watching TV in the guesthouse. I felt joyous witnessing my two children having so much fun.

It was also an opportune time to get some dirt cheap pain-free dental work done on my broken teeth and after a few appointments I left the private clinic with a sparkling set of pearly whites. I was now at the ready to give a quick flash to any fair maiden who caught my eye.

A psycho of geckos gobbled up mosquitoes on the wall at the front of our guest house. A lounge of monitor lizards was on the prowl in the undergrowth and a school of fish splashed in the lily-covered pond on this magical moonlit night. I hear you loud and clear as you remark, "A 'psycho of geckos', that can't be flipping right?" Well, keep your hair on because in fact geckos don't have a cool collective noun since they don't form groups. Therefore, being a bit of a smart arse, I decided to name this mob of insect gulping creatures a psycho. I have always been strange and blame it on the magic mushroom trip I had as a long-haired teenager. So be a good sport and play along.

The three of us were sitting on a wooden bench by a small pond at our remote Bangkok guest house, which was located on a gorgeous slice of greenery far away from the busy roads. An army of noisy frogs disturbed the night as the geckoes continued feasting on the bastard of mosquitoes under the wall lights. In fact, the correct phrase is a scourge of mosquitoes, but after being buzzed and bitten during my tropical travels I renamed these bloodthirsty blighters, bastards.

We had been here almost a month, so it was high time we got a move on. Tickets for tomorrow night's overnight express train to Nong Khai in the north-east were safely stashed inside my wallet. I held Eric Jay closely, explaining how much I loved him and of course, promising to see him soon.

***

Eugene and I sat facing each other on the massive comfy seats in the air-con carriage as we both waved to Eric Jay. The train slowly pulled away as the vision of my firstborn waving goodbye pulled on my heartstrings. Life is often painful but at least visiting him would be easier now that I was in his part of the world. Sleeper trains in Thailand are an awesome 'must do' experience when visiting the land of smiles. Inexpensive too.

We sat in the restaurant carriage slowly eating fried rice whilst observing busy Bangkok at night through the window. Tomorrow we would be in the charming laid-back city of Nong Khai, which sits on the banks of the Mekong River just across from Laos. Upon returning to our seats we were met with ready-made-up beds, prompting us to grab some shuteye.

We arrived in Nong Khai just after sunrise and dumped our bag into a fan room at the Mutt Mee Guesthouse. It cost just £2 a night. We relaxed in hammocks in the magical garden overlooking the mighty river. This well-established backpacker-friendly establishment offered meditation,

The following morning, we bumped into Emma and James, a smart young English couple who were spending a month backpacking around Thailand. We all jumped into a tuk-tuk to visit the very strange Sala Keoku; a bizarre park of massive sculptures. This mishmash of over 100 quirky statues of Hindu Gods, smiling Buddhas, many-headed serpents and multi-armed goddesses amidst delightful trees and gorgeous flowers was spectacular. This spiritual wonderland had been created by Sulilat; a mystic Laotian monk.

My favourite sculpture was the thought-provoking Wheel of Life. We entered through a tunnel representing the womb and walked in a circle past statues depicting the stages of life from childhood to death. However, the final sculpture wasn't death but a fully enlightened Buddha crossing over to the other side, pointing out the way to escape the Wheel of Suffering. We returned to the 'Mutt Mee' for a beer and a curry as we lived in the moment, breathing in the magnificent sunset and the tiny silhouetted boats on the Mekong River.

We spent a magical week with our two friends, visiting towns and villages in the north-east. They both made a fuss of Eugene: Emma held his hand while visiting attractions and James played chess and Jenga with him in the evenings. We also took a strenuous hike to a viewpoint for stunning views of the mountains of Laos in the distance. Eugene was once again spoilt because Serena, a young athletic Canadian girl who joined us, gave him a piggyback to the top. We watched Manchester City defeat Manchester United 3-1 in a German guesthouse in the sleepy village of Sangkhom. Lots of beer, cheering and dancing I'll have you know.

Although we did have a couple of unpleasant incidents during that week. The German owner at the guest house had two pet monkeys who he insisted were very tame and didn't bite. However, one jumped up and gave Eugene a slight nip on his arm; a dab of antiseptic cream and a plaster and my brave soldier was as right as rain once again. The other event occurred when a transvestite sneakily stole a small purse containing $50 from James' pocket. James shrugged his shoulders and declared, "Shit happens." We said farewell to Emma and James in the city of Loei. (Remember...that's the city we visited in Chapter Three where the young student met the man who'd spiked his drink.)

***

I was shocked at discovering online that two Swiss cyclists had been shot dead in Laos. "Should I Stay or Should I Go?" I sensibly decided to spend a further week in Thailand and monitor the situation. We took an air-conditioned bus to the large city of Udorn Thani. Upon arrival I was surprised to see a female tuk-tuk driver wearing a Manchester City shirt; it was usually Liverpool or Manchester effing United! She drove us to a resort with a small swimming pool and gave me a dazzling smile after I handed over double her asking price because she was wearing my team's colours.

After a couple of days of splashing about in the pool, Eugene finally learnt to swim. That's my boy. The friendly owners had a couple of kids and Eugene would often play with them and watch cartoons in their house while I chilled out reading a book by the pool. I got chatting to a tall slender girl while I was buying some fruit at the market. She was a primary school teacher and out of the blue invited us to see a movie. I was on the edge of my seat in the modern cinema watching a Thai film called *Ongbak*. It was a martial arts film that made Bruce Lee movies look like *Alice in Wonderland* and I loved it. My new friend visited every day after school, and we went for dinner together each evening followed by a walk in a park where Eugene would have fun in the playground and feed the fish in the lake. Another lady mothering my lad.

What about his poor old dad? Well for a change his dad got a bit of loving and some hugs and kisses too! We became intimate most evenings while Eugene was watching cartoons with his friends. The friendly owners knew what was going on and winked and smiled as they happily looked after my son. It was wonderful tasting erotic pleasure again after spending two lonely years as a housebound single dad in Blackpool. Sadly, it was time to hug and kiss my ladyfriend for a final time because our visas were expiring, leaving us no option but to cross the Mekong River into the People's Democratic Republic of Laos. There had been no further violent incidents, so I judged that it was safe to enter.

***

At the end of February 2003, we checked into a guest house in Vientiane, the capital, and got our passports stamped with Cambodian visas. I rented a motorcycle for a week to see the sights before we set off for our "Holiday in Cambodia". We rode around the city visiting temples, museums and markets. It was so relaxing just doing as we liked. One afternoon I spotted the Honour International School and instantly enrolled Eugene. A gut feeling told me it was the right thing to do so our "Holiday in Cambodia" was put on the back burner. I swiftly rented a small detached house for just £90 a month, employed a part-time nanny and started work at Vientiane College, the top place for teaching in the city.

I was a "Wild Thing" for a while and had a few flings with local ladies but still hadn't found the elusive soulmate I was seeking. Life was fantastic, and I loved Laos and adored the beautiful Lao people. This was where I wanted to live and die. My son was happy and doing well in school. I spent every morning at the gym running on the treadmill, lifting a few weights and swimming for an hour; then I taught in the evening.

After work I would have a couple of beers in my local; the Samlo Pub. I changed the music from the Eagles and more Eagles to an amazing mix of classic tunes, mainly focusing on Indie stuff such as: The Stone Roses, Radiohead, Muse, Oasis and The Killers. I also sprinkled in classics such as "Bohemian Rhapsody", "I'm a Believer", "American Pie" and "Riders on the Storm". My goodness, what a change from feeling sorry for myself in Blackpool. I was now sparkling as I lived the dream.

In June we moved to a huge fully furnished detached house with a massive tropical garden for just £150 a month. Goodness gracious… you couldn't rent a shithouse back in the UK for that! I bought a Chinese motorcycle and employed a new live-in nanny. I recall cheering in my local when England defeated Australia in the rugby world cup final.

On Christmas Day 2003 I was given the perfect present. My wife telephoned and asked if I would like to see my daughter. I grabbed the opportunity with both hands. My wife was still in New Zealand and Francesca was being raised by her aunty. I put the phone down elated as tears of joy filled my sky-blue eyes.

The 27th December my heart danced with happiness as I met Francesca Emma for the first time in over three years at an indoor play centre in Nong Khai, Thailand. She was now four years old and very smartly dressed, wearing a white floral dress with a pink bow in her long hair. At least she was well-fed because she had a bit of puppy fat but was not obese by any stretch of the imagination. It warmed my heart watching the kids play together once again. I thanked my wife's cousin for bringing my daughter. I hugged and kissed her goodbye and returned to Vientiane with Eugene, with happy memories in my heart.

***

The following year continued with teaching, swimming and Eugene doing well at school. I adored living in this beautiful country. I had found the place I wanted to live forever but had not yet met the woman I wanted to love forever. Dates with local ladies proceeded as they should but I still hadn't found the one I was looking for. "Nice and Sleazy" one-night stands were not my cup of tea. I yearned to drink in true romantic love with a "Together Forever" best friend and lover. And then towards the end of 2004 I came face to face with the Wicked Witch of the East.

A beautiful, tall, slender and large-breasted female floated up to me through the thick cigarette smoke and flashing disco lights, putting her hand on my crotch before whispering, "Hello, handsome man". I smiled and brushed her hand off and continued through the smoky haze. A ladyboy! I was in the Chess cafe, a seedy nightclub opposite the hospital. I had polished off a few beers at the Samlo and decided on one last drink before bed. After ordering a bottle of the tasty 'Beer Lao' I saw an even tastier female sitting at the bar. I drifted over and handed her my phone number, smiled, winked and slurred, "Phone me sometime". I then staggered out of the club, stumbled onto my Chinese motorbike and somehow got home to dream about another amazing day in Laos.

She phoned the following day which was May 1st, 2004, and I invited her to see Manchester City play Newcastle United in the Samlo Pub for a romantic first date. Proper Mancunian charmer, me. Only one problem - I was so drunk the night before that I couldn't remember what she looked like. Well, my beer goggles hadn't failed me as a very attractive lady smiled and sat next to me. We watched the game (City won) and went to a nightclub. We didn't become romantic partners but remained friends, meeting for lunch occasionally.

On one occasion in October a very pretty young girl joined her and started flirting with me. I explained that she was beautiful, but far too young for me at just 19 years of age. I didn't want to be one of those sad old Western men with a teenage girlfriend. However, she phoned a week later and asked to meet me, and we ended up doing the inevitable.

For a couple of months, we'd meet once a week until December 2004, when she arrived at my house with a bag, announcing that she was now my girlfriend and was moving in. I was stunned but didn't protest. At first, I felt self-conscious and uncomfortable at having a girlfriend half my age but after a while the age difference disappeared. She could have been older, younger or the same age and it wouldn't have made the slightest bit of difference because I had fallen deeply in love.

The first year was absolute bliss as our beautiful relationship blossomed. We were inseparable. I met her parents who were poor but good honest kind people. I also bumped into an angry ex-boyfriend who warned "Be careful, she is very, very bad and will destroy you." I felt sorry for him and put his warning down to sour grapes. We got engaged; we were one and "We Were Gonna Live Forever." I always bought her a new item of clothing every week because I loved watching her pretty face light up. She was happy and took great care of Eugene. What more could a man ask for? Luckily, she had a very high sex drive like me so mornings, evenings and sometimes afternoons were spent in a fever of hot adventurous passion; usually instigated by my better half.

My goodness, after two lonesome years in Blackpool as a stay-at-home single dad, dedicating myself to my son, karma had finally rewarded me with a loving partner and as much lust as my greedy libido could wish for. What goes around comes around.

***

In 2005 we moved to Gnommalard in Southern Laos, as I started work on a hydropower project. The money was much better, and we had amazing holidays in China, Hong Kong and Thailand. I bought a quality 4x4 SUV which made life a lot more interesting because we could spend days out visiting nearby attractions.

We finally got married in early 2008 and baby Jo was born in December that year. Next, I spent all my savings on buying a house and by January 2012 we had been together for over eight years. I loved her more deeply than I had ever loved anyone before. Although, she wasn't always the angelic girl I had been with during the first year of our relationship. She had a hot temper and would either explode in a crazy bad-tempered frenzy or I would be given a few days of the silent treatment. I hadn't a clue what I had done wrong, but I was so besotted that I just waited for her to apologise and receive her remorseful love.

I did everything I could to change her life for the better. I sent her to college to learn English, helped her family, remained totally faithful and gave her everything she had ever dreamed of. I ignored her bad moods and worshipped the ground she walked on. When I am in love, I love with all my heart and I had never been this deeply in love before. I was so proud of my gorgeous Lao wife but as the saying goes; pride always comes before a fall.

Welcome to Paradise

(January 2012)

All was not so quiet on "New Year's Day". The countless cocks in the idyllic leafy suburbs of Laos' capital City, Vientiane, cockily cock-a-doodle-doo-ed the birth of 2012. So, I did what comes naturally and opted to 'wash the chicken's face'! Washing the chicken's face is a Thai idiom which translates to, make love at the crack of dawn! I am scratching my baffled bonce as to why, but it always makes my mucky mind chuckle. Equally, the locals itch their brainboxes in confusion at the British expression 'the dog's bollocks'. How can a dog's testicles mean the best of the best, they chortle! To be perfectly honest I can't recall whether my morning glory had its satisfying vegan oats during the first sunrise of 2012 but erected, sorry, elected to do a Finbarr Saunders (look it up if you don't know) and slip it in! The idiom, that is!

"Welcome to Paradise". I now lived the life of Mr. Riley in a modest two-bedroomed bungalow with a magnificently lush equatorial garden; complete with eye-catching tropical fruit trees bearing their delicious heavenly gifts. The jungle was on my doorstep, which was a far Tarzan cry away from my old council house with its tiny lawn and flowerbed in Manchester. Jane was usually chilling indoors in the air-conditioned atmosphere, living the life of Mrs. Riley as the servants cooked, cleaned and washed clothes. Eugene who'd reached the age of fourteen played computer games in his room while three-year-old Jo watched cartoons in the living room.

An organic vegetable plot and sweet-smelling herb garden spiced up and flavoured this exotic lifestyle. Skin-tingling, mind-revitalising power showers were blissful in this steamy wonderland thanks to the refreshing cool water from our very own spring water well. This luscious Oasis was finished off to perfection with wild-growing, deep-green creepers, vines and plants camouflaging the "Wonderwall" encircling our ambrosial garden of Eden.

Most weekends our potent turd-brown Hyundai Santa Fe 4x4 went like shit off a hot shovel along dusty trails, ultimately dumping us at a remote jungle temple, an isolated riverbank or a magical mountain a few hours away from Vientiane. When we didn't take to the skies to *Billy Whizz* to another country for our holidays, we undertook longer expeditions, speeding in our powerful A-OK wheels to out-of-this-world hidden gems around Laos and Thailand.

One such unforgettable adventure in Laos was the visit to one of southeast Asia's 'must see' geological wonders; the spectacular Konglor Cave. The awe-inspiring experience of jumping into a tiny boat to follow the Nam Hin Bun River on its remarkable 7.5 km underground journey through dramatic caverns to a sleepy rainforest village at the other side left me breathless. Put it on your bucket list.

As Laos is landlocked, many of our odysseys in Thailand were to dreamy islands in the warm blue sea. I regularly reminisce about renting a beach bungalow on the unspoilt island of Ko Kood in eastern Thailand near the Cambodian border. I played the part of the stereotypical beach bum to perfection as I frittered away hours on the sun-kissed white sand. The gentle lapping of the waves was occasionally disrupted by the high-pitched call of a sea eagle. I would periodically cool off by lazily swimming with the psychedelic fish in the crystal-clear water. I gazed in deep love and admiration at two beach babes; my gorgeous wife and my adorable two-year-old son. It was just "Another Day in Paradise".

Once a month we would while away a couple of nights in the metropolis of Udorn Thani in north-eastern Thailand. Udorn, as it is commonly referred to, is a busy city with an abundance of shops, hotels and restaurants, as well as hundreds of coffee shops, bars and nightclubs, recalling a bygone era when it catered for American GIs during the Vietnam War. It was just an hour's drive across the border and as a rule we crashed out in one of the spotless spacious rooms at the Irish Clock Pub. It was centrally located and had everything we could ask for, including wi-fi, a pool table, live football and a varied selection of western and Asian dishes. I would get stuck into cheese on toast, chips and baked beans, with a pint of Kilkenny Bitter, as my better half happily polished off a spicy Thai meal while sipping Coca-Cola. The kids usually gorged on a pizza or two.

The primary purpose for our weekend getaway was shopping in the modern superstores, which were non-existent in laid-back Vientiane. My wife would hungrily devour the latest fashionable clothes at the Central Plaza shopping mall during the day and grab a few bits and bobs from the busy night market after dinner. The children got new clobber and a few toys, but I rarely bought anything for myself. I was more than happy treating the ones I loved to their heart's content. Finally, we would stock up with food from Tesco Lotus and the Big C Department Store. Little did I know that I would be receiving an unwelcome free gift from this bizarrely named retail outfit in the very near future.

I had bought the house, land, car, a zippy Yamaha scooter, flat-screen TV, computer and all the furniture with the dosh I had earned whilst working on a hydropower project. Night school was attended twice a week to study Chinese, which together with my fluent Thai and Lao language skills would give me extra brownie points at future job interviews. In fact, I had already been offered a position with yet another hydropower project, due to begin in the summer of 2012, where my Mandarin would be put to good use.

In the meantime, I was working as a primary school teacher at the unfortunately named PIS! (Panyathip International School), which followed the British education system. I thought about opening SHITE – Syd's Higher International Teaching Empire – to compete, but sensibly decided against it. A bonus for being an employee of the school was that I didn't have to cough up any tuition fees for Eugene who was studying there. As a multilingual Mancunian, I had never had a problem securing lucrative work in the Far East.

I was still deeper than the deepest in love with my drop-dead gorgeous Lao wife. She was slender with long cascading hair and a sweet angelic face, but I only had to peep into her dark brown eyes to see the endless nights of frenzied lust she had up her devilish sleeve. I was as proud as the proverbial peacock as we walked hand in hand. My rose-coloured specs were glued to my smiling love-struck mush as I floated on air with my dream girl.

As a cheeky Caucasian I had frequently received offers of love and lust from young Lao females, but they always came to nothing. I only had eyes and other parts of my anatomy for my stunning wife. When I was footloose and fancy free, I was a skirt-chasing charmer, but once I had tied the knot, I became a faithful, besotted hound dog. My friends agreed that she was pretty but quickly added that there were a multitude of pretty girls in Vientiane. "It is your spoiling her with new clothes, weekly trips to the hairdressers and expensive make-up that make her look a cut above the rest", they laughed. I was having none of it. She was my Mrs Universe.

***

I was living the dream and Vientiane was paradise. It was the capital city of Laos PDR but felt more like an extensive village due to its relative lack of scale, and its intriguing mix of French colonial architecture and ancient Buddhist temples. Breathing in the atmosphere of the timeworn French villas and sacred sanctuaries during a lazy cycle along the tree-lined boulevards at sunrise was an atmospheric start to my day. I bought fruit and veg from one of the colourful outdoor markets, bread, tea and coffee at a local minimart and treated myself to cheese, baked beans and Marmite from a store catering for ex-patriots.

Like a mirage shimmering in the midday sun, the monumental golden stupa known as Pha That Luang was a truly magnificent sight to behold. I stood mesmerised by the golden spire, before my jaw dropped with the realisation that I wasn't gazing at sparkly paint, but 500 kilograms of pure gold. Nearby, Patuxai, Vientiane's version of the Arc de Triumph, reached up to the sky too. I slogged to the top of this high and mighty structure for a bird's-eye view of my favourite city in the world, pinching myself to make sure that I wasn't dreaming before retracing my steps back down to the bottom.

In the evening I contentedly sat beside the Mekong River with an ice-cold 'Beer Lao' watching the sunset over in Thailand. Yellow, tangerine then deep orange until the mighty Mekong flowed like blood. "Another day in Paradise" ended as millions of diamonds sparkled in the night sky.

Though it seems I have waxed lyrical about life in Vientiane I still haven't revealed the primary reason why it is such a fabulous place to lay down your hat. And the answer is simple; it is the extraordinarily kind and gentle Laotian people. You are greeted by smiling happy faces all day long. You rarely see anger. Peace and contentment shines from their joyful eyes. This relaxed lifestyle is like an infectious yawn as you begin to chill right out and smile too. Similarly, the pace of life is super-slow. There is always time to think, chat, take a nap under a tree or just sit back for a few hours and watch the world go by. The locals laugh as they explain that PDR stands for 'Please Don't Rush.'

Compare that to a city in the west where the programmed hordes of deep in debt zombies race around chasing a dream they will never reach. Their unhappy faces frantic with worry, stress and anger. They are far too busy to chat; in fact, they are far too busy to enjoy life as they sprint towards a happy future that doesn't exist. Moving to Vientiane is like escaping from a crazy nuthouse to sit in a tranquil temple garden where you have time to live like you were always meant to.

But did I forget to mention the full delights of the cuisine? Foodies were in mouth-watering dreamland in Vientiane too, sampling food from almost every part of the planet at the large collection of restaurants which had sprung up catering for the ex-pats, a steady flow of tourists and curious locals.

I nostalgically recall having dinner with my family, amongst the tropical plants on a breezy veranda at the elegant Cage du Cog. This upmarket French eatery, housed in a charming old villa, was hidden away in a picturesque leafy side street just a stone's throw from the Mekong River. At the opposite end of the scale we would visit the plastic chairs and cheap foldaway tables for a spicy Indian curry at the very basic Taj Mahal. Japanese, Italian, Korean, German, Thai and Lao establishments were visited when the mood took us, and the prices were ridiculously cheap.

However, the ultimate dining experience was indulging oneself in an all-you-can-eat buffet lunch at one of the vegan cafes. My best-loved was a hard-to-find tiny shophouse down an alley where for less than two pounds sterling I could eat like a vegan king. In Buddhist Laos vegans were revered because of their compassion towards all sentient beings, which made a welcome change from being portrayed as a tree-hugging oddball back in the west. I had my choice of curries, noodles, rice, soups, spring rolls, steamed buns and a variety of fake meat dishes.

My eyes were always bigger than my belly as I attempted to scoff the bloody lot, inevitably ending up well and truly stuffed. I ate a minimum of four deep-fried sticky rice rolls, which I loved but had to be on the lookout for a Prik Kee Nu (mouse shit chilli) which was cunningly concealed inside. These tiny red chillies, resembling a mouse dropping, were off the charts when it came to hot. One bite would have me exploding into sweats and screams before drinking copious jugs of icy cold water, much to everyone's amusement.

In fact, the word shit (kee) is not considered a profanity in Laos, so you can confidently ask for a mouse shit chilli without worrying whether you have committed a cultural faux-pas or not. If someone is stingy you would call him a sticky shit (kee neeow) or if extremely drunk, he would be a drunk shit (kee mao.) All in all, I was as happy as a pig in kee, eating to my heart's content at the ubiquitous dirt-cheap establishments in this wonderful city. It was a delightful surprise to see that fast food chains such as KFC or McDonald's had not yet arrived to peddle their junk, but I am sure they soon will because I am sad to report that the international franchise chain 'the Pizza Company' has just opened a branch.

Weekends were spent in our new local, a British pub called the

Hare and the Hound. It was run by John from Milton Keynes, who was a dead ringer for *Freddie Mercury*, and his beautiful Indonesian wife who looked like a Balinese Queen. It was a one-roomed affair comprised of two large slabs of wood for tables, with long benches beside them, and a few chairs at a small bar in the corner. It was packed solid when live Premier League football was shown on the large screen television.

One memorable night in 2011 was Manchester City's 6-1 thrashing of Manchester United. I jigged with another blue while the Man United fans gazed in astonishment as they finally realised that their noisy neighbours had arrived. I found myself singing "Another One Bites the Dust" followed by "We are the Champions" on that remarkable dreamy evening. I also had my soccer needs sated at budget prices, having live Premier League, European, international and cup games on the goggle box at home through Lao Cable TV, for the princely sum of £2 a month.

So, you can visualise an idyllic happy life and I felt like the mutt's nuts living this utopian existence. I had found what I was looking for; the perfect partner and the perfect place. Prince Siddhartha Gautama teaches us that nothing is permanent, and it was just about my turn to learn this painful lesson in the most harrowing way you could possibly imagine.

Run

(January to March 2102)

A shiny cherry-red Doc Martin boot thudded into my jaw and from that point in time I had difficulty speaking or masticating. I felt uncomfortably numb. Of course, I hadn't been booted in the kisser by an angry bovver boy or smashed in the gob with a pool ball concealed in a sock by some scumbag but was wishing I had. At least there would have been an explanation for the troublesome symptoms.

The only possible logic my numbed skull could put forward for my aching mandible was the rotten molar which was painfully extracted at the French clinic a few weeks earlier. I arrived hand on face with biting toothache before the throbbing yellow-green ivory was brutally ripped out in one aggressive wrench, which must have taken all of 0.00001 seconds. I departed with the same hand on face, gigantic startled eyeballs, a Formula One racing heart and lines of blood, sweat and tears overtaking and crashing into each other on my gobsmacked Mancunian mug. It was a far scream from the kind, softly-softly Thai and Laotian dental surgeries I had previously had the great pleasure of visiting.

I quickly hunted down the Hare and Hound pub and poached a litre of Tiger Beer to sedate my jangling nerves. My boozy drinking buddies howled with laughter, almost falling off their comfy bar stools as I reported my distressing episode at the merciless *Chamber de torture Française*

"Sit down," I mumbled.

"You visited the bloody frog butcher; you fucking idiot!" they yelped with glee. As the magical healing qualities of that exotic tropical brew started to take effect, I joined in the fun and laughter and almost fell off my bar stool too, as my chums recounted tales of other unlucky ex-pats who had foolishly made the same hilarious painful error as me.

"If I ever write a book, I will include this tale for sure," I slurred to my chuckling companions.

Thankfully I could at least still chew things over in my mind and concluded that the savage extraction was the cause of my discomfort. Unless, God Forbid, it was that vile thuggish hooligan CANCER, goading me with "Come and have a go if you think you're hard enough!"

January was the cool season in Laos, evoking memories of glorious summer days back in the UK. After nine months of sweltering sticky hotness and furious tropical rainstorms the cool season was welcomed with wide open arms. I even had to don a pullover whenever we were hit by a rare cold snap. It was nowt like the nut-freezing brass monkey weather back home in northern England, though!

During the first week of the month an old school mate I hadn't laid eyeballs on for over 35 years paid me a visit in Vientiane. She was bearing typical British gifts such as Marmite and a Terry's Chocolate Orange. It was incredible to see her after so long. She looked older and had put on weight. She no doubt thought the same about me because the last time we met I was a skinny, baby-faced youth. She sketched out in black, grey and white the sorrowful picture of a lonely life in England for a single woman in her fifties. She felt invisible.

My God, I couldn't think of anything worse than being back home as *The Invisible Man* in the UK. All my H.G. Wells nightmares rolled into one. To be sat alone and ignored during an icy-cold winter, with not a moggy in hell's chance of attracting a pretty femme fatale. Just another old codger who nobody takes any notice of. That would never happen in a million lifetimes. Over my dead body!

Here I was in a tropical paradise and here my Mancunian arse would stay until I drew my last dying gulp of jungle air. I reflected, I have my beautiful wife, my house, my work and my lovely kids. Even if I were single, I would be eyed-up here because as a multi-lingual Caucasian I am different. People smile and chat with me when I walk into the pub or go into the shops. And pretty ladies by the bedful would be happy to be my partner in Utopia and laugh and dance with me through this magical life. And there's as much well-paid employment as I want, too. No way will I ever be a lonely old man with no name in Blackpool. I would rather be dead.

Three wonderful dreamy days were enjoyed with Janet and her travelling companion Carol, visiting temples, markets and eating out at the many international restaurants. In an Italian favourite we had a vegetarian western-style spaghetti together whilst reminiscing about *The Good, the Bad and the Ugly* old days. I loved it. Eventually it was time for her to disappear, finish her backpacking trip and return to invisibility in cold, rainy England. With sadness in my heart I realised I would never see her again.

***

I was still teaching primary three at the international school but finding it increasingly problematic to talk and concentrate because of the ache in my jaw. Eating was no picnic either. So, I sheepishly returned to the frog butcher and explained the problem, but he brushed me off and arrogantly snarled, "Not my concern, go and see a doctor". My first inclination was to visit the doctor at the same clinic but after the harrowing episode with the dentist, quickly decided to give this house of pain a miss. So off I toddled to the private hospital near the airport and coughed up $100, to be informed it was a severe infection of the tonsils and given a plastic bag full of mega-strong antibiotics. The young doctor laughed when I mentioned the word cancer. "No way," he chuckled, "I would have seen it." Phew, well thank Buddha for that.

February arrived but the pain in my neck hadn't been cured by the ultra- expensive rip-off medication and was in fact getting bloody worse. However, I still tried to hide my fears and soreness and lovingly took care of my family as I wore the mask of happiness, without a care in the whole wide world. Jo started his first day of nursery on 1st March and we had a brief holiday in Thailand with me and the kids clad in Manchester City shirts. We could even win the Premier League this year! As we rambled around Phu Prabat Historical Park taking snapshots, I was starting to struggle with the fight against the discomfort in my face and the dreadful suspicion of cancer in my mind.

So, the next "Magical Mystery Tour" was to the private hospital in Udorn Thani in Thailand. I was given the diagnosis of swollen tonsils and had the image of them being cut open and drained tattooed on my jittery mind. The young female doctor also laughed off the possibility of the big C. I left the teaching job because I could hardly speak and found it futile attempting to focus on grammar, maths and homework.

I went midweek for this frightful little operation given under local anaesthesia. Unfortunately, my darling wife threw one of her frequent whirlwind tantrums from hell and refused point-blank to accompany me. I found this unbelievable under the circumstances: it gave my "Achy Breaky Heart" a proper bashing. I battled to keep my aching mouth open as the young doctor injected, sliced, cut and drained. Once finished, she insisted that I stay in the hospital overnight. I think the greedy bastards just wanted the money.

Day by day the pain just escalated. I quit the cancer sticks, but the agony didn't quit tormenting me. I started work as a business development manager for a bomb disposal company but had to stop after a couple of weeks because the pain was getting unbearable. So, as a last resort and with some trepidation I opted to visit the doctor at the French clinic.

What a wonderful surprise. He was warm, kind and gentle; the total opposite to the sadistic, heartless, arrogant dental butcher. This elderly Belgian physician treated me with compassion. At first, he couldn't see anything amiss but then he thought he spotted something at the back of my throat and stated that my facial shape didn't look quite right. He immediately organised an MRI scan in Thailand across the Mekong River for the following evening.

The hurricane-force-10 temper of my moody missus had now quelled, and I was joined by a bright, sunny, loving wife on the hour-long drive across the border. Into the clinic and into the machine which required me to lie flat in a narrow tube with banging noises going on around me. And it was so claustrophobic and noisy that I started to panic a bit. And me an experienced potholer with tons of experience of squeezing through the tightest-of-tight low wet tubes; so, you can imagine how bloody awful it was! Even worse was the extremely effeminate male nurse, who kept gripping the top of my thigh while I was stuck in this fucking machine. He whispered, "Be brave, I am here with you." *Well, thank fuck for that*, I mused. I was wishing it could have been a cute, slender, sexy female Thai nurse in white uniform and white stockings, but on second thoughts, maybe it wouldn't be such a good idea after all. Being trapped in this contraption with a Blackpool Tower on would have been rather embarrassing to say the least. (I just realised there is a ballroom below Blackpool Tower - lol.)

I was eventually released with massive beads of sweat on my brow and felt a gigantic feeling of relief, only to be told that they were going to inject a dye into my vein to make the results more visible. Ten more minutes stuck in that clanging machine almost sent me insane and it seemed more like 10 hours. I felt like climbing the walls but couldn't because I was trapped in this brain-battering apparatus. My swirling mind was gripped by terror while the male nurse's hand was gripped far too close to my knob.

Eventually I was released and given a large plain brown envelope to hand to my doctor and relieved of about £300 for the mind-numbing experience. Of course, I ripped it open it as soon as we got back to the car to discover a large tumour had been found in my throat. I gazed at it wide-eyed and in absolute horror as my wife hugged and kissed me.

The following morning, I drove like billy-o to the Belgian doctor at the French clinic and passed him the torn brown package. In hindsight,

I thought about the French dentist and realised I had been overcritical of him. He had just extracted a tooth, but the mollycoddling of the previous Lao and Thai dental surgeons had made a normal extraction appear brutal. The doc advised me to get to the cancer hospital in Khon Kaen, Thailand, a three-hour drive away, as fast as humanly possible. My now sympathetic wife accompanied me once again and we stayed overnight in a guesthouse next to the hospital. At night my worries didn't allow me any shuteye, so I attempted to read a book on Buddhism but could not still my thoughts and fears. Nirvana seemed 10 lifetimes away, but hell was just around the bend. And so was my screaming, terrified mind!

Into the hospital for an endoscopy; a tiny camera which was pushed up my nostril and down my throat, causing me to panic and gag. Of much greater concern was the gaggle of doctors focusing on the monitor, saying it was massive, aggressive and very serious. They didn't know I was fluent in Thai! I understood everything. They told me to return for a biopsy and if it was malignant, I would need chemotherapy. Lord have mercy; the gates of hell are opening, and I can feel the heat already. I was fully aware that life was a roller coaster but wasn't prepared for this sudden scary ride on a ghost train.

***

Upon returning to Laos I recall my mates being aghast with shock as they screamed at me to get back to the UK NOW. *"You will just die here."* Some even suggested that I dash back alone but I thought I would rather die here in agony than be away from my wife and children. So, a plan was swiftly thrown together to get me and my family to the UK as soon as possible. I had to get visas for my wife and Jo, who only had Laos passports. So, the first port of call was the British Embassy in Bangkok, about which I had read horror stories online regarding the difficulty of obtaining visas for ex-pats' wives or girlfriends.

The next few days were just an agonising blur. I managed to sell my car to a friend. My jaw was getting worse and worse. I was starting to spit big lumps of blood out of my twisted gob. I would scream out loud in agony when no one was close by. I was in extreme pain and was having difficulty in speaking or eating. The target was to get myself, my wife and kids back to the UK pronto. I was scared to death that I would be too weak and ill and wouldn't be allowed on the plane. I can recollect saying goodbye to my wife's family and with immense sorrow realised I probably wouldn't see them again.

Down to Bangkok and a small hotel. To the British Embassy to apply for visas for Jo and the Missus. Pain, confusion, weakness and lumps of bright red blood, spat from my gob and splattering on the pavements, were the norm. One night when the kids were asleep, I gazed adoringly at my beautiful wife and said, "It isn't good sweetheart, I think I am going to die."

She cried, "I love you, don't die, you have taken care of me since we met." Yes, I had done everything for her and her family and solved every problem that came along. How would she cope without me? We cried softly together and made tender love.

The next day the pain went stratospheric and my bloodstained jaw wouldn't move so my spaced-out mind decided there and then it was time to take off. I couldn't wait any longer; I had to fly NOW. My family would have to follow if their visa applications were successful. With tears in my eyes, on 31st March 2012 I left them at Bangkok airport and got on the plane to Doha. I used to hate flying and would be panic-stricken at the slightest bit of turbulence, practically crossing off each minute of the journey on a scrap of paper with a tick and getting totally pissed but never being able to pass out. Now I didn't give a shite, this cancer was far scarier than a bumpy trip through the sky.

I got to Doha and had a four-hour wait for my flight to Manchester. I recall lying down on a very uncomfortable bench shivering and in terrible pain. Of course, the flight was delayed for another three hours. I was in agony, bringing up blood but doing my best to hide the pain so I could get on the flight. But the pain of being away from my wife and kids hurt so much more and I felt so alone and helpless in this cold, air-conditioned airport lounge. At long last I got on the plane and off we flew to Manchester. Going through arrivals, I was pulled out by customs and my bag was thoroughly searched, which delayed me another 30 minutes.

The customs officer was a City fan who still believed the Sky Blues could win the title. I wasn't so optimistic and believed that they had thrown their chance away and our biggest rivals would take top spot. All clear at the customs and out into the reception, where I met my brother Jeff and his wife Ann. And guess who was with them; the very visible Janet, who only two and a half months earlier I had thought I would never see again. "Isn't Life Strange".

Psycho Killer

(April 2012)

"Thought you would look thinner," my brother mentioned.

"Soon will be mate, I can't fucking eat," I quipped.

I was so jaded and as sick as a dog, so it was a supersonic relief to be near people who cared whether I lived or died. The people who didn't, I would have kicked in the head if I had had any energy! Helen, my tall niece was there too. They proposed that I should dart as fast as my flagging body would arrow me to Wythenshawe hospital and throw my crippled self at their mercy. It didn't quite hit the bullseye with me, so I insisted on going to Blackpool with my brother and his wife and visiting my quack the following day.

On the car journey from Manchester to Blackpool I gazed with wonder at the bright sparkling green fields of spring. My face was scarlet as I struggled with the pain and my heart sank in deep blue sorrow, as I longed to be with my wife and kids. At that moment I decided I would take my loving wife and gorgeous kids to visit as many places as possible in the UK before I finally ended up as a line between two dates on a gravestone. If I wasn't trapped in some Godforsaken hospice from hell, that is. I shuddered as I pictured myself in palliative care as I faced death all alone in a small room. The horror of wasting away and howling in agony with psychedelic tears in my eyes, knowing I would never see my beautiful spouse and offspring again. Bloody scary times, I must say!

At long last I conked out in pain, misery, confusion and exhaustion in my brother's spare room. The following morning, I popped my aching head into the docs and was given an appointment with an ENT consultant in two weeks' time! Good job I only had a tumour in my neck and not something less serious, such as a broken leg, otherwise I would have had to wait for at least six months! I left disheartened and outraged at the hold-up in securing the urgent life-or-death support I needed NOW.

Fuck that! So, I pleaded with Jeff to whizz me to the A&E at the hospital and was granted an appointment in three long days' time. Phew - a bit better, I suppose. I held my jaw in torment, with fearful daymares of death, pain and gloom bouncing around in my deranged skull, and with no escape at nightfall either, coz even worse bad dreams were endured when the sun went down. Believe me, once the word CANCER wallops your eardrums, your whole existence transforms into a fiendishly scary

24-hour blurry nightmare.

I heard that 1 in 2 males and 1 in 3 of the more deadly sex of the species will be stunned and see stars when they hear "sorry, you have cancer" during their time on planet Earth! So, if you wish to dodge the hair-raising (before the chemo - lol) bad trip along the cancer "Highway to Hell", then you'd better do something about it "Right Here, Right Now". Prick up your lugholes and quit the cancer sticks, cease the intake of dead animal flesh and chicken's periods, all processed foods, sugar and especially the dangerous, tumour creating bloody dairy.

The good news is that you can scoff all the delicious fruits and vegetables to your heart's content and a massive lip-licking bonus is you are still permitted bucket loads of dirty sex too. Therefore, because you will now be full to the brim of amazing power boosting vitamins and nutrients and devoid of artery and vein-clogging shite from the junk food, your sex life will be hard to beat! An extra incentive is that you won't be a lethargic fat bastard either. Right, I will climb down off my cruelty-free vegan soapbox but heed my warning, before it becomes your turn to have a chinwag with the Grim Reaper!

I was phoning my loving wife a few times a day telling her how much I missed her, worshipped her, needed her and loved her and of course, my beautiful kids too. I was not only sick with cancer but also sick with worry about the visa applications. I decided at that painful moment in time that if the visa applications were rejected, I would fly back to Laos and die with the family I loved so much. I couldn't live without them!

I borrowed a Bear Grylls survival book from the library. This super hard ex-SAS hard man could overcome any death-threatening situation, but I bet he would shit his fleecy camouflage four-season trousers if he were walking in my cancer riddled slippers. I would much prefer to be facing any of his life-or-death survival adventures than battling with the big C. I would even drink my own piss and eat my own shit but would draw a line at murdering an animal and eating it. That is just downright sick and disgusting.

Into the hospital for shedloads of unpleasant tests including the dreaded MRI scan. It wasn't as harrowing this time around because I knew what was coming and I didn't have an effeminate male nurse feeling me up. The long and the short of it was that a tumour was confirmed, and I would have the pleasure of a biopsy to see if it was malignant. Still in pain, I was given oral morphine to gulp. Thank God for that, otherwise

I would have had to seek out a local dealer and score a wrap of smack to ease the symptoms!! I had difficulty eating and was rapidly losing weight. I didn't think I would ever be a fat bastard again.

Then at long last I got the news I had been longing for. The visas had been approved. I had an "Uncontrollable Urge" to dance but my dying body wouldn't allow a session of pogoing or headbanging, so I went to the spare room and sobbed 4,000 disco tears which bopped from my psychedelic eyes down my now gaunt cheeks. What a relief! I swiftly arranged the flights and my loved ones would arrive in two days' time, on 7th April. Soon I would hold my wife's hand, be hugged, kissed and cared for as I battled for my life. I would see my two kids. I loved my family so deeply and these few days were the longest we had ever been apart. Each minute seemed like a day as I fought the pain and the fear of death, waiting to be united with the ones I lived for. It felt like I was in the monkey house serving the last two days of a sentence for a crime I did not commit. Old Father Time is a proper bastard as we all know too well; making the good times flash by and the bad times drag on for a fucking eternity.

***

Time crawled by until at long last I was at Manchester airport with my loyal friend Janet. We had a coffee as the butterflies fluttered madly in my tense stomach. My eyes were glued to the monitor, counting down the minutes, seconds and milliseconds waiting for the flight to arrive. At last it landed. Then about 30 long minutes later a chilling announcement echoed around the reception lounge: Would Mr Sydney Barnes please go to desk number three immediately. Oh my God, they are going to be refused entry, my mind cried. The dancing butterflies suddenly died a grizzly death as they were strangled by the knot in my belly. I felt gutted! Luckily it was just for a confirmation of address and a few minutes later I was reunited with the people who were my world. My beautiful wife smiled, and my kids hugged me. I felt like crying but boys and sad old men dying of cancer don't cry, do they?

My brother Jeff had kindly booked and paid for some holiday flats on the Prom, but that was from tomorrow, so we stayed a night in a dingy B&B in Chorlton, the area of south Manchester I grew up in. My family and I had a wander around my childhood haunts. Would I be haunting this place in the near future, I mused. I was as happy as Larry but ill and not at ease with my achy breaky jaw. The following day Janet picked us up and took us to Piccadilly train station and soon we were in Blackpool residing in the Granada holiday flats. It was lovely being hugged and held by my wife and being close to my children.

My wife loved watching a programme called *Cheaters* on TV. The camera crew followed and caught a cheating partner, causing uproar, tears and fights. There was nothing like that on Lao or Thai TV, so I fully understood her fascination. I was lucky, I had a loyal, loving wife who would never do that to me in a million lifetimes.

I was given the date of 27th April for my biopsy to see whether the tumour was malignant. In the meantime, I took my wife and kids out every day. The missus loved the shops in the town centre and we would go on buses and trams to local places such as Fleetwood, St. Anne's and Poulton-le-Fylde. I knew I was weak and very ill, as the trail of bright red blobs of shiny blood I spat out confirmed. I just wanted life to be a holiday, treating my wife and kids to days out while I still could. Holding my wife's hand and being with my kids was heavenly, but for how much longer, before I fell to hell?

I went with the missus and kids to have a PET scan to see if the cancer had spread to other parts of my knackered carcass. They injected a dye into me and I was informed that I may feel as if I was urinating, but I wouldn't be, so not to worry, and I could have an itching sensation in my anus too. Well, the test went ahead and just to let you know, I didn't feel like pissing my two-year-old ripped jeans or scratching my God-given Mancunian arse. And even better news was the fact that no further cancerous growths were discovered. Every dark cloud has a silver lining, I suppose.

We were forced to move out of the Granada holiday flats coz some candy floss, Blackpool rock, toffee apple devouring, obese, slobby arsehole in a Kiss Me Quick hat (bloody quick in my opinion) complained that Jo had disturbed her by making too much noise in the flat. And Jo wasn't that noisy. I was livid. Normally I would just accept the situation and feel sympathy towards another fellow being. Was this tumour changing me from a laid-back Mr Coolio into an angry Mr Billy Fury?

The new landlady at the Seaview holiday flats we moved to, looked aghast when she came within breathing distance of my yellow-grey, sunken cheeks and deathly decaying face. But then everybody did when they saw the coffin dodging look of death, before swiftly averting their shocked eyes. This was what it must be like to be disfigured, or to have been one of the first black people to immigrate to the UK.

Remember, I had had a similar feeling when visiting remote areas of China. People just looked at me with dropped jaws and stared and stared at the foreign devil. So, to combat this I would just focus my gaze at a point 1000 yards into the distance. I was using this method now to avoid the looks of shock, the whispers and pointing fingers. Nosferatu was alive but not so well, living like a death-warmed-up ghoul in rainy Blackpool, Lancashire.

My wonderful brother and his wife took us all out for a meal at a Thai restaurant in the town centre and I even managed to sip a bit of veggie curry. Well, the 27th arrived and I was out cold for the biopsy, coming around a few hours later. I begged to go home so I could be with my wife and kids, but the doctor insisted I stay overnight. I was drowsy and slept like a corpse, rising the following morning. The young doctor came to see me with a sad look in his eyes and said softly, "I am very sorry Mr Barnes, your cancer is malignant, very large, very advanced and very very serious. It is stage four, and we have taken your tonsils out because they were riddled with cancer. I am so sorry to deliver such bad news."

Fuuuuuuuuuck! My darling wife please help me, hold me, kiss me, love me. I have terminal cancer. I am going to fucking die!

Jump

(May 2012)

I lay in a nauseating dreamy blur struggling to live with the fact that I was dying and that my involvement in the game of life was nearing the final whistle. Before long I would be worm food six feet under. "Ashes to Ashes", dust to dust. *Will my psychedelic life pass before my sky-blue peepers at the moment I finally pop my Lancashire wooden clogs*, I mused. I closed my eyes and stared at the gruesome grinning face and dark soulless eyes of Death, knowing that my given tarot card foretold an impending painful finale.

A nurse punctured my unreal trancelike state. "Hurry up and get ready because you will shortly be going home by ambulance," she instructed. For some uncanny reason my distressed psyche jumped to football and the vile threatening taunts of "You're going home by fucking ambulance", chanted by mobs of goading hooligans. I cannot for the death or life of me comprehend how someone can obtain pleasure from kicking ten tons of shit out of another person because he happens to support a different football team. My peace-loving hippy mind just cannot suss it out, man! Although I do admit to once calling the referee a no-dad.

The ex-Liverpool manager Bill Shankly once said, something about football being far more serious than life and death. Well my "Live or Die" situation was super serious as my terrified mind knew full well. If my life were a football match it would be an FA cup tie and I would be losing by a single goal to the evil unbeatable Death United. They would be coached by the very special one: The Grim Reaper. The tie would be in the dying seconds (lol) of injury time (lol - yet again) and I would be fighting for a last gasp (and once more...) miraculous equaliser to take the match and my life into extra time!

Back to the Seaview holiday flats by fucking ambulance to break the sad news to my wife. We held each other close and tight. The tormenting reflection that I wouldn't be holding my elegant loyal partner for much longer or be able to watch my adorable kids grow up hurt far worse than the tumour, as you can well imagine.

***

My ex-wife contacted me to say that my daughter Francesca Emma would be arriving at Manchester Airport in two days to visit me for a week. I had been in constant contact with Francesca and she had visited me in Laos and had joined us on holidays too. She was now living in Lille in France as the ex had tied the knot with a French bloke. I knew full well that this trip was arranged so she could be with her father one last time before he snuffed it. I took my dying body and a bottle of liquid morphine on the train with me to meet her at the airport. On the return journey to Blackpool I remained chirpy and happy, making her smile as I hid my dreadful fear of pain and death from her 12-year-old mind.

The next unwelcome visit to the "House of Fun" (Blackpool's Victoria Hospital) was an appointment with the oncologist. I was informed that the cancer was stage four and too large for surgery. It would mean cutting half my face off, which would improve my looks but not my survival time because it would no doubt kill me. So, three sessions of full-on chemotherapy were proposed in an attempt to shrink this massive deadly tumour. My panicking mind couldn't put forward any other method of delaying my inevitable final ending, so I readily agreed.

After the appointment I held my wife's hand tightly as I was led into a small "White Room" with a lovely caring senior ENT (ear nose and throat) nurse called Jo Ashton. She passed me a DS1500 form to hand into the benefits office. I knew full well that this note was for terminally ill people with a prognosis of less than six months, so they can receive full benefits and bypass all the usual interviews and questions. I looked into Jo's eyes and whispered, "This is a note for people who are close to death."

She softly replied, "I am so sorry Syd, your tumour is very large and very advanced." I walked out of the hospital in a zombified blur. I was the walking dead soon to be the eternal dead. I held my pretty wife's hand and trembled as the cancer was eating me alive while the thought that I would soon be parted from my sweetheart ate me up inside too. Vaughan, a friend from Norwich who I had worked with in Laos phoned as I was walking to the bus stop and was shocked by the news.

As well as the pain and the shock of having inoperable terminal cancer I had the problem of money. What little cash I had left was starting to run out after flights and relocating to the UK. Staying in the expensive holiday flats was out of the question so I had to cough up nearly £4000 to rent a house for six months. It was a two-up two-down terraced house in the centre of Bispham village, north Blackpool. It was clean and tidy with a large kitchen and dining room and a small back yard. My amazing brother Jeff helped by getting me some second-hand furniture.

I had no option but to throw myself at the mercy of the benefits system and the DS1500 document plus a phone call from my local MP who I had contacted for help ensured all benefits were paid and I was even refunded all the money I had spent renting the house. Great, but I would have preferred not having cancer to be perfectly frank.

My friend John, who had bought my car in Laos, visited me and paid for Eugene and Francesca to go on some rides at Blackpool Pleasure Beach. They even went on the Big One; a huge white-knuckle roller coaster. They loved it, but I didn't join them because I was still stuck riding the cancer ghost train to hell.

Francesca Emma went back to France and there were tears in my eyes when I realised that I probably wouldn't ever see her again. On 7th May we stayed in a Premier Inn for a night before moving into our tiny house the following day. This was now home until I moved into my next place of residence: a wooden coffin. Ha-ha. *What a change from my house in tropical paradise,* I sadly pondered.

***

The first adventure of the chemo trip was to have a PICC line fitted. PICC stands for Peripherally Inserted Central Catheter. It is put into a vein in your upper arm during an outpatient appointment. The line runs up the vein inside your arm and ends up in a large vein near your heart. This is where they would attach the different poisons, to travel straight to my jam tart (heart) and be pumped around my system, hopefully shrinking the tumour but unfortunately destroying lots of healthy cells and giving my immune system a proper bashing, leaving it left for dead.

So, I lay on yet another hospital bed with two nurses beside me and a shiny steel tray full of scalpels and other instruments of pain. The younger of the two was preparing for the cut and holding the line to be pushed up the vein in my arm, towards my shoulder and from there down to my tick-tocker, which was now pumping like the bloody clappers. She looked a tad nervous, so I joked, "You alright love?"

She stuttered, "Yes but it is the first time I have performed this procedure." *Well, fuck me!* my mind screamed. She was fit and sexy but a session of the 'old ins and outs' (*Clockwork Orange* speak for sexual intercourse) was the last thing on my startled, terrified mind, I can assure you.

The elder nurse speedily and loudly piped up with authority, "Don't worry - I am supervising her."

Well, thank fuck for that, I thought as I breathed a sigh of relief. If I was frightened and apprehensive before this minor operation, I was now shitting myself. Well, my arm was cut, and the line was pushed along my vein to near my rapidly beating ticker and a contraption was fixed to my arm, onto which the poisons would be attached next week. It was unpleasant and did hurt but I didn't flinch as I focused on my wife and kids. I was getting used to pain. It was the norm. I smiled at the young nurse and praised her for the excellent job she had done and thanked her for being gentle while taking my PICC line virginity.

A week later the ambulance arrived to transport me to Preston Royal for my first session of poisoning. I gazed in deep love at my beautiful wife and little Jo waving goodbye at the window as we pulled away. My God, I really wanted to live and be with them. Into the hospital for a blood test, then into the chemo lounge to sit with my Chemical Brothers and sisters. Comfy armchairs were filled with sad-looking faces being given the so-called lifesaving, or in my case life extending concoctions. I held my arm out as the first of three bags of toxic fluid were attached to the uncomfortable contraption and sang, "Hey guys, Hey Gals Let's go," Let the madness begin.

I read the *Lancashire Life* magazine, looking at the massive country houses I would buy if I won the lottery, until reality kicked me in the knackers, leaving me in pain as I realised that a tiny coffin was my next place of abode. The boring six-hour session continued until at long last a glass bottle full of poison was strapped to my stomach, to continue pumping the toxic potion into my claret for a further five days to shrink the fucking tumour. I was speedily transported home to my loved ones. So far so good.

I had a heavenly kip in the land of nod and awoke in hell. "Welcome to my Nightmare". I was vomiting, choking and my mind was not in this world. District nurses would visit me daily administering huge injections and handfuls of drugs to swallow in an effort to keep infections at bay and numb the bloody pain. I was counting down the days until the horrendous pump would finally be taken off, releasing me from this terrifying, cloud cuckoo land. I would sit on the sofa in complete madness.

At times I thought I was sleeping on the beach under the pier. I was desperate to escape this insanity. I looked through the window at the pub roof across the road and my unsound mind chuckled, *Jump off the roof and this bad dream is over.* The tiny bit of sanity I had left warned, *Bad idea Syd; you may not die and just imagine the horror of being mangled or paralysed and having to struggle with terminal cancer too!* Or even worse, I might end up mentally retarded, with my unhinged mind not permitted to decide whether I would agree to further painful treatments for the cancer. Phew! Just having the minor problem of only having to battle with terminal cancer didn't seem so bad after all. Although I was totally pissed-off with being off my psychedelic rocker, living in madness, with this bastard bad trip-inducing pump attached to my dying body.

Well, ultimately the day arrived when the abominable apparatus was at long last to be detached, freeing my deranged mind from the toxic nuthouse from hell. The district nurse arrived with more drugs and injections before finally taking the no-dad contraption off. "Thank God, Allah, Buddha and Krishna for that," I chanted. Then, oh no, the very last words I wanted to hear: "It will continue to get worse before it gets better," the nurse warned. Spiritual chanting screeched to a halt as I realised that there can't be a God but there must be a devil and Lucifer was laughing his evil head off in his fiery palace at this very moment.

Shit, is there any escape from this crazy nightmare? Maybe I should have jumped after all, I reflected.

And believe me it just got worse and worse. I was insane, couldn't eat, was choking and vomiting, with constant diarrhoea and rapidly losing weight. I hurriedly made an appointment to see my oncologist and got a taxi to the hospital. My broken bag of bones couldn't walk so my caring wife had to push me in a wheelchair. Another first on this cancerous bad trip. My brother and his wife swiftly came to join us, and their shocked eyes nearly popped out of their skulls when they saw my dying skeleton. My brother later informed me that I looked just like my dad, days before he died of cancer. The oncologist took one look and admitted me pronto to a small isolation ward.

My doomed frame was placed on a bed and punctured with injections, fed pills and foul-tasting liquids, and I had a drip in each arm in a last-ditch effort to keep me at fingernail's length from death's door. I knew full well that I had one foot in the grave as I struggled for my life. My wife, brother and kids visited my fading bod. My super-fit drop-dead gorgeous wife kissed, held and loved my super-unfit, soon to be drop-dead form. However, I refused to give up the ghost because the vision of being away from my loved ones was a fate worse than death.

I read a book about a young lad who sailed alone across angry oceans, but it was all dreamlike in my foggy, drugged-up mind. No more adventures in foreign lands for me; my next trip would be when I broke on through to the other side. If there was another side?

Then about six days later I awoke feeling as right as rain and was told I could go home by effing ambulance. Wow, it would be blissful being with my wife and kids again. Wonderful. I felt so happy that I even forgot that I was dying for a second or two.

***

From August 2011, before the cancer-mare, I had watched every game played by Manchester City live on the goggle-box, right up to the final must-win game against QPR to secure the title for the first time in 44 years. It had looked as if they had thrown it away to our biggest rivals but a couple of bad results for United and a pair of victories for City gave us a chance of winning the long-awaited prize. Even while I was ill, I still managed to hobble to a local pub to watch my team. An eventful match against United was watched with a cup of tea in the crowded, shouting pub. City won by a single goal and the pub went wild. I couldn't jump and cheer but did raise my painful arm a little and put a smug Cheshire cat's grin on my gaunt face. I chuckled to myself as I thought of my team's acronym, CTID (City 'Til I Die). Even though I was in my nutty dreamland during the good old chemo trip, I did know that I must somehow watch the final game which was being played tomorrow.

Out of the blue I saw on the news that Manchester City were the Premier League champions. Great and shit. My confused tree had got the dates mixed up and this was the first game I had missed this season. I watched the game on *Match of the Day* that evening and it was probably a good thing that I had missed the live game because I don't think my ticker could have withstood such drama. Typical City, they were dead and buried and had lost the title but in the final five minutes had scored two goals to win the league and achieve the impossible. Sergio Aguero's last-gasp goal is the most iconic goal ever scored in the history of the Premier League. I was elated and dared to dream that I could achieve the impossible too, and beat this bloody cancer?

I was in blue moon heaven but was brought swiftly back down to planet Earth with the realisation that I still had two more bad trips to red-hot scarlet hell and total toxic madness to come. To have an iota more than a cat in hell's chance of doing a Sergio Aguero and achieving the impossible by defeating the big C I had to dream, fight and be strong. *Superbia In Proelio*; pride in battle. I shuddered as I felt the icy fingers of death on my shoulder and the hot fiery breath of that red devil Beelzebub burning my mind. But I was ready for the next round and these two evil cocky bastards would soon be laughing on the other sides of their ghastly faces when my gaunt mug laughed last and loudest. I could not die yet; my family needed me. Bring it on!

Highway to Hell

(May-June 2012)

I felt as joyful as a swine in shite as I fooled around with my gorgeous wife and kids. Holding, hugging, loving and playing. I was tickled pink as I let what little hair I had left down; treasuring the magical moments with my loved ones as I sluggishly awakened from the chemical fire and brimstone netherworld. Sadly, I failed to snog goodbye to the grim spooky image haunting my troubled tree, which was unremittingly trumpeting that there were still two further journeys to the centre of venomous madness to be endured just around the next dark psychotic corner.

With my skinny back against the impending hospice wall I had no alternative but to come out fighting, but what could my now streak-of-piss slim body do to increase my even slimmer chances of survival. I had been sipping two litres of fruit and vegetable juice a day thanks to my friend Janet, who donated her juicing machine. Apples, pears, pineapples, carrots and beetroot were just a few of the natural foods that were liquefied and fed into my body to try and give it some ammunition to fight the big bastard C. I was now a raw vegan. I was wise to the dim prognosis that the time-honoured conventional ritual of poisoning the tumour didn't appear to permit me the time to live happily ever after on planet Earth. Under these dire circumstances my only option was to clutch at straws and think from outside the mind and immune system destroying chemo box.

Therefore, I declared war on this pernicious enemy. I will fight it in my hospital bed, I will fight it at home on my second-hand cream sofa and I will fight it on Blackpool Beach too. I will never surrender. However, this wasn't some brash jackboot-wearing, goose-stepping foreign invader but my own sneaky cells slyly mutating and attacking my sick and dying body. Welcome to the 21st century war of the roses. My Lancastrian red rose knackered immune system battling the rapidly advancing warmongering black rose cancer cells of the Grim Reaper. A bloodthirsty civil war to the death! It was imperative that an ally was found pronto to give me an outside chance of repelling and defeating this mushrooming rebellion. But where would I find my magic Trojan horse?

So, I did what any poor sod would do if they were limping in my dead man's slippers - I searched the internet. Big mistake. I went from tales of horror, doom, gloom and pain ending in certain death to fairy tales of mystical herbs that would cure me in seven days. It was soul-destroying. But eventually I found my ally in Chris Woollams and his website www.canceractive.com. It was a charity run by Chris, a biochemist whose daughter had died of brain cancer. It was loaded with information about conventional and alternative methods of fighting the big C. I ordered two books - *Everything You Need to Know to Beat Cancer* and *The Rainbow Diet* to help me plan the strategy for winning this war. "Onward Psycho Syd's So-ol-diers. Marching Off to War!"

I also got in touch with The Swallows, a local head and neck cancer support group run by Chris Curtis, who had also battled the dreaded disease. I went to a meeting to chat with fellow sufferers who had fought or who were fighting the frightful affliction. It was good to meet people who had been through or were going through the same fearful nightmare, but I still felt so alone and so afraid.

***

My wife, kids, my brother, his missus and my skeleton entered the oncologist's room. "Welcome to the Barnes Army," the doctor smiled. Well at least he got into the spirit of things by recognising that it was all-out war. He confirmed that the chemo had shrunk the tumour. And a further plus was that I realised my gob didn't have the foul stench of death anymore. I'd been mulling over why my better half had suddenly ceased snogging me! Thankfully other parts of my doomed frame didn't stink like a murderous tumour, because we were still at it! The trivial inconvenience that I was soon to kick the bucket wasn't about to put an end to our highly sexual erotic relationship. We had made love daily for the last eight years and nowt was going to put a stop to that while I was still on planet Earth. I knew full well that I was in Dire Straits and that there was sod all chance of "Dancing by the Pool" but at least we were still capable of being "Romeo and Juliet".

The Buzzcocks tune "Orgasm Addict" rang a bell but their more famous hit, "Ever Fallen in Love (With Someone You Shouldn't've)" certainly didn't as I gripped my loving wife's hand, awaiting further news from the doc. The main man agreed that the initial bout of chemo had given my body a proper kicking, so he proposed a lower dosage with different chemical poisons. Who was I to argue? I hadn't yet had time to come up with any alternative battle plans.

The ambulance transported my nervous skinny frame down the

M55 "Highway to Hell" for the onset of the second session of madness at Preston Royal. Once again there was a blood test, three bags of poison, magazines in the comfy chemo lounge, a glass pump attached to my stomach and I was sent home by yet another effing ambulance. So far so good and I dared to dream that the lower dosage and different poisons would not send me to toxic la-la land once more.

"Sweet Dreams" were not made of this as I awoke in *One Flew Over the Cuckoo's Nest* for a second time. Pure lunacy. My head was here, there and bloody everywhere. I could still talk to my wife and kids as I sprawled on the sofa in the living/dying room! The screaming toxins played havoc with my foggy mind and my squealing body. Gigantic jabs administered by the district nurse were the norm. There were plenty of pills and bellyaches but alas, no thrills on each unhappy Monday, Tuesday and every other day of the week.

On this subsequent chemical bad trip to Hades I wasn't glaring at the horrific poison pump with loathing, eager for the swine to be detached from my pitiful body, just in case I collapsed once again. Well, after five days the contraption was finally separated from my toxic frame and off I crawled to my sick sofa and into the land of nod. "Sun-a-riseEearly in the Morning" welcomed me to my next nightmare as my body folded in torment. I was gagging, trying to regurgitate the deadly toxin sprinting amok inside my temple, shitting all over the brown carpet, keeling over in extreme agony and battling to control the alarming noisy hysteria screaming inside my bald brainbox.

In a panic-stricken frenzy I phoned my brother Jeffrey Lewis Hamilton, who pit-stopped at my house, then raced to the imaginary chequered flag at Blackpool Victoria Hospital's Accident and Emergency department. It was no "Champagne Supernova" moment as I waited in dread and despair for them to source me a bed. I was spewing up bright green alien vomit, while glow-in-the-dark liquid emerald shite was squirting from my suffering sphincter. My brother gasped in shock and couldn't believe his eyes as he informed the nurses of my desperate struggle for survival. I was rapidly placed on a bed, pumped with drugs, drips were put in my arms and I was wheeled to yet another isolation ward. What the fuck had they been pumping into me, I wondered, because it was fucking killing me! If this was my karma, I must have been a right evil bastard in my previous life.

Eating and drinking was almost impossible and then came yet another new experience on the cancer trip; I couldn't walk without a fucking Zimmer frame! I was deteriorating and going downhill fast. "How the hell am I going to climb back up if I can't even move without a sodding frame," I asked myself. Looks like I'm never going to see another Christmas because this war is over! I almost gave up the ghost and surrendered.

The nurses egged me on to eat but it was no chicken's periods for me, just bits of bread, veggie soup and mashed potatoes. Alas, any food swallowed was painfully spewed up over the bed before one could say "Always Look on the Bright Side of Life". I still had a special case of the runs but in my condition, I couldn't even walk to the loo. In my Madness I would struggle with my frame to reach the bog, which would always be "One Step Beyond", resulting in me shitting my baggy pyjamas. Bad Manners I know, but I couldn't bloody help it. If it got any worse, I would end up busting a blood vessel and haunting a black and white "Ghost Town".

My wife and my brother would visit me every day. She would kiss me and love me. I was so lucky having such a caring and loving partner, which inspired me to fight on when all hope seemed lost. I just wanted to be home in her arms, away from this cold and lonely isolation ward. My body had reacted very badly to the chemotherapy and I was in a bad way, fighting for my life.

There was this vile red liquid potassium that I had to drink. It was like slurping hydrochloric acid and had me writhing in torment, gripping the side of the bed, gritting my teeth in a sweaty torturous hell for a few minutes. I would avoid it for as long as possible then gulp, followed by mind-blowing shock that this off the chart mega level of pain even existed.

***

Out of the clear blue sky I was given the unwelcome news that it was crucial to have a peg tube attached to my stomach because in the not-too-distant future I would be in such a state that I wouldn't be able to eat. To survive I would need to feed myself calorie high sweet sugary milk through a tube in my belly. Not my idea of a liquid lunch I can assure you. Bloody hell, whatever next, I mused!

I was pushed to the theatre in a wheelchair and instructed to lie on a bed in a room with six corpses. My jaw hit the floor as I gazed in shock, fear and terror, until I realised that they weren't dead after all but still breathing and clinging on to mortal life by the skin of their decaying teeth.

I released a welcome sigh of relief until a dreadful realisation snatched the rest of my breath away. Shit, I am a death warmed up cadaver too, barely alive, waiting for my turn to be a stiff in an ice box in the shadow of the morgue. Tears filled my eyes as I visualised my wife and kids.

A plump, smiling nurse held my sweaty hand as my bed was wheeled into the torture chamber. Three serious-looking men in white coats stood near a monitor and a cold-hearted tray of shiny instruments. I was informed that until recently, this procedure was performed under a general anaesthetic, but it wasn't a major operation so was now completed with the patient wide-a-fucking-wake. This really was my lucky day. Must check my lottery tickets. Is this what the NHS has come to? I was injected with a drug to make me drowsy but believe me, my eyes were almost popping out of my skull.

Two of the men forced my painfully locked cancer ridden jaw open as wide as possible and jammed a contraption in to keep my gob open. Another taste of agony. And there's more. They then pushed a camera which just about fitted, down my cancer throat and into my hopefully cancer-free stomach. I was gagging and struggling to breathe as rivers of hot panicky sweat cascaded down my quivering cheeks.

The third man grabbed the knife! He carefully proceeded to cut a hole in my middle. I felt each and every sharp jab and stab as he pierced my flesh and sliced through my stomach lining. A tube was pushed through the hole and the other two men struggled for over 20 minutes to attach and secure it to my trembling belly. One operated the camera while the other manoeuvred a tool as they both focused on the flickering monitor. My eyeballs bulged like an insane, scared-to-death Marty Feldman as I tried to ignore the screaming pain and dread.

One day in the future I would meet a man selling books at a vegan fair who informed me that he once worked as a nurse in a theatre where the PEG tube procedure was performed. He stared at me sympathetically upon learning that I had undergone that horrifying operation. He confessed that he still had nightmares about the appalling terror the poor patients had endured.

Virtually 2000 petrifying light years later I landed back on planet Earth; my excruciating out-of-this-world trip was over. I was wheeled back to my isolation ward, astonished and more than slightly dazed, for more stinging injections, distasteful liquids and shed loads of multi-coloured pills. I felt so alone and vulnerable and desperately needed to hold and love my beautiful wife and lovely kids. My shell-shocked mind raced over that torturous soul-destroying experience, hardly able to grasp that it had actually happened. Thank God it was over, but things were soon to get even worse.

***

After seven days I started to recover from my harrowing trip to toxic hell. I even managed a smirk when the doctor informed me that I could go home the next day. I was still very weak but could just about manage the few steps to the throne, saving me the embarrassment of shouting, "Nurse, sorry, I've shat my pants again." I was a proud, crippled, cocky, council estate Mancunian as my gorgeous wife on a visit walked my broken bag of bones through the main ward and along the corridor for 10 minutes.

The other inmates - err sorry, patients - must have been gobsmacked, wondering why such a good-looking lady could love and be with such an ugly old Hammer House of Horror monster. What they didn't know, of course, was that I had transformed her life from poverty, bought her a house and land, car, beautiful clothes, taught her English as well as taken her on holidays to foreign lands. But more than this, I had adored her, treated her with love, kindness, warmth and respect, also being completely faithful in a land where the Caucasian male is inundated with daily temptations from the opposite sex! Now it was her opportunity to help me during this desperate battle as I fought for my life. She would "Stand by Me" as I fought tooth and claw with the bastard cancer for a happy-ever-after ending.

I didn't bat an eyelid at their astonished faces because I had always had super-fit, head-turning, stunning athletic women on my arm for as long as I could remember, much to the confusion of Mr Joe Public. Would my cocky arrogance come back to bite me on the arse?

Just one more night in "So Lonely" isolation. I looked on in fear as the dreaded red liquid potassium was placed on the cabinet next to my bed. A devilish grin slowly spread across my cheeky face as I realised that I was going home tomorrow. Therefore, I crept to the lavatory with the evil drink in hand and gleefully shouted, "Fuck off," as I poured it into the toilet and flushed it far away from me. I felt like a naughty schoolboy with the empty plastic container next to my bed and smiled as I drifted to sleep, knowing I would be with my loved ones the following day.

The warm-hearted nurse took my temperature, blood pressure and a claret sample just before the friendly doctor examined me and informed me that I looked better and would be able to go home now. I was so happy but then there was another shock out of the sky blue! A short while later the doctor arrived with a concerned look written across his worried face and said, "So sorry Mr Barnes, but your potassium count is low so you will have to remain in hospital for at least another night." My mood sky dived from the heavens and the parachute failed to open as I crashed to the hard floor and mentally screamed, *Noooooooo, Syd, you fucking idiot, you have thrown your chance of being with your family down the shitter.* I lay on the hospital bed feeling as sick as a parrot and convulsed in agony as I gulped the vile potassium drink before eventually getting some shuteye later that night.

The next day I was sent back home to my family for hugs, love and kisses. I lay on my sofa as weak as a kitten, recovering from the latest battle with cancer and suffering from the effects of the mustard-gas chemotherapy drugs. I was losing this war and knew full well I needed a new battle plan to have any hope of victory. But I was certain of one thing; if I agreed to the final proposed trip to toxic madness, it would kill me. My broken body wasn't capable of withstanding another chemical onslaught. Death would be the only outcome. They say it isn't over until the large female bursts into song, but I was shitting myself because I had just spotted the fat bastard making her way to the microphone.

Beat It

(May-June 2012)

I slouched on my one and only sofa, once again struggling to recuperate from the harsh hammering my dying body had had to live with during the previous grand tour of chemo land. When the word cancer bites your mind, you are instantly zombified and transformed into a member of the walking dead, starring in your very own "Thriller" music video. In this state of terror and dread, you're transported on the conveyor belt of conventional medicine, blindly dancing to the cutting poisoning and burning along the way. Like my living dead comrades, moving in a ghostly trance, I was mesmerised into believing that this was the only feasible method of having any hope of avoiding impending death. But I mused, "Is everything so "Black and White?" as "Shades of Grey" flickered across my ghoulish Visage. Any alternative way was just plain quackery and doomed to failure. Or so I thought!

My chemical-addled head was in a state of utter confusion this "Paranoid" Black Sabbath as I contemplated the cancer industry. Now don't go getting your grey matter or your Ann Summers see-thru knickers in a twist as I don my army surplus thinking cap and chemo-brainstorm the whole caboodle of engrained concepts. The well-established viewpoints I had the spherical spheres to question at the time would result in eyeball-rolling at best and blind rage at worst. Therefore, I became bosom buddies with the countless so-called Charlatans and Kranks. And so would you if you were marching in my second-hand combat boots on a quest, not for the elusive fountain of youth or the even rarer elixir of eternal life, but for any old damn thing which would bestow a little more oh-so-precious time with my wife and kids.

Do big pharmaceutical companies really want a cancer cure? If a cure was found, would they be willing to give up the trillion-dollar chemical golden egg for the good of mankind? Would they snuff out and ridicule a natural product that could help to prevent or even cure the big C because it couldn't be patented and make them any wonderful cash? Do they control the world to such an extent that all doctors are only trained to dish out their money-making chemicals for every ailment? Do the powers that be promote and feed us junk and dangerous chemical rich processed foods to make us ill, then sell us the drugs to keep us alive for as long as possible, to make the greedy heartless bastards even richer?

Has the chemo made me totally stark raving bonkers or has it opened my eyes to the truth?

Well, first things first. I knew full well my immune system needed a shed load of tender loving care after being bombarded and almost destroyed by the chemo nuclear bomb. So, the full-on mega juicing with the food of the gods was continued with a psychedelic rainbow of fruit and veg entering my system daily. This had to be the main focus as I chased the distant pot of gold hidden in far-off survival land.

The army surplus cap was put on one side as I covered my bald brainbox with a mad scientist's safety helmet, and researched drinking water. Nothing healthier than a cool refreshing glass of thirst-quenching council pop straight from your tap, I concluded. Well, not really because it is full of chemicals and metals including liquefied chlorine, which is associated with higher cancer risks. It is contaminated with high levels of oestrogen which returns to the water system from the millions of women using the contraceptive pill or on hormone replacement therapy. And some water even contains fluoride; a hazardous waste which is used as a rat poison.

Our well-meaning dentists bang on about the benefits of fluoride after being fed misinformation during their training without ever researching the list of negative effects including neurological problems, thyroid problems, cancer and a weaker immune system. So, I immediately stopped supping the tap water and bought large glass bottles of spring water before fitting a reverse osmosis system to my water supply. Now I could drink from my tap with peace of mind.

The next port of call was Beverley, a herbalist who worked with Peter at the Natural Choice health shop in nearby Poulton-le-Fylde. She reminded me of a new-age hippy as she carefully mixed a magic potion of cancer-fighting and immune-system-strengthening herbs. Black Walnut, Red Clover, Burdock, Nettle, Dandelion, Milk Thistle and Wormwood were just a few of the bullets in this strange brew, to help me in the war with the Grim Reaper.

Now it was time to bring in the heavy artillery to wipe the smug grin off Mr G Reaper's ugly mug, coz the cocky bastard was starting to piss me off. A massive plastic basket of secret weapons was swiftly secured and stored at the side of HQ - my second- hand cream sofa. Vitamins, herbs and minerals were consumed daily as I decided to pull a fast one and attack the bastard big C by strengthening my troops, who were ready to have a right old go at the enemy. There were about 30 different pills and potions to take including; a selection of vitamins, magnesium, astragalus, echinacea, aloe vera, selenium, potassium, co-enzyme Q10, chlorella, to name just a few. Father Time hasn't given me the two thumbs up to explain the benefits of each one, so you'll have to google them if you wish to become a smart-arse like me.

I had an overwhelming feeling of well-being, not only from feeding the pigeons but also by suddenly terminating the trancing to "Thriller". The song didn't remain the same because I was now moonwalking to "Beat It" By not blindly following the mindless brainwashed zombies and at least attempting to fight this deadly disease with every method possible, a song and dance was put into each step when all hope seemed lost. Hi-ho, hi-ho, it's off to war I go!

Another vital step was kicking sugar in its sweet head, because cancer cells need glucose to grow and prosper. And as they continue to mutate and spread, they need more and more of their favourite sugary treat and I was not going to feed the greedy, deadly fuckers. Of course, the cancer industry will tell you this is a myth, but I was not a zombie anymore, remember, so I would question everything. Patients continue to die by the millions after countless years of research and billions upon billions of dollars of cash being spent. For decades we have been urged to donate because a cancer cure was just around the corner. Are they taking the piss? Shouldn't they be educating us about lifestyle changes rather than making piles of filthy lucre flogging us their expensive treatments?

They put radiated sugar in the PET scan to see if the cancer has spread in a person's body, coz the super energetic cancer cells grab it to feed hungrily, giving our normal cells little chance of having a snack. Meaning they can spot the piggish swine's, slyly scoffing glucose wherever they may be hiding in the body. They could stick their myths up their brainwashed arseholes cos I was having none of it as I fought for survival. And the NHS dieticians feed the poor souls who have been on the chemotherapy trip sugary sticky cakes, ice cream, chocolate, Coke and biscuits because they don't want them dying of cachexia, which is serious weight loss caused by the chemo. Better to die of cancer than chemotherapy for god's sake! It is like pouring petrol on the fire. They are feeding the cancer the oncologist is trying to cure.

Now one little thing that should be easy-peasy for anyone with even half a brain to comprehend. Cow's milk is meant for baby cows. Not rocket science is it, Mr Einstein? It has everything needed to transform a 60-pound calf into a 400-pound cow. It is not intended for human consumption. You may as well drink monkey's, dog's, pig's or cat's milk. What other animal drinks milk as an adult? Think about it, you big cry baby! And we are drinking another species' milk!! If we should drink any milk as adults it should be human milk. Ewww, you vomit with disgust, yet you happily slurp the milk from another species. Open your eyes, because you are even crazier than me. Even worse is that your glass of milk contains dangerous substances such as growth hormones, pus, antibiotics and is linked to - yes, you've guessed it, obesity. So not only does it make you a jolly fatty but as an added free bonus it supplies breast cancer, man boobs and diabetes too.

Does the bloody dairy industry give a monkey's if it makes you ill? No way Jose, it only wants your hard cash, just the same as my favourite heroin dealer on the street corner. Don't be fooled by the poster of the titillating large breasted female looking healthy drinking a glass of milk. Don't ogle with lust or admiration at her sexy boobs but stare with x-ray vision at the very unsexy tumour forming beneath the skin. Don't be a big tit. Give up this foreign milky invader for your health and for compassionate reasons too, which will be explained later.

Now I am not a revolutionary psychedelic hippy living in a cave meditating and eating just fruit and berries but sometimes I wish I was, as I gaze at the madness of our artificial society. Facing death has opened my mind and helped me see how brainwashed and controlled we all are. I was the same as the masses as I scoffed my four-cheese pizza and blindly allowed them to inject vaccine after vaccine into my kids without even checking what was in them and the possible side effects. Hands up who thought that they must be good, because the government and the National Health Service wouldn't promote these fortune-making vaccines with wonderful pretty marketing campaigns to get the population protected if it wasn't for our own good? Surely, they wouldn't be conning everyone, from doctor to nurse to man and woman on the street, just to make gigantic profits, would they? Don't be a prick and research what is in them, the possible life-changing injuries and if any government around the planet has banned them. And believe me, you are in for a big surprise.

Everything is up to you of course, but I do recommend that you do your own research on everything rather than following that Big Brother big pharma and other organisations spoon-feed us to line their pockets. Is it 1984 already? Or is it June 2012 and the chemo has sent me totally doolally? But what do I know? I am just a Mancunian council estate div! Anyway, don't start ripping your hair out in outrage at my toxic

"Anarchy in the UK" ramblings, otherwise you will end up with a bald chemo skull just like me. And believe me it was no "Holiday in the Sun" as I did things "My Way" but at least my psychedelic Sex Pistol was still banging and shooting with my colourful better half! "Happiness is a Warm Gun"! Was Psycho Syd becoming Sid Vicious as he confronted the bastions and bastards of society? "God Save the Queen" and me too, "Pretty (Vacant)" please!

The Prettiest Star

(June-July 2012)

A "Holiday in Cambodia" or dancing to the "Zulu Beat" in "Destination Zululand" appeared far-flung and far-fetched but I had to provide my adventurous intrepid spirit with the belief that more breathtaking, intoxicating escapades lay ahead when I finally fucked off this bastard cancer. So, I ventured online and ordered book after book of long-distance walking trails in the UK. Laughable really, because I struggled to even limp 10 painful steps. However, I could abscond from my cream sofa detention centre and liberate myself by dreamily trekking along each of these paths with my wife and kids. They were my world.

As each guidebook arrived, I would plan the adventure, studying maps, viewing photos, landscapes, villages, waterfalls and much more. I walked through romantic forests hand in hand with my perfect pretty partner, we'd snog at each kissing gate, go up misty mountains and across wild desolate moors, shooting videos of the kids running and playing. We'd have hot soup and half a real ale by dancing open fires in remote country pubs and sleep at charming quaint village inns. I walked trail after trail, carefully outlining the places to view, scoff food at and get some shuteye in. Of course, I always focused on the happiness of my beautiful wife and kids. I delighted in purchasing my loved ones treats and surprises in the village shops and markets and showing them fantastic sights, taking heaps of snapshots of the happy family. I even visualised the clothes we'd wear on each day's trek.

Alas, most of the time was spent in the very cruel real world of terminal cancer, but it was magic to be able to flee with my loved ones through an enchanted wood, across a fairy-tale bluebell meadow, and inside an otherworldly medieval castle whenever the Grim Reaper's taunts became a little too much to bear.

I had frequently spotted lucky people with massive mansions and expensive luxury cars, but I never once turned green with envy because I was the wealthiest man on the planet, living heart in heart with my priceless soulmate and I loved her more deeply than you or she could ever imagine. What a "Lucky Man" I was.

The Barnes army once again trooped into the "White Room" with dark curtains and met the smiling oncologist at Blackpool Victoria Hospital. I sat on a comfy Cream chair holding my dream girl's hand.

The main man apologetically informed us that I couldn't have any further chemotherapy because my broken body wouldn't be able to take it and it would be the death of me. I was singing 'A*ye, aye yippee, yippee aye*': no more journeys to the centre of chemical insanity for me. "So, what's next?" I inquired.

"I regret to inform you that without any further treatment your maximum life expectancy is now just 12 months," he explained professionally. Shit, shock, horror. The Grim Reaper has got me by the short and curlies and I am in very deep shit. "However, there is one glimmer of hope of extending your life," he remarked with a frown across his serious forehead. He then clarified that a full-on six-week course of radiotherapy, with weekly doses of small amounts of chemotherapy, could possibly extend my life. He sternly warned that this would be the most agonising and terrifying experience of my life, which would have horrific lifelong side-effects. And if you gasp in shock and fright at that offer, there was even worse to come. It only had a 20% chance of success.

The toxic trip to Hades wasn't a walk in the park but it seemed like a piece of piss compared to this proposed journey to the burning fires of hell. After the radiation it would be a year-long nightmare of torment, pain and disability and it only had a 1 in 5 chance of succeeding! As if I hadn't suffered enough already! I would spend what little time I had left loving my wife and kids, not collapsed in agony for a year on my sofa. Bollocks, bollocks and even more fucking bollocks.

As well as not opting to burn my neck, I also elected not to burn my bridges and informed the main man I needed a week or two to play things over in my terrified mind. Talk about being between the devil and the deep blue sea. On the one hand a slow painful death from cancer, and on the other an agonising year of disability with an 80% failure rate. Syd, would you like a steel toe capped boot in your right testicle or your left testicle? There was the third option of ending it all and topping myself but my deep love for my wife and kids meant that that choice was a non-starter.

***

I was still very ill when my friend Janet and her sister Jackie paid me a lovely surprise visit. We all dilly-dallied on a slow walk to the promenade to see the sea. *And all that we could see see see was the cold grey Irish sea sea sea*! And it really was a very slow walk, in fact at snail's pace because I was so weak and fatigued, recovering fraction by fraction from the poisoning. Every 50 yards I had to stop for a couple of minutes to catch my breath and regain my strength. At the prom, oodles of pics were snapped of my wife holding and kissing me. I felt so lucky and proud having such a beautiful caring lifelong partner; '*till death do us part*.

We spent a dreamy hour by the seaside before hopping on a bus to the Bispham Rock Gardens, a landscaped park with beautiful flowers and a playground for the kids. I felt so warm and loved this marvellous day and mused what a "Wonderful World". I was chatting with two smashing friends, my wife was holding me and loving me, and my children were laughing, running and playing. It was a memorable "Day in the Life" which I will treasure until the day I snuff it, which if you read the news recently doesn't seem too far off; does it?

***

"Day after Day" I lay on my sick sofa battling to regain my strength. Juices, herbs, vitamins, potions, distilled drinking water - but no magic mushrooms - were fed to my damaged body. I had already experienced enough colourful hallucinations during my two previous bad trips to chemical La La Land, thank you very much. At that very moment the universe delivered the next earth-shattering event in the death and life of Psycho Syd. Fling your memory back to chapter three when I promised that my eldest son Eric Jay would blow everyone's minds. Well, keep a tight hold onto your jaw coz all will be revealed now.

I had kept in constant touch with him, visiting whenever an opportunity arose. I recollect that he was always dovelike, gentle and effeminate from the age of eight. It did of course cross my mind that he could be gay, but I thought nothing of it and left his sexuality well alone. In 2007, he eventually came out of his Bangkok closet, informing me that he was indeed gay. He said "Daddy, I am afraid you won't love me coz you like football, beer and girls."

I hugged him. "Jay, I love you with all my heart, don't worry about anything," I tenderly reassured him.

In July 2008 I had driven to Bangkok to collect Eugene, who had a week earlier flown from Laos to Thailand to take a short break with his mum and his sister, Francesca. I had driven down in my shit-hot turd-brown four-wheel drive car with my wife, who was four months pregnant with our first child. We had taken three days to slowly travel to the Thai capital, playing together and visiting temples and waterfalls on the journey. Perfect bliss. We were picking up Eugene and my daughter

Francesca to go on a holiday, visiting islands off the east coast. I asked Eric Jay if he would like to join us, but he sadly explained that he was busy studying at university!

However, I arranged to meet him at Pizza Hut near Don Muang airport in the north of Bangkok. My gorgeous better half sat inside with our bun in the oven, scoffing a pizza while I stood outside, excitedly waiting for my son. As I lingered, a stunning tall fit blonde with legs up to her armpits and large eye-magnets got off a scooter. She walked towards Pizza Hut, mesmerising me with her swaying hips and bouncing breasts. I felt a deep connection with this Miss World, which was strange coz I had only ever had eyeballs for my gorgeous wife! I was even dreaming of suggesting a threesome to my sexy missus.

My breath was stolen as she walked straight up to me and softly said, "Hello Daddy." My semi-erection and ménage à trois fantasies vanished before you could say, "Well, fuck me!" (On second thoughts, well don't.) Over pizza she informed me that she had undertaken a full sex change and was now female in every sense of the word. I put my arms around her, explaining that I loved her but warned her to be careful and not to mix with the wrong people and that I was always here for her. After lunch I kissed her goodbye and was still gobsmacked as I enjoyed an idyllic holiday in paradise with my perfect family.

Back to June 2012. I was slurping my beetroot, apple and carrot juice when my wife looked up with mouth wide open from the laptop and shouted, "Syd, your daughter is in the news and on TV in Thailand. She has won Miss Universe and the TV channels want to interview you." I nearly spilt my kaleidoscopic fruit juice over my baggy blue and white striped pyjamas in astonishment. I gazed in wonder at the pictures and videos of my daughter winning the ultimate prestigious transgender prize, transforming her into an instant celebrity in the land of smiles.

I phoned her to congratulate her and tell her how proud I was of her amazing success. Unfortunately, I had to break the sad news that I was dying of cancer and wasn't in any fit condition to do TV or newspaper interviews. It was a "Bittersweet Symphony", but I was determined to knock everyone and everything out of my path as I fought for my life the natural way, coz the conventional drugs just didn't seem to work!

***

So, it was hand in hand that I went with my pretty partner to a Swallows Head and Neck cancer meeting where I met Simon and his good-looking, caring wife. Simon had been on the harrowing chemo/radiotherapy trip approximately 10 months previously and was still in pain and recovering. He warned me of the torture and horrors and that he wouldn't have survived the terrifying, agonising ordeal without the support of his wife. "It is impossible to do this nightmare alone, it is far worse than anything you could possibly imagine," he forewarned.

I gazed with deep love into my wife's beautiful eyes and asked her if she would support me if I elected to grab a ticket for the wretched voyage to hellfire. She replied, "Of course Syd, you know that." I felt awfully guilty for even questioning my wonderful loyal partner. She would never abandon me. We were together forever. What the hell should I do?

At the eleventh hour, 59 minutes and 59 seconds I unenthusiastically volunteered to go to inferno land. A voice inside my tree screamed, *Don't do it Syd, this is not the answer, this will really fuck you up.* I ignored my inner being because I was prepared to face all my demons and "Scary Monsters" for just a little more time with the ones I loved. With a million nagging doubts in my skull, I gave the good/bad news to the oncologist and was informed that the jolly jaunt to anguish would depart on 21 July 2012 and I had my seat reserved and confirmed. I was shitting myself but decided to try and make the most of things before the frightful journey began.

I bought bus passes and visited local places with my family, trying to have fun before the hellish adventure took off. Eugene went to France for a couple of weeks to stay with Francesca, his sister. Each week I bought my model missus an item of clothing, the same as I had always done since we had met. t-shirts, coats, skirts, dresses, boots, shoes. I loved watching her face light up as she dressed in her new fashions.

I opened a Facebook account for her, so she could post pictures of us in the UK and show her family and friends her new fashions and the places we visited. The kids and wife were always well dressed but I looked like a bloody paraffin lamp (tramp). I hardly ever bought anything for me because I just wanted to spend any spare dosh on the ones I loved. It was fun, and I was getting stronger, but the upcoming ordeal was at the back of my mind. I was afraid, terrified and shit-scared all rolled into one!

***

At long last I was finally strong enough to see my mum, who was in a care home in St Annes-on-Sea suffering from dementia. I didn't visit her earlier because I didn't want to cause distress by exposing my cancer-ridden bag of bones. I went with my brother Jeff and his wife Ann to meet her. I was so excited. When I saw her for the first time in about 10 years I was devastated. She just stared into space, with her head tilted to one side. Not sure if she even noticed me.

I made an excuse and walked outside to the park across the road and collapsed behind a tree, sobbing my heart out in sorrow and shock. A few weeks later I went to see her again with Eugene and Jo. I invited my wife but was astonished that she decided not to join us. She was busy on her new Facebook page. My mum seemed a little more alert and even whispered my name when she saw me as we pushed her around the park in her wheelchair that sunny afternoon. This was the first time she had met her grandson Jo and I saw the pain in her eyes as she hugged him after he had fallen over, grazing his knees on the gravel.

I knew full well that I may not see her again for a while because I was just about to enter the gates of hell in the next haunting episode of *Tales from the Darkside*, but I am grateful for this very precious day. As I write this I am choked up and there are tears in my eyes, but I won't cry because once again, remember, boys and sad old men dying of cancer don't cry, do they?

I continued taking my family out because I knew I probably didn't have much longer to live and wanted us all to be a happy family in the here and now. The hospital delivered about 200 small bottles of liquid milk to build me up, but I didn't touch it as I continued juicing and having the odd plate of mashed spuds. On 16th June the family went to Lytham for a walk and a scoff in a Thai restaurant. I even managed to yet again sip a bit of curry! We had trips to Fleetwood and Poulton and took lots of photos of us together. It was great.

One brilliant day I walked with my wife to our local church and had a walk around the graveyard. The sun shone as I accepted that death was as natural as birth, visualising my name chiselled on stone. 'Here lies Psycho Syd 1956-2013 Aged 56.' He lived a colourful adventurous dream worshipping his beautiful wife and his four adorable kids.' On this amazing day my wife kept taking selfies of us together. I felt I had already snuffed it and was residing in heaven, happy and lucky that I had my lovely wife by my side as I was about to undertake the most frightful journey of my fast disappearing life. I felt so warm, cared for, safe and loved on this "Perfect Day": another special time I will take to the grave with me.

A trip to the oral and maxillofacial unit at Preston Royal, my soon-to-be-home-from-home. A kind friendly dentist with bright blue Frank Sinatra eyes informed me that he would have to extract two teeth that were decaying. He warned that any extractions, fillings or root canals during or after the radiotherapy could cause osteoporosis. This would mean my jawbone disintegrating and they would have to cut bits of bone from my legs to build me a new one. A long and very painful process. Fuck that for a game of soldiers! "Rip them out, old blue eyes," I instructed. I didn't blink one of my bored eyelids at the needles or the ripping, twisting, tugging and pain. This journey has changed me from a timid scaredy-cat to a hard as nails, fearless tiger.

The next exciting little adventure to Preston Royal occurred a week later when I went to get my radiotherapy face mask sorted. My head was clamped to a table and the nurses covered my face with warm sticky plastic which they moulded to the shape of my face. It was a suffocating unpleasant experience. But unpleasant experiences had happened almost every other day since the cancer diagnosis. Eventually the mask was ready for the radiation to hit the areas needed but I wasn't ready; I was dreading it.

As it got nearer to my trip to burning hell I continued to go out with my family. We went to Blackpool carnival with Jeff, his wife Ann and my niece Helen and her boyfriend Scott. Jo played on bouncy castles and had a donkey ride - his last, because I would never allow that to happen again, with my new compassionate eyes wide open.

Next, I went with the missus and Jo to a transport festival in Fleetwood. Jo insisted on going on the ghost train. I tried to deter him by explaining it was scary, but his three-year-old mind refused to take no for an answer. So, I reluctantly agreed, and we sat in a chair ready for the ride. The instant we went through the doors into the ghostly darkness Jo started screaming, so I told him to close his eyes and held him close. It was soon over, and he cried, "I never want to go on the ghost train again."

"Neither do I," I reflected. But in just a few short days it would be my turn to take the bloodcurdling, spine-chilling locomotive ride to my worst nightmare. I hoped my wife would "Hold me Close" when I shut my eyes and started screaming!

Welcome to The Machine

(July-August 2012)

I was clad in ripped and faded old blue jeans, a 50p crimson t-shirt acquired in Laos many tropical moons back, a green canvas jacket donated by my brother, and on my plates of meat (feet) were a dirty pair of trainers that even a vagrant with snot running down his nose would turn his conk up at. There wasn't a flask of meth's slyly stashed in my hobo coat pocket but something even more hardcore: a bottle of liquid morphine! I wasn't ogling girls coz I only had eyes, heart and warm gun for my gorgeous partner. I was a poor old scruffy sod ready to pick up a few dog-ends and sell the odd copy of Big Issue on a bleak street corner in Blackpool town centre.

No, you are not as "Thick as a Brick" as you scratch your confused head, because I am only pulling your plonker; I was cloaked for something rather less frightful than that. I was casually attired for my inaugural rendezvous with Lucifer, who was grinning madly as he warmed-up in preparation to zap me with his new-fangled hell-fire sizzling ray gun at Preston Royal Inferno. I just couldn't see the point of getting dressed to the nines in shirt, tie and designer suit to scream in agony during my red-hot "Dance with the Devil".

I smooched my striking wife and kissed little Jo adios as the spew-coloured yellow and green ambulance drew to an unwelcome standstill outside my tightly locked front door for the first of my 30 daily visits to hell. I joined the other sorrowful frightened sods who had been rounded up in Blackpool for the nervy half-hour ride to perdition. I unenthusiastically clunk clicked my trembling body in, with sporadic teardrops exploding from my shiny sky-blue waterlogged eyeballs. I was "Drowning in Love" as I gazed at the ones I worshipped as they waved and blew kisses from the front window of our humble abode.

The lion's share of patients were supported by one or more loved ones but not me. There wasn't a big pussy cat in hell's chance that I would give the green light to the ones I worshipped having even the slightest taste of the painful dishes being served up at Preston Royal. I had faced the chemo nightmare in solitary for starters and now just me, myself and my shadow would sample the radiotherapy main course. Well done, please!

However, I wasn't really a one-man band because my missus and kids were singing in my heart, trumpeting in my mind, dancing in my psychedelic eyes and drumming in each individual cell of my dying body for each and every second of this tear-jerking sad song. So, the red lights were on as I cried, "Stop - in the Name of Love", and sheltered my wife and kids; keeping them in Supreme ignorance, safe and sound at home, putting a halt to any possible unpleasant experiences. Protecting my loved ones from this relentless nightmare was paramount.

I felt more like a lamb to the slaughter than a courageous big cat as I bleated meekly into the hospital for numero uno of the weekly heart-to-heart, face-to-face chinwags with the oncologist. I was sternly cautioned that the name of the radiation game was to fill my cancerous cakehole thick and fast to avoid the severe weight loss which many deteriorating cancer warriors suffer. Easier said than done though, when you have an agonising tumour in your throat, meaning swallowing is on the brink of impossible and bloody painful too.

I did sample a few of the peg tube liquids through the tube in my abdomen. Alas, I just couldn't stomach the plastic bottles of sugary fruit juices they supplied coz they kicked off an unpleasant, burning reaction. As sod's law would have it, the sweet-smelling strawberry, chocolate and vanilla-flavoured milk drinks produced no unpleasant foul kickback. As I was bent on giving the big C creating dairy the Spanish archer (el-bow), these pungent milky liquids would only be fed into my dying skeleton in a last-ditch effort to keep my death warmed up body alive on this spinning lump of rock in cosmic space.

The gruesome announcement that they were preparing full-on morphine to relieve the fast-approaching mega agony echoed around my petrified but not yet lost marbles. This was to supplement the gobfuls of liquid opiate I was already gulping. Gulp! The ultra-serious no-nonsense pain would launch in just one month's time and must be suffered for the terminal two weeks of this torturous treatment. I had to grin and bear it with my happy-go-lucky, never say die attitude.

A stiff upper lip was required to go with my stiff lower organ! Yes, we were still indulging in a bit of slap and tickle coz my one-track mind had resolved that if I was going to meet my maker then I was going out with a fucking bang! Ha-ha. My better half must have been head over heels in love and lust with me or her head had already lost its blooming marbles, to be intimate with my hideous bag of bones!

The next unwelcome bit of nerve-jangling info was that once the treatment finished it would be blast-off time as pain levels rocketed, taking me off the chart to the outer limits of outer space. "Is there Life on Mars" or in any other distant galaxy in the universe? Well, it seemed my future scorched "Starman" body would soon have the answer to that little "Space Oddity". FFS - once the burning hell is over it gets even worse. Flashbacks of the no-dad chemo-pump nightmare made nauseating appearances in my frightened mind.

Next, my frail, puny body tiptoed nto the hospital scales to gawk in astonishment at the rapid weight loss from partaking in the awfully unbeatable cancer diet plan. My weight was going down faster than a girl I once knew from Macclesfield! Fatties worldwide eat your chubby hearts out - and a sneaky bag of cheese and onion crisps too. I was then sent on my unmerry old way to the radiotherapy waiting room where the thin men with bulging, jittery eyeballs sat.

I flipped through the *Lancashire Life* magazine, with its ads for massive fuck off mansions and luxury funeral services. I couldn't focus as my eyes bulged and jittered too. My bony feet lightly tapped the polished floor as I nervously waited in apprehension for my introduction to the machine. At long last my name was called, and my shaking skeleton followed an overweight radiologist into a treatment room. I scratched my scalp as thoughts of *Laurel and Hardy* sprang to mind and almost expected her to turn around and admonish, *That's another fine mess you've got yourself into,* but she didn't. And I am relieved she didn't coz the last thing I needed at this scary moment was some Stan and Ollie slapstick catastrophe involving the deadly, dangerous piece of equipment I was about to face. That just wouldn't be funny. A piano yes, but a radiation gun - no fucking way.

The radiologist sang, "Welcome Mr Barnes; "Welcome to the Machine." She really instructed, "Please remove your coat and t-shirt and lie on the table under the machine." I did as requested, and scrutinised the icy cold automaton, menacingly looking daggers just above my panic-stricken cranium. A young student lad from Liverpool was assisting with the preparation. I almost quipped, "Bloody hell, a Scouser, I better keep my hands on my wallet," to the youthful trainee, although I quickly thought better of it. This wasn't the time or place for urine extraction.

I was made aware that each session of radiation persists for approximately 15 long minutes but on this inaugural occasion it would be double trouble coz a 15-minute warm-up was necessary to ensure that the cold-hearted robot was in full evil working order before the real zapping could begin. Warm-up! FFS! Maybe this is the piss-taking room after all. I was also informed that the pain would not begin until at least a fortnight into the treatment. Well, finally a bit of good news in the here and now.

The final frightful dollop of information was that the experience is extraordinarily claustrophobic, and no end of suffering patients panic. If this sensation raises its ugly burnt head, then just raise your hand and we will stop the machine. However, be advised that if you select this course of action then any time endured under the machine is forfeited and we will be compelled to commence the treatment from the very beginning once more. Shit! I will keep my mucky 'Manc' paws firmly by my side next to my wallet and my mobile phone in my faded blue jeans pockets. Before long, the unfeeling, faceless mask which would subsequently smother my head and shoulders showed its unwelcome visage. Let my Alexandre Dumas nightmare begin.

Now drag your soul to that cold, shadowy cellar, dark and grim, where "All the Madmen" scream. You know, the place with monstrous spiders, thousands of creepy-crawlies, scurrying rats and evil whispers from dark corners. The basement where the vile scary blackness grabs you by the throat and squeezes the life out of you. The room with the childhood scary monster under the bed or the thin nasty 'Grumbly-Grimblies' who have escaped from "The Land of the Grey and Pink" to get you as you hide and tremble under the blankets. That's right; the spooky room with the cobwebs hidden deep within your conscience, where your worst fears and nightmares are safely obscured from your cloudy day-to-day life. They are usually outta sight, outta mind unless a gruesome movie scene, a paragraph in a spine-chilling novel, a grizzly news story or a true-life experience from *The Death and Life of Psycho Syd* sadistically opens the rotten creaking door and shoves your screaming, terrified psyche inside.

Visualise being alone, clamped to a metal bed, unable to move, in a cold dimly lit room. In the background you hear the obscene whirring of an unfeeling mechanical torturous device. Then some loathsome grinning maniac places his dirty murderous hands over your mouth, smiling as he nonchalantly suffocates you to death. You are struggling to breathe through the tiniest of gaps between his beastly sweaty fingers as you battle for dear life.

Well, if you are not screaming yet then start now, coz the treatment at Preston Royal Inferno is far worse than that! Horrific! It's no wonder many sorrowful head and neck cancer victims panic and struggle, raising their thin skeletal arm to stop the terror, before their eyes bulge and jitter as they realise, they have to start right from the very beginning all over a-fucking gain.

The mask was squeezed tightly over my alarmed head as I was clamped to the table beneath the machine. I was masquerading as its next torture victim. My mind screamed in terror like an Edvard Munch bad dream as I battled to breathe. The closest (pun intended) analogy I can paint is being enclosed in a collapsed building covered in rubble with a 100kg bag of dry cement bang smack on top of my smothered face. I was powerless to move even one tiny millimetre, fighting for air. It was like I had been petrified by having had a sneaky peep at Medusa's hideous venomous head. The experience was so restricting coz it was imperative that my upper body was completely immobile, to ensure that the mechanical monster blasted precisely where it was programmed; at the cancerous tumour. The protective mask pressed hard into my face, neck, nose and mouth.

I lay there panic-stricken with darting eyes as the radiologists left the room and the lights dimmed. One small consolation was that I didn't have a male nurse gripping my upper thigh whilst whispering, "Be brave", to my now cowardly, cowardly-custard shaking mind as I tried to keep my eyes averted from my only companion; the machine.

Suddenly, the merciless metallic monster awoke from its slumber; moving, whirring and zapping. I struggled to control my frenzied thoughts as my "Senses started Working Overtime". I certainly didn't experience any pain but emotionally I was already bats in the belfry raving bonkers. I attempted to carry my hysterical mind to a peaceful place in the countryside far away from this chilling dark room. Alas, I failed miserably…not hearing any birdsong, church bells or babbling brooks because they were drowned out by the commotion of this machine.

As my almost dead skeleton lay comatose under the noisy apparatus my very alive mind frantically searched for some long "Lost Mantra" to take me away from the land of hell to "The kingdom of God." So, I mentally chanted *Om Mani Padme Hum* before progressing to *wife, Jay, Eugene, Francesca, Jo*. My combat with this obnoxious deadly disease was for my loved ones and it seemed only right and proper that my mantra should be their names, which were mentally repeated as I visualised their images one by one. (my wife's name shall remain anonymous; you'll understand why later.)) The only way to go through this crazy unbearable torment was to repeatedly chant the names of the people I was dying to live for.

For 15 eternal minutes my distressed unhinged mind grappled to hang on to my sanity as I withstood this relentless, suffocating horror. Each time I felt an uncontrollable urge to raise my bony right arm I would focus on my mantra and visualise my loved ones. My escape and relief would last only a few seconds as my thoughts would quickly return and welcome me back to my nightmare. I struggled on until the noisy machine stopped, the lights came on and the radiologists appeared. They walked over and released me, giving me what seemed like the greatest sense of relief I had experienced since drawing my first gasp of air as a screaming babe. Even Sergio Aguero's last-breath-winning goal had nothing on this.

Well, the warm-up was over, but the burning issue was: would I be able to withstand the subsequent bona fide heart-stopping segment of this mind-bending ordeal?

With only a couple of minutes respite, the mask was once again jammed over my fainthearted skull, clamping me right back into my scary movie. The radiologists departed, the lights dimmed, and the machine returned to life. It was just as hellish as the warm-up. I almost threw in the towel and lifted my bony arm demanding release from the mask, before thereon bellowing "fuck it" and flying home like a "Bat Out of Hell". But I was a brave soldier and fought on in deadly combat with my terrible nemesis; my very own mind.

Eventually I was released from Hades and left the room in XTC as the "Generals and Majors" of the radiotherapy department were making plans for their next sorrowful victim (probably Nigel!). Then it was back home by effing ambulance into the hearts and arms of my loved ones. One down, just 29 more terrifying daymares to go.

**

By the first week of August, ten trips to the "House of Fun" had been endured. However, I courageously battled the torment by continuing to chant my mantra. It was no "Walk in the Park" but on the 27th July, I had taken my wife and two kids for a walk in Stanley Park. We enjoyed a motorboat on the lake and a drink in the art deco café too. However, my pretty better half was a bit distant and moody because she wanted to be 'her indoors' back on her new Facebook page. Fair enough, coz it gave her something to focus on while the radiation gun focused on me.

I endeavoured to get some sense back into my life by focusing on the present, but heaven knew I was miserable then, coz my deluded mind kept flashing painful visions of the next twenty satanic journeys. I was counting them down, eager to get them done and dusted, but on the other skinny hand I was apprehensive because I knew full well that the naked to the visible eye edge of the universe level of agony was about to big bang my broken life. And this dreadful unbearable treatment had only a 1 in 5 chance of extending my sad existence!

What have I done? Please wrap me up in a straitjacket and cart my "21st-Century-Schizoid-Man" crushed mind off to the nuthouse because without a shadow of a doubt I must have lost the plot by agreeing to buy a ticket for this no-hope downward spiralling ride to red-hot pandemonium.

Burn

(July-August 2012)

Heavens no! Hell yes! The terrorising therapy never ceased, leaving me struggling to make headway with my mantra in a futile attempt to escape the suffocating nightmare. I felt like a frayed tennis ball being smashed between mantra and horror for a breath-taking heart-stopping 15-minute rally. My terrified mind screamed, "You cannot be fucking serious!" At long last it was game, set and match. My exhausted much relieved psyche caught its breath as it was unclamped from the claustrophobic head crushing mask. On a couple of soul-destroying occasions, the radiologist, role-playing as an umpire, called a tie-break. It is with regret that the 15-minute rally must be replayed because of a technical problem.

Well, that really was a pain in the neck. I did feel like smashing the machine but took the ace from up my sleeve and boldly smiled, saying "Hit me Baby One More Time" to the bastard apparatus. I had to be brave and play the game of my life to stand any chance of reaching the promised land of "I will survive".

Day after day I would be transported to the machine by ambulance or a volunteer in his own car. These volunteers were friendly kind-hearted chaps who received a mileage allowance for supplementing the overworked ambulance service. I got on like a house on fire with these amiable guys as they conveyed my flaming neck on fire for further sessions of scorching at Preston hothouse. We chatted about the news, football and of course the evil big C. These compassionate blokes sympathised with my scary journey, but I proudly and defiantly stressed that I was going to kick the Grim Reaper's arse coz I had the most beautiful wife and adorable kids in the whole wide world and they really needed me as they began a new life in the UK.

However, one bad-tempered, grey haired arse wipe, who had the barefaced cheek to call himself a volunteer, drove off, leaving me stranded because he refused to wait just a couple of minutes while I got my things together. He obviously didn't get paid for waiting and this greedy piece of shite was just in love with his milometer and the lovely cash he could make; the seriously ill patients were just money-making objects to this uncaring monster.

I frantically phoned for another car and went to the burning machine in a fiery rage. Luckily, I never laid eyeballs on this scumbag again so my screenplay of giving him a taste of poison and fire with a large glass of bleach, before burning the bastard alive with a blowtorch, never came to pass. Therefore, he missed out on playing the starring role in the now cancelled, *Death of a Volunteer* movie, but karma is waiting for this piece of dog shit, you can be sure of that.

Of course, I let go of my fury shortly afterwards because rage and anger are not part of my non-confrontational, easy-going non-violent hippy nature. I suppose the stress and fear of fighting for my life and maybe the mix of toxic chemicals swimming around my dying body could be to blame for these rare outbursts. Anyway, I had more important things to focus on than some hard-hearted knobhead; fighting for my life and my loved ones. "Que Sera Sera". The future doesn't seem to be mine to see!

I got close and chummy with my radiation comrades as we travelled by effing ambulance or car to "Danger, Danger High Voltage" sessions of "The Heat Is On". Virtually all these sorrowful souls were obtaining radiotherapy for prostate cancer, which was a piece of piss (pun intended) in comparison to the asphyxiating horror of donning the mask. A strange cocktail of oddballs joined Psycho Syd on these journeys to the heart of fear. There was an ex-comedian who told jokes, a jolly man who owned a tailor's shop and one crazy fool stepping off a cliff who was also living the wide-awake bad dream of wearing the mask. He was smoking and getting pissed every day. That was his way of dealing with this smothering hell, but I had kicked the cancer sticks and booze into oblivion at the very beginning of this bad trip.

As well as enduring this I had to focus on the mundane issues of daily life. Paying the rent, electricity, gas and phone bills. Shopping for food, clothes and household items. I managed to get Eugene and Jo into local schools. Closely followed by school uniforms, sports kits and free school dinners. I was now on benefits; how the mighty have fallen.

My wife's visitor's visa expired in October and it couldn't be extended but a right-to-stay visa could be applied for under exceptional circumstances. Being alone with two kids, both British nationals and a British husband dying of cancer seemed pretty exceptional to me. This problem could be put on the back burner until October while my neck faced the front burner in the here and now. I also had to make plans to enrol my better half into college to study something like hairdressing or beauty therapy so she could find work when I lost the battle with the dreaded big C.

Painful visions of my soul mate living and loving a new partner when I was six feet under floated across my sorrowful mind and stabbed my heart but I just hoped and prayed he was kind and loving and took care of her and my kids. Bollocks to that scenario, I was going to beat this pernicious illness. I gazed deep into my gorgeous partner's eyes and thought, *Listen here baby, we're gonna "Live Forever".*

***

"The Final Countdown" continued. I was heading to Mars, Pluto and the edge of the universe. Maybe I'd come back to Earth, who could tell. The end of this harrowing treatment still seemed light years away. My weight was still rapidly going down, which unlike Miss Macclesfield's pleasure tasting experiences was something I could well do without. So, I reluctantly opted to pour six small plastic bottles of sweet sickly pungent milk into my stomach through the peg tube on a daily basis to avoid the dreadful experience of having another face mask moulded. I was still slurping a rainbow of fruit and veg juices plus all my herbs and supplements to give my broken body the nutrition necessary to survive my "Supersonic Rocket Ship" trip to uncharted territories of pain.

I continued to hide my fears and pain from my loved ones as I donned my 'at home mask' of happiness, hope and love. Psycho Syd, a master of disguise hey! I knew full well it was very unlikely that I would survive so I had to make the most of what oh so precious little time I had left as I took my family out.

One sunny day we visited the Sealife centre; something I would never do again, since my compassionate eyes have opened. I now detest Sealife with a vengeance and the blind uncaring morons who visit these poor imprisoned beautiful creatures that rightfully deserve to be free in the ocean, not money-making objects for the cruel and heartless Charlie Uniform November Tango Sierras who own the centres.

Worryingly, the missus was once again moody and impatient to return home to Facebook! Every day through all the frustration, pain and despair the sparkle in my wife's eyes had kept me alive. However, just like the lights that dimmed in the radiotherapy room, the shine in my partner's eyes was starting to dim as she spent 50% of the time upstairs alone on her fucking FB page. This was even more scary than the mask, because I needed her full-on support to have even an outside chance of winning this seemingly hopeless battle.

My daily jaunts to Preston Inferno continued. Car or ambulance, banter with my fellow cancer-fighting warriors, step on the scales, suffocating mask and burning before returning to "She (who hopefully still) Sells Sanctuary". These little jollies would last between two and three long hours. A weekly 45-minute drip of chemo poisoning which magnified the effects and pain by zillions was part of the dark humour. This time for a laugh included a blood test and chat with the oncologist. However, the punchline of the gag was that I still had to face the dreaded mask on this day too. I was crying in pain, not laughter as my gloomy mind failed to see the funny side of the sick joke. I did have something to smile about though, because this time round I didn't have any adverse effects from the chemo, meaning the mental anguish of residing in chemical La La Land was given a much welcome miss.

Well, it took 20 shots of radiotherapy and 3 blasts of chemotherapy (they forgot to give me chemo the first lucky week) until the touch paper was lit and the intense pain blasted off. There was "Instant Karma" coz it was me who was the star in the horror film, being burnt alive by Lucifer's evil blowtorch from hell. The flesh on my neck and shoulders was black and shiny crimson as it started to melt. That wasn't enough for this devilish ghoul because he constantly poured boiling water down my swollen scalded throat too.

I never realised pain levels like this existed on "Planet Earth", but I wasn't on solid ground; I was "High in the Sky" on morphine. My scorched and blistered mind screamed out for the Grim Reaper's bony hand to take me away from Satan's tormenting agonising torture right now. Alas, my dark shadowy stalker had left me just when I needed him most.

The final 10 treatments slowly screamed by. The morphine hardly dimmed the pain. Laxatives were swallowed because opiates cause terrible constipation, as I found out on a couple of hard to get through teeth gritting occasions. Some may say I am full of shit, but I really was at those painful times. I had tramadol and other drugs to get down my burnt neck including a liquid to stop me getting mouth thrush because my immune system was knackered, leaving the door wide open with a welcome mat for all the nasty bugs and shitty infections.

I still fought to hide my agony from the ones I lived for. We would venture out for an hour to the park or the shops. Eugene would stay home and take care of Jo while my burnt skeleton with bulging eyes took my pretty wife to the shops to buy some fashionable items of clothing, which she had been addicted to since we had met. Even though I was screaming inside I was not going to allow my soulmate to go "Cold Turkey". The angel from my nightmare was going to get her fix. Her life and my life depended on it.

Unfortunately, I was too frail and weak to walk around the shops while she scored the latest t-shirt, skirt or pair of jeans so I hid in a corner of the nearby Waterstone's book shop and sat on a chair clutching a walking book. Alas, I was in far too much pain to abscond with my loved ones across a moor or through a forest, so I just sat there in agony and deep sorrow that I couldn't be holding my wife's hand, helping her select the next item of clothing to adorn the body I so worshipped. Eventually she arrived with a massive smile lighting up her gorgeous face, with a couple of wraps of trendy gear in her arms. She was buzzing and even higher than my morphine-soaked head.

There'd be a painful trip home on a red double-decker bus before she disappeared upstairs to try on her new outfits and take loads of selfies. An hour later she would come down to visit me on my sick sofa and ask me to upload the pics she had selected onto her FB page before vanishing back upstairs. I did worry that my pretty wife could be getting a lot of attention from other men, but I was far too ill to deal with the unthinkable nightmare that my angel could become the devil in my bad dream. So, I stashed these niggling doubts in the dark grim room hidden deep within my soul and focused on my fight to survive.

I was crashing out on the sofa to avoid the painful climb up the stairs. My wife did assist me by helping me go upstairs for a bath and sometimes pouring some of the sickly fluids into the tube in my stomach. However, she seemed to be becoming more distant which was very worrying at this time when I really needed her support. Maybe this was her way of dealing with this frightening period, so I left well alone.

The last week was totally indescribable. The pain really did skyrocket. My friends on the ambulance trips just stared in horror. I was close to death. A skeleton with shell-shocked staring eyes, unable to even speak or take notice of anything as it tasted the pain of "Being Boiled" alive. At home I would sit on my sofa and hide my agony from my beautiful wife and kids but when they all went to bed and all the night was warm and quiet, I would whimper and yelp to myself as I gulped my sachets of morphine. The final five treatments passed in a blur of torment and pain. Blood tests and needles were almost impossible because my veins just collapsed at each jab, with the hammering my poor dying body had already gone through.

Eventually my broken bag of bones went for the final session of smothering and burning. I didn't notice anything. I was in a hazy agonising daze. My skin was black and angry-red, peeling and dripping in painful weepy rivers of puss. That was nothing compared to the swollen, blistered scorched inside of my mouth. It felt like I was sucking on a red-hot glowing piece of coal. I really was at the outer limits of outer space and I felt like screaming but couldn't, because even the tiniest movement meant a jolting, agonising flash of white-hot pain.

They asked me if I would like to keep the mask as a souvenir. I shook my head from side to side and if I could have spoken would have asked for a bottle of Nembutal, so I could peacefully euthanise myself and become a happy, pain-free flatliner. I blurred back home by ambulance in painful silence as my friends gaped in sympathetic shock; they must have been thinking that death was just around the corner for poor Syd and I was hoping they were right.

Then my mind jumped back to the first chat I had had, at the outset of this painful radiotherapy trip, six long torturous weeks back. "Be warned, the real pain starts after the treatment has ended." Lord have mercy! My agony was going to scream into the next dimension. I decided there and then that tomorrow I would buy a gun from some dodgy underworld geezer and lift my head up high and blow my fucking brains out coz I could not take any more of this.

I arrived back home to my loved ones. I saw my beautiful wife and kids and realised that the pain was for them and they were worth it. Yes, I had to accept this agony and terror, and dream of the time when it would all be over and visualise holidays and love; I would rebuild my broken body and life and help the ones I lived for to be happy and safe. Even so, I was bloody terrified about what the next few weeks would throw my way.

But believe me, everything experienced up to now on this scary cancer trip was nothing compared to the horror, misery, pain and confusion I was about to taste! And yes, if I had known what the future had up its evil sleeve for me, I would have bought a shooter and blasted my grey matter into tiny little pieces. And if you, dear reader, had known what was going to take place next you would have given me the money and your blessings to do it!

Too Sick to Pray

(August-September 2012)

I was "High in the Sky" and felt that I could touch the moon and the stars above me. My spaced-out mind was running on rocket fuel; massive doses of morphine "All of the Day and All of the Night". My opiated godlike psyche gazed down from the heavens to the confusion on planet Earth. For once I had to turn a blind eye to wars, cruelty, poverty, starvation, the extinction of numerous unique species, global warming and the destruction of the rainforests as I zoomed in and focused on my dying burnt skeleton "Being Boiled" alive.

I floated in a strange way during the "Flying Saucer" trip inside my skull, while my doomed scorched frame writhed in torment. The ferocity of the agony increased daily as did my morphine, laxatives and other colourful medications. I was sick to the back teeth of painfully regurgitating gooey sticky splodges of slough into my bright yellow hospital bucket on the brown carpet by my sick sofa. Slough is a slimy, gluey mass of dead cells, in my case murdered by the radiotherapy. I observed my contorted body choke, tremble and twist in pain as it endlessly spewed and spat into the bucket. This distasteful, foul gagging struggle was aggravated by the soreness of the swollen and on-fire inside of my mouth and neck. The outside of my shiny scarlet neck continued to blister and peel, open wounds seeped puss. I felt like kicking the bucket as I lay in silence behind "Pale Blue Eyes" while the torture lingered on.

Both my children started school as each day dragged cruelly in a morphine-induced blur. "I'm so High"! I constantly phoned Simon, who was much further down the excruciating line on this relentless ordeal. He attempted to inspire me by pointing out that things got better and told me to be bold, before reminding me that you cannot endure this "Eternal Flame" alone; you need your wife's support. Shit, while the cancer treatment sent me to hell, my Lady Godiva was sending me to Coventry, and I hadn't a clue why. I was all alone in tormenting agony fighting desperately for survival without even one droplet of help, comfort or love. What the effing hell was going on? I dabbed the weeping wounds on my neck, mopping up the thick yellowy liquid which was oozing out. I also wiped a couple of tears from my weepy eyes. I felt so lonely. You may be the most broken person in the world, but you'll never be as broken as me.

I made a weekly trip to the ENT department for an endoscopy to see if the treatment had made just a teensy-weensy scrap of difference to my chances of surviving more than 12 caustic months. As they pushed the camera up my nostril and down my swollen burnt throat I knew by (faint) heart that the odds were stacked against me. The main man didn't have a clue if Mr Big C was "Hanging Around" coz he couldn't see a bloody thing, as my throat was plastered with the repulsive sludgy slough. I would have to wait a couple more inflamed months to see if the bastard Mr Big C would raise his ugly head before taunting, "Na na na na na; didn't touch me".

I still managed to take my "Dedicated Follower of Fashion" missus out once a week to score yet another trendy item to pile next to her full to the brimstone wardrobe. Of course, there was the usual scenario of going upstairs for selfies before uploading them to her FB page. She went out once a week with some Thai girls she had met, to eat and chat, while I survived on my sofa choking out gobfuls of gunky dead cells while taking care of Jo.

***

On the 22nd September 2012 my frail bony skeleton was 56 years old It was not a dead certainty that it would make Christmas, never mind the ripe young age of Heinz Varieties; 57! I was still pouring six bottles of sweet, sugary milk through my peg tube into my stomach as well as stingingly imbibing the fruit and veg juices, herbs and supplements in a scramble to continue as a mortal being. I took my family to the town centre for an arduous blurry walk as my mind toyed with the harrowing hypothesis that this could well be my terminal birthday in this dimension.

At home we had a small cake and snapped a few pics. Worryingly, my so-called better half refused to upload any images of her hubby onto her beloved FB page, coz she didn't want anyone to feel sorry for him. Was this the truth or was she ashamed and perturbed that his hideous monstrous face and body would blemish her FFB (Fuckin' Facebook) page and the beautiful pics of her pretty self in her brand spanking new up-to-the-minute outfits?

It seemed beauty and the beast wasn't her thing. I almost took my ugly broken carcass to the local church before scaling the outside to sit with the gargoyles, then screaming, *Esmeralda, where the fuck are you? The cancer, the cancer, it made me this way.*

Without warning a shuddersome notion booted me in my Quasimodo bollocks, snatching the breath from my grotesque form. Could she be play-acting as a single woman? FFS Syd, don't even consider visualising that heartbreaking drama. It would be final curtain time before this tear-jerking tragedy had even started. I couldn't deal with the pain of fighting terminal cancer and being betrayed by the woman I lived for.

***

I woke up one morning on my lonely sick sofa and thought, *Just because I'm dying of cancer baby, it doesn't mean I'm "Too Sick to Pray."* And my imaginary friend answered my prayers. The all-powerful one's whispered wise words were: "Don't "Let it Be!" If you make camp on your sick sofa you will be yet another one to bite the dust. Stand up and fight. Get your dying body outdoors if you want to live. And start planning it "Right Here Right Now." Well "Praise Me"! Time for yet another dollop of pure tomfoolery in the death and life of ex-fat boy; the now extremely slim Psycho Syd.

Of course, this was out and out Madness but it's nice to be a lunatic. The Barnes family was equipped with walking gear, but a misty mountain, a desolate moor or a remote forest were non-starters for my broken burnt frame, so a two mile schlepp along the seafront from Lytham to St Annes was the expedition that got the nod from my gaunt, "Up in the Sky" cancer head. I had undertaken numerous jeopardous escapades in my mad as a March-hare life in an endeavour to quench the eternally thirsty daredevil in me. Super severe caving trips crawling around the icy waters underground for miles in tight tubes prone to flooding if it rained on the surface, jungle treks in the far east, and high-altitude shenanigans in remote snow-covered mountains of Western China; but this was by far the foolhardiest undertaking, on the grounds that I was now a death-warmed-up corpse.

So just a meagre 27 days subsequent to the painful grand finale of the horrifying four-month cancer treatment, I attached hiking boots, walking trousers and a 3-in-1 mountain coat to my poisoned burnt skeleton. A bit over the top for a two mile traipse along the seafront, but I was alive to the fact that this was a walk hopefully not to the death. I had to recognise this as the ultimate perilous trip. This was serious risky business. I ingested my morphine, assortment of drugs, sweet sickly milk and a fruit and veg juice to get my broken body ready. There wasn't a Kendal Mint Cake energy bar safely tucked inside my coat pocket for emergency use, but a bottle of liquid morphine in case my flagging skeletal frame needed a boot up its bony arse.

On the 45-minute bus ride to Lytham, my cooked, sizzling swollen neck unceasingly cautioned that I was playing with fire. My fragile and weak-as-a-kitten frame protested as each bump and jolt rattled my on-the-blink bones. Nonetheless, I camouflaged my discomfort and trepidation from my beautiful wife and Little Jo; the other team members on this jolly jaunt. I was smiling, humorous and confident in front of the ones I lived for. Their well-being was first and foremost.

We lazed in a swanky café in Lytham Square for 30 minutes before I finally laughed and embarked on this madcap trip. Slowly and gingerly we went, from green storm shelter to green storm shelter, where I could plop down my dog-tired body and grab back my breath. I delighted in viewing my wife and son smile and play to a background of grey sea and travelling clouds, with the salty wind kissing my fatigued face. It was a painful but welcome change from my sick sofa and four walls.

After an exhausting mile we reached the halfway point, Fairhaven Lake, with all its swans, ducks and visiting seabirds. I plonked my ready-to-drop self in the café and sipped a bit of herbal tea. I felt knackered, but I would NEVER give in; I wasn't ready for the knacker's yard just yet! I had to fight through the pain barrier to be in with even a smidgen of a bloodcurdling scream of a chance of winning this battle royal.

The second mile was far more intimidating and one hell of a slog for my flagging bag of bones. I had to fight the urge to hold a white flag in my fist and phone for a taxi. As an alternative option I took a sneaky gulp of morphine and struggled on like a broken man with a thorn in his side. I gazed in adoration at my two giggling loved ones running up and down sand dunes, masking my discomfort by encouraging their play with a laugh and a few of my time-honoured off-the-wall quips. At long last we accomplished our mission; I zonked out in a white plastic chair in yet another café at our destination, St Annes Pier.

I felt as proud as Punch that I had fought tooth and nail to complete this initial Herculean task. My companions tasted seaside fish and chips as I tasted sweet victory in yet another daunting skirmish in my fight for life. My smirk concealed my private pain, as I kept my loved ones happy and smiling.

Heaps of photographs were snapped to record this first adventure since the cancer had knocked me for six. Even more distressing than my tender neck and burnt-out body was the cold-hearted fact that my partner was reluctant to have any pics of husband and wife together, coz any shots containing Mr Eyesore couldn't and wouldn't be uploaded to tarnish her FFB page. Every silver cloud has a dark lining!

My opiated and stubborn, high as a psychedelic kite mind refused to give any benefit of respite to my broken body, forcing it out of sick sofa land for another walk. No rest for the wicked, they say. So only two days later Eugene joined the three intrepid adventurers for a two-mile saunter along the seafront in Blackpool. My better half started getting moody after about a mile as she was missing her FFB. The promise of a bit of fashion shopping when we reached the town centre put a smile on her face and a dance in her step but not enough for photos with the thin ugly man! She was visualising wearing her new garments, then taking selfies for her admirers. Her husband's feelings were completely irrelevant, he only served the purpose of supplying the costumes she could wear to flaunt her pretty self online.

I had a massive smile and would have danced if I was able when my wife invited me and Jo to go to a play area with a Thai girl and her husband on the last day of September. Up until this moment, as well as refusing to upload my pictures on her FFB, she had also put her foot down, insisting that I wasn't presentable enough to meet any of her friends. I was really gutted and shocked to say the least and felt like the bloody elephant man with my gaunt cancer face and dying bag of bones. In just the blink of an eye she had transformed from a wife who was supporting her dying husband to a partner who only acknowledged he existed when she wanted something.

On one unfortunate occasion my 'happy go lucky' mask slid off my twisted face as my broken body doubled up when the white-hot agony intensified. I involuntarily let out a spine-chilling scream, oblivious to the fact that my wife was sitting in the armchair just a few feet away. Mrs FFB nonchalantly averted her eyeballs from the laptop screen, glared at me with repulsion and icily inquired, "Does it hurt?" Then it was eyes back down before smiling at her FFB page.

An additional warning sign that something was seriously amiss was the fact that she was now concealing the monitor and turning the screen away whenever I walked nearby. And if that didn't set the alarm bells ringing in my confused skull, there was the fact that she had had the unbelievably hard-faced cheek to ask her husband to spell words such as romantic and handsome as she sent messages.

Talk about taking the piss! Gleefully chuckling inside as she spitefully twisted the knife. Jesus Wept and so did I! Was Mrs Barnes changing her name to Mrs Judas Iscariot? I had no option but to take it on my helpless chin as I fought against all the odds for my life. The frightening possibility that my better half would renege on her vow to be by my side for this one year's hellfire fight for survival was too much for my sick mind to even imagine. If I managed to survive one year, that is!

The most appalling incident of September 2012 transpired one rainy grey afternoon as I was sprawled on my sick sofa while my partner was comfortable in her armchair close by, but not close enough for me to observe her top-secret screen. I had polished off my morphine, juices, herbs, supplements and sweet sickly milk and flopped down in burning agony after gobbing out lumps of sticky dead cells. Out of the corner of my eye I caught my missus peep over the top of her laptop for a split second, glare at me with loathing and evilly whisper the word, "die" before focusing on the monitor again.

My loving wife's wish was almost granted instantly as the shock nearly killed me right there and then. I thought I had sampled the outer limits of agony by being burnt and poisoned as my battered body battled advanced cancer for survival, but I knew nothing. That short three-letter word mouthed by the one I trusted made the harrowing big C treatment seem like a doddle, coz now the hurt was screaming inside my very inner being.

The one I was dying to live for was living to see me die. The sooner the better it seemed. I felt like not only gobbing in the bucket but "Gobbing on Life" too. I would have given up the ghost there and then if I only had my snake in the grass missus, but I didn't. I had my mother, two brothers and four kids. If I had stood up to her and thrown her out, then she would have had her visa cancelled and had to return to Laos and I was too ill to care for little Jo alone. The thought of dying without being with Eugene and Jo was totally unbearable and out of the question. I was trapped, and she knew full well I couldn't fight back as she delighted in cruelly tormenting me, like a cat with a mouse. I lay quietly on my sofa in complete shock, despair and terror. I was not only crippled outside but "Crippled Inside," too!

Are you feeling depressed, lost and suicidal? Welcome to my life. Has the sparkle gone out of your world? Welcome to my world.

My name is Psycho Syd and my home address is hell! Or so I thought! However, I had only reached the red, devilish front door of Hades. I couldn't for the death or life of me fathom out what sins I had committed to warrant this banishment to the land of eternal torment. The door to wretchedness slowly opened and I stepped inside and instantly began falling into the bottomless pit. Fucking hell! This really is the pits. Good Lord! Surely things can't get any worse.

Then Lucifer glared at me with them big red fiery eyes, and laughed, "Ps-Ps-Ps-Psycho you just ain't seen n-n-nothin' yet."

Wish You Were Here

(October 2012)

I used to live in heaven but now my home address is hell! Morphine, a kaleidoscope of drugs, pungent sweet milk, vegetable and fruit juices, herbs and supplements were the de rigueur to keep me alive to the fact that I was dying. I was now my own "Personal Jesus" coz the angel from my nightmare had without warning remodelled herself into my very own bad Samaritan as she walked on by leaving my broken mind and body squaring up to the Grim Reaper all alone.

All I needed was a miracle; not water being turned into wine, coz alcohol was off limits in this brawl to the death, but the dream that this was just a blip and the woman I adored would return and pick my dying body up off the roadside and "Stand By Me" as I fought for my life. Sorrowfully, this appeared awfully implausible as Mrs Judas Iscariot seemed to be so distant, unconcerned and oblivious to my grave circumstances. I felt helpless and squashed, just like a dirty smelly piece of dog shit on the sole of one of her brand new shiny black boots which walked all over me. I found a reason for living; every day I would die.

I had no option but to walk this "Boulevard of Broken Dreams" with only my gaunt shadow beside me. In this mood of despair and despondency I took a stab at viewing things from my better half's perspective. What in heaven's sake had given birth to such a brutal, drastic transformation. Maybe the cancer had kick-started the abrupt flip-flop from devotion to repulsion. Possibly the bottom line was that beauty is skin-deep in her pretty, critical eyeballs and my hideous monstrous look of death had exterminated any drop of love she may have had for me - as she now loved to hate me. The naked truth was bewildering because she was still intimate with me on a daily basis for fuck's sake (pun intended). Why? The mind boggles. Sympathy? Lust? She hated me but still wanted her daily session to continue like nothing had happened.

Now you may be thinking that if she was happily enjoying carnal pleasures with me maybe there was still some kind of spark and perhaps, she wasn't that bad after all. Like you I was confused. The only explanation I can provide is that the physical side of our relationship had been full-on from the moment she had asked to move in with me all those years ago. She had a strong appetite and would often instigate the no-holds-barred passion. I had fallen on my feet marrying a highly sexed partner to match my addiction for hot lust. Therefore, it seemed that she would have sex with the monster she hated rather than going without. Probably closing her eyes and imagining someone else, I sadly mused.

Even though I was in agony and at death's door my broken body was well up for it. I soon discovered that being intimate with the woman I loved with all my heart, knowing that she no longer felt the same way, was soul-crushing. Even so, I tried my hardest and gave it my best shot in the hope that we were just going through a sticky patch and that her romantic love would soon return. Heartbreak will be my "Epitaph."

This wretched period in my life when I was defenceless, dazed and weakened was the perfect opportunity for her to let the 'I don't love or give a shit about you any more' cat out of the bag because I was far too ill and fragile to protest and question why the undead was now the unloved. I just lay on my sick sofa, sad and befuddled. Maybe she had never really loved me, and Miss Venus Fly Trap had only enticed and held me captive to improve her and her family's economic situation. After being bought a house, taken on holidays overseas, clad in the latest fashions and spoilt rotten, she had delighted in living the high life. But lo and behold, I suddenly couldn't work my skinny hands to the bone and keep her in materialistic Utopia because I was at death's door! My once-upon-a-time piss-poor partner now held her snotty toffee nose to the heavens as she looked down her snobby conk at the broken man who she wouldn't piss on if he was on fire as our romance became a funeral pyre.

She was blind to the fact that this lowlife unemployable dog turd was the reason she could now proudly strut along easy street, living out her wildest high-class fairy tale fantasies and live happily ever after, yet had no qualms about biting the hand of her husband who was crawling along the dark stormy road to Mordor all alone.

A little bird with worrying news flew into my perplexed tree and landed in my flustered nest. Surely, she couldn't be one of those Asian femme fatales that ruthlessly dumped her partner once she was in the UK, as soon as a wealthy, better-looking target had been smitten? Jeez! We had lived together for eight years and had a child. I didn't meet her in a go-go bar on a three-week holiday to Pattaya FFS! Could the sudden admiration from men on her newly opened Facebook page have caused instant blindness to my soft faithful heart and sparkling adventurous mind, but 20-20 vision for my unsightly face and loathsome body?

Undeniably there was a large age difference, which was the reason I ignored her at first, because I didn't want to be yet another repulsive old western male with a young Asian partner. I should have listened to the advice I had given countless heartbroken skint old codgers I had encountered in the Far East, who had been dumped by their much younger dream lovers. "Don't be bloody daft mate; she doesn't love you; she only loves your money, because you are far too old for her."

However, love is as blind as a white cat with blue eyes, so I went against all S*ense and Sensibility* once I was "Spellbound" and mesmerised into believing that she loved me to death. Well, please keep your promise Mrs Wicked Witchy Poo of the East and hang on for a few more months, my "Black Magic Woman", before standing around weeping a few crocodile tears as they lower me down into the ground at the bitter end. But please don't put flowers on my tomb when I have snuffed it, coz you detested me while I was living.

We have all been there, worn the straitjacket and cried our eyes out in madness, despair and disbelief, when our *'til death us do part'* soulmate suddenly does a runner from the romantic together-forever love story. Endure sleepless nights replaying the whole relationship over and over and over a-bloody-gain, while never finding the answers needed or any glimmer of hope. At the sound of the dawn chorus your exhausted mind slurs, *Oh no, not another day made of tears.*

Or there's a restless sleep of tossing and turning only to eventually open your blurry eyes to the nightmare that she no longer needs you. Then your mind crumbles and your heart wails as you sob, "Oh, shit, "Here I go Again." Well, thank God my neighbour didn't have a bright red door, otherwise it would have been painted jet fucking black already. The time-honoured old clichés such as 'plenty more fish in the sea' and 'light at the end of the tunnel' fail to inspire much hope when you have one foot, one hand, one ear, one eye and one bollock already in the bloody crypt!

Living with terminal cancer, hand-in-hand with being ditched by your trusted lifelong partner, was a proper bastard, no kidding! If she had given me the boot prior to the onslaught of the cancer I would have been distraught and out of my tiny mind with my achy breaky tick-tocker smashed to smithereens. On the other hand, I would still have had my friends, my job and my exotic lifestyle in the tropics and not been here in cold rainy Blackpool all alone, except for my shadowy stalker, the Grim Reaper, breathing down my burnt neck. Although, I very much doubt that my smart-arse she-devil would have drop kicked me into touch then because a Caucasian male was a rare catch and there would have been plenty of dishy Angelic Upstarts ready and willing to dance into her place and heal my broken life.

However, a sad old man dying of cancer in the UK wasn't wanted or needed by anybody, including Mrs Wicked Witchy Poo, masquerading as his loyal loving missus. But now she was an attractive oriental girl in the UK and it was her turn to stand out from the crowd and be in demand! Would she be loyal and faithful just like I had been throughout our marriage and avoid the many tempting offers from the opposite sex like I had always done? It doesn't bloody look that way, does it! "Reasons to be Cheerful" are none!

I had no alternative but to hold my scrawny hands up to the distressing reality that she was under no obligation to love me as she smiled and jumped for joy in her sparkling new life in the UK. It was just a mega bummer being in perpetual physical pain grappling with the big C in solitary confinement, and even more of a shitter knowing that my final few months on planet Earth had to be endured with taunts, hatred and if-looks-could-kill glares from the one I had trusted and believed in. In moments of anguish I dreamed of becoming the Grateful Dead I'd wish the cancer treatment would have finished me off, saving me from the misery and torment of discovering that my wife had been keeping her fingers crossed in the hope that her husband Mr Barnes would soon become Mr Flatliner.

I gritted my fangs and snarled with my bony back against the wall as I stood steadfast in my seemingly impossible fight. I still had my kids, my mum and my two brothers, who hoped and prayed that my broken heart continued pumping my chemo-infested claret around my poisoned bloodstream. And my poor mother was very sick too! I yearned to visit her but that was out of the question in the here and now because she had lost her father and her husband to cancer, and the last thing she needed to witness was her first-born dying of the big C too! I must fight like a warrior to regain my health, so I could see my mum again.

Therefore, the subsequent crusade against the sodding cancer was put into action; a couple of days' rambling to keep my dying body out of sick sofa land. At half-term we journeyed on a big bright crimson double-decker bus to the historic city of Lancaster and checked into a basic family room at the city-centre Travelodge. My black and yellow backpack was brimming with copious amounts of herbal tonics, supplements and plastic bottles of yucky strawberry-flavoured milk.

We had a dawdle by the River Lune and dropped anchor at a Thai restaurant for dinner; I even managed three spoonsful of veggie curry.

My wife was civil but there was no sign of love or affection in her eyes and the only time she smiled was when she said cheese, as a photo was snapped for her admirers on her FFB page. Then it was back to the hotel for some much-needed zeds.

Prior to snatching a bit of shuteye, I gave a swift call to my brother to check on my mum's health. His wife Ann answered, and softly whispered, "I am so sorry, Syd, your mum passed away." She explained that my mother was at the funeral parlour and there was no point in returning to Blackpool coz I couldn't see her. My mind stood still in horror. I swivelled my dazed face to my wife and kids and stammered, "My m-m-m-mam is d-d-d-dead." There was an additional shock as my wife displayed a speck of sympathetic emotion for the first time in weeks and held my hand just before the darkness came.

I slowly opened my sleepy eyes the next mourning as the sun had begun to rise in a golden sky, but everything seemed black for me. Yes, the sun had got its hat and shades on this morning but my whole world was black. Last night I had collapsed and passed-out upon learning of my mother's death. I stood to attention at the window and gazed at the dazzling orange coloured dawn making the rooftops of the Lancaster skyline sparkle, then up to the heavens and like a good boy saluted my dear mum. I silently sobbed with rainbows of psychedelic tears running down my bony Mancunian cheeks and mouthed, "Hi Mam, well, your journey is done and dusted, and it looks like I am living my final daze here on "Planet Earth", so see you soon, my dear mother. And please do me a favour and have a natter in St Peter's ear, letting him know I am a decent lad who always said his prayers and went to Sunday school every week, as you well know." I stood there broken as the grief marked in red circles surrounding my sky-blue eyes reflected my sorrow from the bathroom mirror. Anyone who has lost their mother knows the very raw, deep despair I was suffering at that moment.

My God, Lucifer wasn't pulling my skinny leg when he said "You Ain't Seen Nothing Yet." What future tortures and torments does he still have hidden up his vile sleeve for me to sample on this deadly satanic trip? I was livid with my wicked tormenter; I had seen my bony arse! I had no "Sympathy for the Devil. "Bring it on you cruel swine, do your fucking worst; I will beat this bastard cancer, just you wait and see."

In this mood of defiance, I awoke my three loved ones with a monster smile and a whopping pair of balls in my tartan boxer shorts as my Braveheart spirit proudly announced that today, we were walking three miles to Morecambe. I felt completely insane, just like a "Madman Running Through the Fields," because I knew with my failing health and black frame of mind, this really was a step in the dark. I was determined to complete this task even if it meant crawling on my skeletal hands and knees. Only death could stop me now.

My missus and the kids had breakfast in a small cafe while I had my sweet sickly milk, herbal tonic and supplements. Next came the morphine, which I knew would numb the physical pain but wouldn't even tickle the deep hurt inside. We visited Lancaster Castle where the Pendle Witches were hanged many moons ago. I looked at the Wicked Witch of the East with a wry smile. Next, the Priory, a beautiful old church. My wife must have felt sorry for me because she even agreed to having a photo with Mr Gargoyle inside this holy building. She didn't say cheese though, because there was not a cat in hell's chance of any pics of the grotesque one being uploaded onto her pretty Facebook page. Of course, thoughts of my mum were in my mind at every moment. We ambled beside the River Lune for a spell before treading the concrete path to Morecombe.

I would chat and joke with my loved ones, point out different flowers and warn little Jo about the stinging nettles. Photos were snapped of a smiling family. Whenever my happy-go-lucky, not-a-care-in-the-world mask started to slide away from my cheery face, revealing the desolation I really felt, I would stride ahead and talk to my mother. Pictures of past times with her, my childhood, teenage years and how she was always there for me would be stabbing my broken mind and cutting my already shredded heart. Our last meeting in St Annes, when she whispered my name. The shock of seeing her with advanced dementia. I was in a dreamlike blur as I chatted to my mam. I experienced the weird sensation of floating above my broken body, observing my poor confused and disillusioned self. "Thank you, mam, for everything, I love you and I miss you." The winds carried my words away. I wiped a tear off my cheek, donned my smiley face and waited for my loved ones to catch up. We eventually arrived in Morecambe just as the rain started to spit on my head.

We wandered along the breezy promenade for a few snapshots next to the famous statue of comedian Eric Morecambe. What do you think of it so far? Rubbish! Nothing funny about today mate, but I must agree with you that modern life is rubbish; I used to be a little boy sat on my mum's knee in the good old days.

A quick pub dinner for my family, then it was back to the small guesthouse we had checked into earlier. I lay comatose on the soft bed in the clean Pretty in Pink room, tasting the hard reality that my life seemed to be cracking at the seams; ripped apart by bad dreams. I was zombified, eyes wide open and stared at the ceiling as I silently screamed.

The following day, we went on a lackadaisical saunter along the seafront to Bolton-le-Sands. I was amicable, warm and sparkly with my loved ones as a matter of course, with brief stints ambling ahead in a trance with teardrops in my stunned eyeballs as I divulged my bottomless aching sorrow to the wind. Eventually, it was a pub lunch for my family again as I watched Manchester City beating Sunderland on the TV, but for once the football failed to distract me from my inner hurt. I could only think of my mum and how I would never see her again on planet Earth. Oh mother, how "I Wish you Were Here." Two buses back to my sick sofa to think and grieve and think and grieve again and again.

Epitaph

(October 2012)

My wife's visitor's visa expired, and I had to cough up the tidy sum of £700 to apply for a right to remain visa because of the exceptional circumstances. I got no thanks from the missus because she wouldn't look at me or speak to me. Just a few days after my mum's death, my wife would scream "Ghost-face" at me in fits of anger, while I just sat on my sofa bewildered, silently howling for a drop of love, a touch of affection and a shedload of understanding and support. I got nothing! I was a ghoul trapped and chained to my tormentor, who detested me.

She obviously felt caged too! She was loving her new life in the UK but handcuffed to an ugly monster who she no longer or had never loved. I was helpless to free her or myself from this prison because it was paramount that I was close to my children before I finally became a stiff in a fridge at the morgue. My partner of eight years was totally disgusted by the way the cancer had changed my appearance and had no qualms letting me know exactly just how she felt. She would bend her mouth to my ear with her face contorted with hate and rage and bark sour nothings such as "Ghost-face, hurry up and die." Sadly, the words didn't disappear as they echoed around my brainbox each sleepless night; she was killing me loudly with her words. Ouch!

Early one morning my peg tube suddenly became detached from my stomach and dropped to the brown carpet next to my cream sofa. I elected not to visit the hospital to get a brand new one fitted, so now it was eat or die! Easier said than done after the radiation damage had left my mouth and neck burnt and swollen to buggery! It had also zapped my saliva glands, meaning after sipping my morphine with my moisture-less gob I was left "High and Dry.

At least I was now 100% vegan. I had taken the calorie rich milks because I was informed that I would die without them. I had no option but to gulp large glasses of water just to swallow the tiniest morsels of food. Most unpleasant, I can assure you. My diet consisted of soggy oats and soya milk plus mashed sweet spuds and of course my juices, herbs and supplements. The chemo radiotherapy had also destroyed my appetite, so I had to be vigilant and force myself to eat. Yet another problem was mixed into this can of worms; the radiotherapy had also damaged my taste buds, so I couldn't even taste the grub I was scoffing. The harsh reality of the terminal cancer trip.

The agony from the chemo radiotherapy was at long last easing off a fraction, though. I was still coughing up blobs of slough. The mornings were the worst, when it would take 15 gagging minutes to choke up the disgusting, slimy dead cells. I would get muscle spasms in my neck and back, then terrible cramp, leaving me clutching my sides in pain. Yet another side effect of radiotherapy. I would beg and plead my missus to massage my back and neck and on the rare occasion she would, but most of the time she refused. Yet, she was still intimate with my skinny Elephant Man frame. She wouldn't kiss my ghoulish face but everywhere else was up for grabs! Heartbreak will be my epitaph!

The dreaded day of the funeral arrived. I was living in a bad dreamworld as I loitered outside the church with relatives I hadn't laid eyes on for years. My brother Stephen and his wife were there too. Inside the small Methodist church, I stood at the front, gripping my wife's hand. I felt unsteady and nearly collapsed when the coffin was brought in. I visualised my mum's body in the box and was "Holding Back the Tears" and the screams of anguish.

Next, it was off to the cemetery in deathly silence to watch my beautiful mother laid to rest. Ashes to ashes. Dust to dust. My wife politely smiled to everyone and I thought my mum would be turning in her grave already coz she knew how cruelly she was treating her son during his desperate fight for life. A quick meal in a pub with my two brothers and their families, and then it was back home to continue mourning.

I knew full well that I had to fight and carry on the herbs, juicing and fitness regime; therefore, a local rambling club was contacted, and I arranged to join them for a short walk with my son Eugene. When I arrived at the meet-up point, about eight old folks in their late 60s and early 70s with hiking boots and walking poles were waiting. I chuckled to myself and thought, even my damaged body can keep up with these ancient coffin dodgers. A piece of piss, or so I thought, but I was left trailing behind breathless, with a stitch in my side. They were as fit as butchers' dogs and I was as unfit as a sad old man dying of cancer. It was a massive wake-up call to just how far I had fallen, and the damage the cancer, the chemotherapy and the radiotherapy had inflicted on my once fit and healthy body.

We celebrated Eugene's 15th birthday on the 18th October with a cake and a wander to have a nosy at the Blackpool illuminations. I sent my eldest child Eric Jay in Bangkok a message for his/her birthday the following day. And I was keeping everything crossed that I would still be alive for Jo's fourth birthday in December and Christmas Day too! Francesca's 14th birthday in August next year was just too far ahead to compute.

***

Towards the end of October, I bought a small Fiat Punto from my brother for £500, which was as cheap as chips. The same day I went to collect Francesca from Manchester Airport. She was staying with us for a couple of weeks. *Hopefully it's not the last time we'll meet,* I thought to myself.

Wayne and his Lao wife, who we knew from our time in Laos, invited us to spend a couple of nights with them in Swansea, South Wales. I decided to take the family to spend two nights in North Wales before heading south. Therefore, we all squashed into the small red car and cruised down the M55, M6 and M56 motorways, ending up in Conwy a couple of hours later. Upon arrival the heavens opened, reminiscent of one of the countless mad tropical storms I had experienced in the Far East during the monsoon. Massive difference though, because this wasn't a crazy warm rain, but a bone-chilling downpour cold enough to freeze the bollocks off a brass monkey.

We spent less than 10 minutes sheltering and shivering, looking at a gloomy Conwy castle, saturated by cascades of wild wild rain under an angry black and grey sky. Then it was back in the car for a slow cautious drive through the torrential cloudburst along the North Wales Coast to the Travelodge in Caernarfon. As "Some Might Say," sunshine did follow thunder, so I took my kids and my fair-weather wife to visit Caernarfon Castle before a nosh in a tiny pub and then it was back to the hotel for a kip.

The following day we visited the magical Italian village of Porthmeirion, where the classic 60s series *The Prisoner* was filmed. Who was number one? Me before the big C knocked me down! Well, I was not a free man now coz the Grim Reaper had me by the balls and I was shackled to my wife who detested me. I really was a prisoner. In all fairness to my wife, she obviously felt caged too but, in my condition, I didn't have the key to set us free.

Picture after picture of my pretty wife in seductive poses was snapped for her FFB page. I hurt deep inside and felt like I was wife swapping with men who were married to their wrists! Back to the hotel to get some shuteye again. However, once the kids were sound asleep in the land of nod, my wife and I made quiet gentle love. Yes, as you know she hated my guts but would never refuse an opportunity to jump my bones. Heartbreak will be my epitaph!

The next day we drove from north to south Wales through the gorgeous spectacular scenery of high peaks, valleys and forests. I greedily inhaled the sights and sounds like a man puffing on his final cigarette before facing the firing squad. When you are close to death your senses are operating at a much higher level of awareness as you savour everything; hungrily drawing in every sensation before you are finally stubbed out; the mighty mountains, a lone bird hovering in the sky, the magical shapes and colours of the clouds, the tunes of the singing rivers and the whistling winds. And I thought to myself, "What a Wonderful World."

The long winding, high and low roads eventually spewed us out on our friends' doorstep in Swansea. It was Halloween and their son and my three kids were soon getting dressed up in ghostly masks and costumes for the trick-or-treat malarkey. My partner casually informed me that she was going clubbing with her friend. I had no problem with that but then she stressed with a big smile, "I am not married; I am single." It seems I had been tricked already. Have a lovely evening sweetheart. Enjoy yourself, my ex-wife.

Of course, I was gutted and shocked but joined in with the children's Halloween fun and games. Fortunately, with my Nosferatu look of death I didn't need a mask and just had to "Act Naturally." It made a nice change just fitting in and being part of the crowd instead of standing out like a sore thumb as a one-foot-in-the-bloody-grave monster. Well, I wish it could be Halloween every day.

The following morning, we wasted a couple of hours kissing the salty sea air while being blown about on an empty windy beach on the Gower, before relaxing, chatting and eating with our friends at their warm and loving family home. My missus was supreme in her endeavour to win a nomination for best actress as she played the role of a heartbroken, caring and loving wife with deep tenderness, conveying tear-jerking sympathy for her very sick husband. When no one was looking I would be given the "If Looks Could Kill" evil eye just to let me know it was an act that was worthy of a shiny sparkling Oscar. How does it feel to have three faces? A devoted wife face for our friends, a seductive sexy one for your Facebook admirers and an angry disgusted one for your dying husband!

After a troubled sleep the wearisome drawn-out foot-to-the-floor motorway drive home to Blackpool was performed to the silent treatment, only broken by the occasional whispered curse. Better take my shades off because the future doesn't look very bright. Things are going from bad to worse I trembled as I pondered what future horrors were around the next dark corner. I felt frightened, unloved and so damn lonely on that journey back to sick sofa land. Heartbreak will be my epitaph!

Living on the Ceiling

(November 2012 to December 2012)

I was a "Lonely Man," with no one to call my own, as I drove my imaginary friends to the hospital for another hour of fun and games; on this playful occasion, hide and seek. Will we locate where Mr Big C is hiding this time? Fingers crossed that he has thrown a childish tantrum and decided to piss off and leave me alone, so I can rest in peace before I am "Dead and Buried."

I gingerly positioned my aching bones in the elbow-to-elbow waiting room, shut my eyes and commenced counting to 100 for the pleasure of the coming ready-or-not, eye-watering endoscope. It would be pushed up my hooter and down my gagging swollen throat. The sensation of loneliness was magnified as I surveyed in sadness, self-pity and a slight tinge of envious emerald green, the other thin men being comforted by their loyal loving partners.

I pictured my wife and thought, "Hold Me Close," and never let me go. The warm, loving vision in my brain continued with my missus smiling as she held me tight and gazed deep into my eyes with love, concern and compassion. I pretty near leapt out of my blistered skin at the unforeseen fright night shock as the image transformed into an angry twisted mouth snarling, "Hurry up and die, Ghost-face" Well, if this chilling tale ever gets onto the silver screen, at least you won't shit yourself, jump out of your cinema seat and shower the poor sod in front with toffee popcorn and Pepsi Max coz you'll know what to expect. But watch your back!

"Hugh Barnes, please," the nurse announced. For some mystifying reason I was labelled Hugh at the hospital and Sydney by my GP and dentist.

I have a sneaking suspicion that my dear mother furnished me with a rather posh middle name just in case I decided to spit the plastic spoon out of my council estate gob and become a smart 'n spiffy pinstriped solicitor or a dull gloomy estate agent. Not a prayer. *The Hobbit, Robinson Crusoe, Lord of the Rings, Scott of the Antarctic, Alice in Wonderland* and many other adventurous tales stipulated that magical journeys were perpetually in motion in the centre of my mind. My far-out soul, wanderlusty eyeballs and ever-itchy feet took me on countless intrepid escapades to exotic lands around the planet. "A Day in the Life," living in a dreary 9-to-5 box under a rainy grey Mancunian sky was not for this northern arctic monkey.

I sat to attention in the large white medical chair, eye to eye with the amiable welcoming consultant. "Doctor, can't you see I'm on fire." Not only from my burnt swollen mouth but also from the regular fiery blasts of rage from my evil-hearted, hot-headed partner. It certainly wasn't love I was feeling.

After the test I was informed that there was no sign of the cancer, but it was impossible to be certain because my gob and throat were painted in sleazy coats of filthy slimy mucus. The subsequent episode of hide and seek would be in three long weeks' time.

I drove home to nothing. I really would have liked a bit of tenderness; maybe a word, a hug, a smile, some happiness but she wasn't the slightest bit interested. Perhaps I should trumpet that the cancer had returned and that I would be wriggly worm food within a week or two, just to get a reaction; in all likelihood a song, a smile and an impromptu "Jig-a-Jig".

I looked ill, frail and fragile as I continued battling to escape my death trap. It was distressing and painful struggling to swallow soft soggy food. I persevered with my organic fruit and vegetable juices as well as herbs and supplements day after day in my desperate fight for survival.

I wasn't going to lounge around on my sick sofa as Mr Couch Potato Head and wait for the angel of death to come knocking on my door. Therefore, I joined the Fat Boy Slim (gym) to keep my dying body active. I didn't buy a new track suit and didn't have an old one either! I made do with a faded t-shirt and an ancient pair of base layer walking pants. l looked like a bloody homeless hobo as I struggled up the gym stairs. I had lost all self-respect. I tramped wearily on the treadmill and broke my back fighting to lift a few light weights till I was blue in the face. I also constantly lost my balance at a couple of Pilates classes over the next few days. The muscles in my neck and back kept locking up, leaving me in tormenting agony. All pain – no gain! A dead loss! Alas, I had to kick my health-fanatic lifestyle in the head because I was just too sick. I was sick of being sick.

I was in Dire Straits but refused point-blank to laze at home waiting for kingdom come so I did the "Walk of Life". On this occasion the walking dead limped with Jo, Eugene and Francesca along the nearby River Wyre. It was cold and blustery, but it made me feel alive as the icy wind bit my face. It was fabulous spending time with my kids before

Francesca went back to France.

We are not very long on planet Earth; life is fleeting. A bit too fleeting when you have been given a prognosis of just months to live. Teardrops of sorrow exploded by my feet next to my sick sofa as I reflected that this final year should be the finest year of my life. I ought to be feeling safe, warm and loved as I treasured my final moments with my wife and kids. Alas, I felt cold, frightened, lonely and unloved as the Wicked Witch was hell-bent on making it a year of endless suffering.

I haunted the Macmillan Centre in Blackpool Victoria Hospital for 30 minutes a week for spells of reiki, aromatherapy and massage. I was ready to take a stab at anything for even a dog's chance of a bit more survival time, however "Hocus-Pocus" it was judged to be by conventional medical science. The attentive, chatty lady from Lancaster administered relieving back and neck massages with essential oils, which made a massive difference. She gave me oils to take home, but the wife refused to massage the ugly one and my arm, shoulder and neck muscles were too locked and tight for me to do it myself.

I jokingly voiced to the lovely lady from Lancaster that I should scribble a book about my gloomy cancerous adventure. She enthusiastically responded with, "You could do a gruesome blog concerning the journey and people would be hooked to see whether you lived or died" This confirmed beyond any deathly-dark shadow of a doubt that I really was in deep shit.

My partner was becoming ever-increasingly obsessed with photographs for her FFB page. Each week she demanded shorter skirts and dresses, skimpier, clingier tops and tighter jeans and shorts. Then it was a frantic mad dash upstairs for selfies to send to her wankers; er sorry, admirers. I was given the icy cold shoulder; yes, completely ignored or at best just tolerated as long as I continued to supply her new outfits.

She had me wrapped around her finger to mock and abuse to her black heart's delight. I was trapped and couldn't fight because I was as weak and helpless as a baby cat. I had to bite my lip and focus on my children. It wasn't easy for them, having to witness their critically ill father being constantly abused, shat on and tormented. I could painfully accept that she no longer loved me but the twice daily scream of "hurry up and die" (yes, it really was that bad) was a jagged bitter pill to swallow.

Even worse, what would happen to my kids if, as medical science predicted, I flatlined sometime very soon? Would they then become the focus of her rage and anger? Jo had already been attacked by his mother on more than a few occasions, when she had flown into a wild screaming rage over something or nothing. and grabbed him and threw him to the floor. Eugene or I would dash over and drag her off him leaving a frightened shocked Jo in tears.

A few hours later, after she had calmed down, she would kiss and love him, but we all knew it was only a matter of time before she exploded and attacked him again. She was now in the UK with hundreds of admirers but was frustrated and angry because she was not yet free and single. Her husband was dragging his feet and in no rush to die. Let's hope the Wicked Witch doesn't decide to poison me.

My head was completely messed up and I was climbing the bloody wall. Yep, I was "Living on the Ceiling," going totally insane with fear, panic and wretchedness.

A week into November 2012, I just couldn't resist having a nosy at my partner's FFB page. I felt nervous, naughty and more than a little afraid at what I might discover. Curiosity killed the Cat and it nearly killed me as I was brought straight "Back Down to Earth" in distress at what I spied with my little mischievous eye. Picture after picture of my wife in the tightest, shortest outfits in the most enticing seductive poses. More worryingly, three-year-old Jo was in many too! There were none of the ugly thin man of course. She had hundreds of male friends drooling over her, telling her how much they loved her and how sexy she was. She was lapping it up with her sweet replies. I felt so loathsome, worthless and unattractive.

Of course, she accidentally on purpose forgot to tell her male fan club that she had a devoted husband who was slowly dying of cancer. I pulled her up about this and remarked, "This is disgusting. It is breaking my heart. Can't you wait until I am dead and buried before you start flaunting yourself online, FFS? All my friends and family can see what you are doing. I was so proud of you and now I feel so ashamed." She laughed: "I don't care; hurry up and die." And then blocked me.

Have I got news for you, my drop-dead gorgeous wife? What goes around comes around and one day you will tremble in terror when your heavenly life comes crashing down to earth. We are all in line, heading towards certain death, including your seemingly immortal self, so wipe that smug smirk off your mush and join the queue. I shuddered as I realised, I was stood right at the bloody front.

We were on two entirely different planets when we went out

119

together. I yearned for warm upbeat pleasurable days with my family before I finally snuffed it. My wife had only one thing on her mind; to hungrily amass oodles of alluring glamorous photographs to prick-tease her Facebook admirers with. What the hell was going on? Where was the life that I recognised?

I felt lonely; small and worthless.

She was now turning nasty if the shots didn't show her in her full glory, portraying her as a milllon-dollar supermodel. She was only focused on how many trillion likes and compliments each pic would get. The time spent with me and Jo was irrelevant because her only target was one more perfect pic. In a fury she snatched the camera off me and gave it to Jo, screaming, "You are useless, even a baby can take better photographs than you." On the way home she spat, "You are a very bad driver." She broke my heart and stole my pride!

My brother invited us to watch a couple of bands in a local pub. One band played 60's music and the other did punk covers. I dared to sip a pint of real ale, which was painful to swallow and left me feeling a bit tipsy. When we got home, my wife snarled, "I felt so ashamed being with someone as ugly as you." She continued, "I heard a girl remark, 'What is she doing with that?' " Ouch and double ouch. I wanted to crawl under my stone and die there and then.

At the conclusion of November 2012, I purchased a Christmas tree, fairy lights and decorations. It was weird coz I never thought I would see the lights of Christmas Day. I reflected that I mustn't count my chicks, because anything could happen in the next 25 days.

As we tasted December things went from bad to worse. I was either ignored, cursed or told to hurry up and die.

I peeped at my friends' wives' FB pages and it cut me deep inside. Pictures of warm, smiling, loving couples holding hands - their children happy too. Yet my wife's FFB page was just her advertising herself online in her quest for a new partner as she waited impatiently for her husband to die. At least I couldn't torment myself further, because I was unfriended and blocked.

On 5th December we went as a pair to watch Jo perform as a sheep in his school's nativity play. The evil hearted one, with the perfect phoney smile, kept her rage and hatred for her ugly husband well concealed. Jo played his role superbly too! On stage he hid sheepishly behind the other members of the flock.

On the 8th we attended my head and neck cancer support group's

Christmas Ball. This was an ultra-posh event at the Hilton Hotel. Faded ripped jeans and my three-year-old t-shirt were out of the question. So, I dug out some shiny black shoes, smart trousers, jacket, shirt and tie. I treated my wife to a beautiful purple glittery mini-dress for the ball. I got no thanks, of course. But she did spit, "Why aren't you wearing a tuxedo, white shirt and bow tie like the other smart men?"

My response, "I could only afford to get one outfit so got yours," left her speechless, with fiery eyeballs full of hate. I wasn't dressed like Lord Snooty but didn't look half bad - in a Bela Lugosi kind of a way. Much to my wife's horror, I was still undead. During dinner she didn't speak with me. I was insignificant; all she was concerned with was more photos of herself in her amazing glittery purple mini-dress to impress the men on her Facebook page! There was pose after pose on sofas in the lounge with sweet seductive smiles before we left.

Beware because a pretty face can hide an evil mind! And just to prove me right, once outside, her sweet photogenic smile turned obscenely sour as she yet again screamed "I hate you Ghost-Face, hurry up and die." It seemed like the only peace I would get was when "Bela Lugosi's Dead."

She continued getting dressed up every weekend to go and meet her mysterious friends. She would always tell me it was some Thai girls she was meeting but my gut told me she was lying through her sparkling teeth.

Another milestone was met on 11th December when I enjoyed Jo's 4th birthday. Presents and a cake and he even sang 'Happy Birthday to Me' before blowing out the candles. I felt quite emotional with pride, but also sorrowful because I knew the odds were against me being alive to see his 5th birthday.

***

I would still take my sachets of morphine two or three times a day. With extra gulps of oral morphine too. When the morphine was in my head, I felt dead and thanked God Almighty, because the morphine nullified some of the agonising physical pain as well as dulling the horrific emotional pain dished out my tormenter. But I had been "Eight Miles High" on morphine for eight long months and enough was enough. It was time to freeze and sweat coz "Cold Turkey" here I come. For five days I shivered, sweated, vomited, squirted diarrhoea, suffered sky-high fever, a bone-aching body, suicidal depression and prayed for death. I did it all alone in a solitary nightmare on my sick sofa. I didn't beg for support because I knew it wouldn't be given. I disturbed no one as I hid the hell as best I could, with muffled screams and cries for help when alone in the early hours of the crazy sleepless nights.

At long last I made it but didn't get a gold star or Blue Peter badge from the medical staff at the hospital. Instead I got a proper bollocking because cold turkey is very dangerous, I was told. I smirked inside because I was as proud as a peacock to have kicked the opiate dreamlike state out of the door and was ready to face stone-cold sober reality like a true Danger Man.

Well shit, shock and horror as my gaunt skeletal frame and flabbergasted brain woke up alive to the fact that it was Christmas Day. I couldn't believe it! I was a limping miracle. The news that there was still no sign of the cancer at the last check-up must have really pissed off the wicked one as Father Christmas hadn't granted her wish of seeing me six feet under. I had bought presents for my kids and some things for the wife. I even got a shitty colourful Christmas jumper for me.

Jo woke up to get his presents from under the tree. I shouted up to his mum, but she wasn't interested in watching him open them. This really hurt me. I reluctantly accepted that she had fallen out of love with me but failed to accept a mother not wanting to share the joy of her son opening his Christmas presents. She seemed to want both of us off her back, so she could be free.

Jo loved all the presents, especially the tablet so he could go online and play games. Eugene was happy with his pressies too. The missus opened her gifts and even managed a brief smile when I gave her 100 quid to get some clothes in the sales. Visions of selfies for her fan club danced in her mind!!

In the evening my brother Jeff invited us out to the local pub for a drink with family. We went but the wife was just interested in taking photos with everyone except me. Of course, she was uploading them on her FB page as soon as possible. My family were polite and happy with my wife - they obviously had no idea how I was continuously being put down and degraded until all hope was gone.

Secret Agent Man

(December 2012 to April 2013)

I was sick and tired of being a feeble puppet, dancing when the Wicked Witch pulled my strings. Although in my serious physical condition there wasn't a lot I could do as I lay half-crippled on my sick sofa, in a state of despair and utter helplessness. But I was sick with terminal cancer and sick to the back teeth of being dominated, controlled, tormented and laughed at. Well, time for a bit of northern monkey business because it was vital that I at least did something to stand up for my pitiful self. But what could I do?

So, I elected to live a life of danger and become a "Secret Agent Man". Yes, I chose to spy on the Wicked Witch of the East. I had set up her Hotmail and Facebook accounts and had the passwords. Time for a bit of detective work as SYD became CID! I bet the neighbours would have been as proud as punch if they had only known that the future James Bond lived down their street. I didn't have an Aston Martin DB5 though; just an old tiny Fiat Punto. Maybe I could get some odd job man.to fit a passenger ejector seat and press the secret button next time the Wicked Witch screamed, "Hurry up and die, Ghost-Face," as I smugly retorted, "After you, my dear."

At least I wasn't just sitting back in wishy-washy self-pity. I had to escape the nightmare by making my own adventures in my messed-up head. And every night before I curled up in bed, I got down on my bended knees and prayed to the Lord above because I was a "Secret Agent Man".

The mischievous grin was soon wiped off my face after entering the password to her FB page. As well as hundreds of male admirers drooling over her photos there were heaps of messages too. The most worrying was from a bloke in Canada who was calling her Baby Girl and saying he loved her, and he loved Jo too. His New Year's resolution was to be with them both very soon. And she was telling him how much she loved and missed him with kisses, and that she and Jo would meet him soon.

Not only sexy pics but now love and kisses to some bloke she had never met while screaming at her husband to hurry up and die. FFS Scotty, beam me up NOW! And this bloke loves and wants to be with my four-year-old son Jo too. Over my dead fucking body. Shit! I am bloody dying. Well, I am going to live long enough to protect my son. At least this admirer is far away in Canada! And if he has the balls to step foot in the UK and come within breathing distance of my son, he will spend the remainder of his romantic vacation eating hospital food through a tube. My world was spinning out of control and I had to get this rage out of my skull before I went insane.

I showed the messages to my brother and his wife and from that moment in time, they never visited or spoke to my wife again. They said it was disgustingly cruel treatment, flaunting herself as a single woman while her husband was fighting for his life. I contacted some of my other friends, who also were already appalled at my wife's unbelievably heartless and callous behaviour. Nobody could accept that she was searching for a new partner online while her husband was fighting for his life! They had been following her FB page and knew that something was obviously wrong but never informed me because they didn't want to cause any extra stress while I battled for survival. They just couldn't believe that she could be so hard-faced, doing this to me while I was still alive.

Well, the new 007 had to approach Mrs Givememoremoneypenny with his findings. She laughed in my face and taunted, "I don't care, I am single and can do anything I like." The world turned jet black once more as the darkness strangled my mind.

All was not happy on "New Year's Day". I escaped my four walls and took Jo to feed the ducks. I was going crazy, slowly dying on my sick sofa inside the living room whilst being sadistically persecuted by my wife.

***

I had to escape with the family for four days. Yes, my partner would be there, but I could at least breathe outside my four walls and spend time on holiday with my children. So, I decided to take the family away for a few days' youth hostelling in Derbyshire. We stayed at the Victorian castle-like hostel in the village of Eyam, famous for isolating itself during the bubonic plague in 1665. My wife isolated herself in 2013 by sulking upstairs in our room as she was forced to spend a night away from Facebook because there was no wi-fi. Her undead husband stayed downstairs in the lounge playing with the kids; doing a jigsaw puzzle, building with Lego and putting a train set together. It seemed like the Wicked Witch wanted a separate life from me and the kids!

Next stop was Castleton Youth Hostel, where the Wicked Witchy

Poo was as happy as a hog in shite because they had computers and the internet, so she could message her numerous admirers and promise to love them and be with them forever. One problem stood in her way; I hadn't died yet!

The following night was spent at Ravenstor Youth Hostel; a 17th-century country manor house. No internet, so it was a similar scenario; the missus upstairs doing cold turkey from her FFB page and me and the kids playing games in the basement. The following day I drove us back to Blackpool in silence.

January ended like it had started, with Jo and I escaping the room and feeding the ducks.

***

She had set up a new Facebook Page but no problem, because Syd the investigator had already installed a spy programme on the laptop, so I could monitor everything. I had to know what was happening because I did not want Jo to meet some weird Uncle Fester (child molester) off the internet! His safety was my main concern. Of course, I still had to know what my wife was up to, however much it messed with my mind. Elementary my dear reader.

Well, the latest from the laptop informed me that my wife was promising eternal love to some bloke who said he was from Liverpool. She was sending shite songs such as "Right Here Waiting" by Richard Marx to someone she had never even met. The man's spelling and grammar were terrible. Either he was a thick Scouser who would nick my car or a Nigerian scam artist who would soon be asking for my bank details. And they had been all lovey-dovey, sending messages since October. Painful and stressful - but there was not much I could do now except protect Jo.

I knew my time was limited and it was highly likely I would soon be laid to rest, so February began with another escape. I was not going to sit in one room being ignored and mocked until the day I died. I wanted to see and experience places with my children. This time we went to the small country cottage which was Earby Youth Hostel, and out for a meal in a local pub; the Craven Heifer. Now Eugene had to translate the menu coz the missus wouldn't look or speak with me.

The next day we visited Bolton Abbey, then on a whim drove all the way to gothic Bram Stoker territory; Whitby. The dark foreboding Whitby Abbey was perfect for my Nosferatu appearance. I almost expected to see nothing when I looked in the mirror before bed, but my ghoulish face was reflected, reminding me that I was still undead. It was a spectacular drive back home across the North Yorkshire Moors with lots of snow.

On 15th February, on the spur of the moment I took us all to Hadrian's Wall for a couple of nights. Well, meals in pubs and walks in Roman soldiers' footsteps, taking loads of pics. We all had a snowball fight near the Kielder Forest which was fun, before the last night at the hostel and the long drive back the following day. Even though I was dying, my itchy feet kept pressing me to take holidays with my kids before I finally broke on through to the other side.

Still no sign of the big C at my check-ups but I knew the first 12 months after the treatment were the most dangerous. I continued with my organic fruit and veg, plus herbs and supplements, in my fight. I was half way there, "Living on a Prayer." Yes, six months since the treatment ended and I was still alive but not so well.

We ran into March in much the same fashion. My wife addicted to Facebook and ignoring me. Of course, she would go out at the weekends but not inform me where she was going or who she was meeting. My brother did mention that I should follow her to find out what she was up to. I did think about it, but I was just too ill for chasing her around town. And if I caught her with a bloke, what would I do? Of course, I could kill them both and spend the last few weeks of my life in hospital or meditating in a prison cell. There was a vengeful *Dirty Harry* style *Make my day* fury starting to eat away inside.

I knew at that moment in time whether she lived or died was entirely up to me! A man who is dying is the last person you want to betray, because he has nothing to lose by taking your life too! I had to focus on little Jo and control my hurt and anger when she next screamed, "Hurry up and die."

We did go for a few day trips out. The most memorable was to the 557-metre-high Pendle Hill, one sunny but cold day, with snow still visible on the tops of the Lancashire hills. This was witch country, infamous for the hanging of the ten people accused of witchcraft in the 17th century Pendle Witches trials. The missus must have felt at home; however, I didn't take the piss, in case the wicked one cast a spell and turned me into a black and white mouse! At the bottom of the hill, Jo insisted on climbing to the top. He just went up and up and we followed.

In my physical state it was a struggle. I just plodded on in pain, sitting down out of breath every 10 steps, but I am a determined mother and if Jo wanted to go to the top, I was not going to stop him. At the top we tramped through the snow and the freezing biting wind to reach the summit. Jo began crying and shivering at the top because of the cold and it took us 20 icy minutes to get back down to the car. The heater was put on full blast as we drove home to sick sofa land. I felt so proud of Jo. He has an adventurous spirit too. Following in his dad's wanderlusty footsteps. A future jet-setting globetrotter. Yippee. That's my boy.

In April life dragged on, with my wife getting dressed to kill each weekend before floating out each afternoon to meet the mystery person. I would obscure my misery, bewilderment and gloomy desperation with a cheery smile and a joyful song as I held little Jo's hand. I would take him to different places such as a lake, a park, a café, a playground or the beach. Of course, I was heartbroken at the abrupt cruel rejection from the only person I had left (besides my kids) but I focused on lavishing heaps of love and care on Jo. Eugene would be with his girlfriend most of the time. Good for him. He needed to escape from the reality of this morbid real-life story.

Out of downright straw-clutching desperation and heavy-heartedness I fixed up an appointment with a marriage guidance counsellor. We openly discussed our relationship problems for an hour with a lovely caring professional woman. The lady explained to my wife that I was battling a very serious illness and had only my spouse to help me in my desperate fight for life. My wife smiled sweetly, and butter wouldn't have melted in her mouth as she promised to love, care and support me in my battle for survival. She held my hand tightly and lovingly stroked my cheek as she vowed eternal love. It felt so strange listening to kind words and I almost had tears of relief in my eyes as I realised how alone and afraid I had been, where I now felt safe and loved.

The counsellor was happy and smiled with satisfaction now that the problem was resolved as my wife and I left hand in hand, as a romantic loving couple. As soon as we turned the corner, she snatched her hand away and screamed, "How dare you take me to a place like that! I hate you! Hurry up and die!" Well, it was exquisite being in seventh heaven even for just a few minutes before crashing straight back down to planet Earth with a gigantic almighty fucking bang!

Shortly before the conclusion of April 2013 I confronted my dolled up partner following another of her numerous days out with her unseen hush-hush bosom buddy. We stood eyeball to eyeball as I asked the question my trembling belly already knew the answer to. "Are you betraying me and having an affair with some bloke?"

She chuckled in amusement as she goaded, "Better get that programme *Cheaters* to catch us in the hotel room."

I could observe the vicious smirk of delight as she feasted in glorious wicked satisfaction. She smugly looked down her upturned snout at the crushed, shocked, dying piece of shite crumbling before her. She sniggered, then danced victoriously upstairs in triumph, leaving a shaken and stirred me, utterly defeated on my sick sofa.

I thought of the Beck tune "Loser" and knew my baby wouldn't kill me physically because she was having so much fun murdering my soul.

In April 2012, following a biopsy, I had been distraught, living in a zombified blurred world after being diagnosed with inoperable stage four neck cancer. Now, one year later in April 2013, I was imprisoned in a deranged walking dead netherworld, with my wife whooping with venomous glee as she gloated and taunted that she was having an affair. I failed to see the funny side and didn't split my sides and die laughing. Although the inhumane mocking from the Wicked Witch left me wishing I was dead. Surely things couldn't possibly get any bloody worse, could they?

You bet your last Lady Godiva (fiver, £5) they could. All hope would soon be lost because Pandora's Box was about to be opened and all pandemonium would be let loose.

Where Is My Mind?

(May-June 2013)

Mayday, Mayday, Mayday, save my soul, I am sinking fast. The first of May wasn't spent frolicking around the phallic maypole at some pagan fertility festival. Instead, an unfruitful day was endured feeling sterile and sorrowful, slumped on my one and only sick sofa. The moments that made up a gloomy day tick-tocked away as I replayed the last year over and over in my troubled tree. The long helter-skelter slide from heaven to hell played havoc with my mind. I was "Dizzy." Was I "Living on the Ceiling", or was I broken on the floor?

Just over a year ago it was "Another Day in Paradise." Since then my head had spun round like a record, baby as my life spiralled out of control, whirligigging further and further down. I had lost my job, my house, my car, my pals abroad, my whole sweet life of luxury in the tropics, my mum, my health and now my wife. It felt like I was losing my mind too. I had lived through the harrowing cancer treatment with the everlasting life transforming side effects. Difficulty in swallowing food, fatigue, brain fog and agonising muscle cramps, plus the soul-destroying depression, with the reality that death always seemed to be just around the very next dark corner.

And to top it all, my missus, the only person I had left, not only screamed at me to "Hurry up and die" but was now also taunting and cackling at me as she bragged and gloated about her ongoing hot affair. And I still only had a 1 in 5 chance of extending my survival! So, what would you do if you were limping in my dead man's slippers?

Well I'll let slip what I did. I yelled at the top of my unpolluted restored lungs, "Fuck it," before marching to the local Tesco Express and scoring 20 Player's Superkings. The dirty deed wasn't done dirt cheap though, because cancer sticks cost an arm, a leg and a neck in England's green and pleasant land. Although in third-world tropical Laos they certainly were dirt cheap; they were going for a song at less than a quid for twenty.

Of course, I had booted the coffin nails into touch over a year ago at the onset of this scary cancer trip, but at this moment in time I had had it up to the very top of my bald chemo bonce. I was sick and tired of fighting day after day only to be knocked down by yet another heartbreaking, cruel twist of fate. That day I didn't feel the greatest, so I stayed down for the count of ten. The whole scenario of this fight to the death had eventually knocked me out. I threw in the white bloodstained towel. Death was the only thing I'd got left to live for. Yes, I was dying to be a stiff in the shadow of the morgue. I wanted to break free and skedaddle Samsara's nonstop, brain-damaging, heart-wrenching, pain-in-the-neck wheel of perpetual suffering.

I felt like a naughty schoolboy hiding behind the bike sheds, sadly not with a naughty schoolgirl but with something far more sinful to press my eager lips against; a nicotine-loaded ciggy. I took my kung fu fighter (lighter) out of my skyrocket (pocket) and lit the oily rag (fag).

I inhaled the cancer-causing smoke, tar and chemicals deeply into my spotless lungs. Seventh Heaven. Once a smoker always a smoker, they say. No coughing or choking and I loved it. All it takes is just one cigarette and you are hooked once again, they say. I promised myself, just this packet, then I'll quit. Well, that's a laugh and a joke (smoke). Anyone who has kicked the habit knows full well it doesn't quite work like that. The joke was on me because once more I was a choking smoker and would have to fight to give up the dirty habit once more.

***

The unmerry month of May was suffered in misery, pain and insanity. My marital duty was to look after the kids while my wife took care of her new bloke's sexual desires. I masqueraded as a cheerful, happy-go-lucky father while my hidden hysterical thoughts knifed my soul. We visited numerous places including the Leyland Transport Museum, a red squirrel walk in Formby and had a stroll along the River Ribble. We even scoffed lunch in a haunted pub, where my ghoulish visage gave some of the patrons quite a fright as they took a second glance before averting their startled faces.

My wife would arrive home before the witching hour late in the evening. In many instances an upset and sympathetic Janet would be there, comforting and supporting a distraught and deranged chain-smoking Syd as he paced the threadbare brown carpet. My mad eyeballs would be bulging out of their Gollumesque skull, focusing on the smudged front window for the first tormenting glimpse of my precious returning from her not-so-secret day of sin.

The unremitting torturous wait would finally end when my dressed-to-kill partner turned the corner next to the pub at the end of the road. She would sweetly greet Janet with an innocent smile, then rapidly disappear upstairs before her halo could strangle her. She was then free to relive and dream of her day of pleasure. I thanked a shocked and angry Janet for being there when I needed her most. It was now my turn to relive the nightmare in solitary downstairs, in a mind-destroying sleepless hell.

I knew the chain-smoking and the stress of the unfaithful Wicked Witch were not doing me any favours in my fight against the big C. The missus was still uploading lots of seductive pics on her FFB page, screaming at me to hurry up and die, but now with the additional boasting of how much she enjoyed sleeping with her new boyfriend added to her weaponry of emotional torture. I gazed into her joyful dancing eyes and asked, "Why are you punishing me this way?" Her eyes sparkled before she spat, "Because I enjoy it." My mind churned in madness at the cruelty of it all. Janet, my brother, his wife and a few old chums in Laos supported me but I was out of control. The confusion in my eyes just said it all. I had lost control.

I can fully understand that in all probability you are outraged at the inhumane abuse the kids and I were suffering at the spiteful hands of the Wicked Witch. You must be scratching your skull in mystification as to why I hadn't exploded and chucked her out. And I asked myself the same question! The sad nitty-gritty was that if the wife was out of my life then so was Jo, my 4-year-old son. There is no way on planet Earth that the powers that be would permit such a young child to remain with his helpless old father, now dying of cancer. He would be put in the custody of his sweet-smiling angelic mother and they would return to Laos and I would never see him or hear his voice again. That scenario was a non-starter, so I had no option but to endure any repulsive treatment the wicked one's sick black heart could dream up. Being with my kids before I died was my reason for living and she knew it. She had me by the hairy spherical spheres.

***

I understood that the pictures in my brain were just like clouds passing across a clear blue sky. They were impermanent. However, the floating visions of my wife with her new man while I was slowly dying of cancer were just too much to stomach as the rain fell from my sky-blue eyes. I attempted to just focus on my breath entering and leaving my nostrils but after only one or two breaths, the picture of the Wicked Witch copulating with her new fit and super-healthy boyfriend just smashed up any possible short-lived relief from this relentless bad trip.

I religiously perused a mishmash of spiritual books in a mad last-ditch effort to flee this present-day lousy dream. I flipped each page praying that the elusive escape route would be discovered in the very next paragraph. I hoped to find what I was looking for before the day I died.

My freaked-out mind movies were still driving me crazy so in desperation I arrived at the door of the local Buddhist Centre for a meditation class. Would I glimpse the truth in this sacred abode?

I sat with seven other utopia seekers in a white room before a massive golden Buddha. I wondered if any of the other chasers of wisdom and salvation were ill and heartbroken with a screw loose, like me. A smiling rotund man with cropped hair and glasses draped in red and orange robes breezed in and sat elevated before us. He reminded me of one of those fat beaming Chinese Buddha idols that I had frequently spotted in Far Eastern markets. Would he be the spiritual guide to show me the light and illuminate the path to happiness?

To start with there would be a 30-minute meditation session to help us still the mind, so we could reside in a place of peace and calm. Yes, that is the refuge I was searching for. We were instructed to sit comfortably, to close our eyes and focus on the breath entering and leaving our nostrils as we listened to his guided meditation.

I followed his gentle southern-English-accented delivery as he spoke softly, continually counselling us to concentrate on the breath. I found it nigh on impossible to focus as thoughts and visions of my wife with her new partner kept jumping into my bloody brain and stabbing my soul. I returned to the breath ad nauseam but before you could chant 'Nirvana here I come', a picture of my wife shagging her new boyfriend, an image of my dear departed mum, a vision of my death from cancer, a replica of my house overseas or a mind movie of my poor kids after my death would scream into my very unstill head. I just couldn't remain present as regrets and painful recollections from days gone by and fears of possible future occurrences repeatedly dragged me away from the right here, right now. After an eternity a bell chimed, and I slowly opened my eyes and mind to the shiny golden Buddha, and a serene and smiling Buddhist monk.

I waited eagerly for the spiritual guidance that would unlock my self-imposed mental prison cell, allowing escape from this place of suffering. Wang Chuk, the monk, continued by recalling a German TV programme he had viewed many years ago. In the programme a hypnotist invited six males and six females to join him on stage. He then put them under his spell and explained that when he touched them on their shoulder, they would have an intense explosive orgasm.

Hold on a minute! What the fuck was going on? A Buddhist monk teaching about orgasms! He continued and revealed that when the hypnotist subsequently tapped their shoulders they would moan and groan in joyous ecstasy. Shit, I was at this class to let go of any visions of past moments of rapture and clear my head of the black thunder clouds drifting across my mind, which boomed that future orgasms seemed highly unlikely unless I decided to become a Manchester United fan and use my right hand. Shocking bolts of lightning highlighting my wife and her new bloke having orgasmic pleasure together flashed in my suicidal skull. I had made a disastrous blunder in reflecting that this could be my peace on Earth, light years away from the black hole of eternal despair. It was just making the nightmare a lot bloody worse.

Well, maybe he wasn't a sex-starved mad monk when all was said and done, because he went on to point out that it is all in the mind; you don't need the external world to taste ecstasy. The hypnotised males and females had not engaged in any physical sexual activity yet had powerful orgasms. He added that the pure tranquil feelings gained from deep meditation are one zillion times more potent and satisfying than a sexual orgasm.

Wow, I'm off on my bliss trip to meditate now and when they finally lay me to rest to join the "Spirit in the Sky" you can have the consolation of thinking about me living in the perfect state of Nirvana. You can stick your physical orgasms up your arse! Now there's a thought!

Another bit of useless info I once read is that pig orgasms last up to 30 minutes. Apparently pig ejaculation is measured in minutes, not seconds. The largest estimate is 15 minutes; then add a possible second ejaculation of 15 minutes, and that might be where the 30-minute number came from. Of course, it depends on the pig!

Therefore, if I don't attain the blissful orgasmic state of Nirvana or fail to build up enough positive karma to return as a human being, I will be reincarnated as a pig. At least I will be able to enjoy lengthy periods of ecstatic and frenzied, long-lasting physical elation with my corkscrew-shaped knob before ending up as bacon on some fat bastard's butty.

It was a further 10 minutes' meditation, where I struggled again to stay present by focusing on the breath, before we had tea and biscuits in the comfy lounge. The Nirvana seekers were a lovely "Heart-Shaped

Box" assortment full of love and peace. We chatted about all things spiritual until the topic eventually turned to music. I asked Wang Chuk what his favourite song was. The holy one replied, "Fat Bottomed Girls" by Queen! I spluttered into my cup of spearmint herbal tea as I retorted, "My goodness, you are a celibate monk. I was expecting a tune such as; "Like a Virgin" by Madonna." Everyone laughed including the monk. Good to see I hadn't lost my sense of humour and repartee skills during these grim dark days.

***

June came busting out all over, but my life was still tits up as I fought to keep my loony thoughts under control. I was walking to the edge of madness and felt like grabbing hold of the nearest stranger and crying, "Help me please because I'm losing the plot." "Where is my Mind?" I went to visit a psychiatrist to see if he could help me find it. The appointment was arranged with a kind gentle shrink at the Trinity Hospice, which specialised in palliative care. Well, I am terminal when all is said and done. I suppose we are all terminal, come to think of it. I sobbed out my tear-jerking tale as he listened attentively. I went into detail about my terminal cancer prognosis and how my wife was treating me like a dog. "Am I barking mad?" I quipped.

"You are perfectly sane," he responded professionally. He was appalled and sympathetic over my pitiful predicament. He understood how trapped I was because of my illness but was horrified at how I was being betrayed and hounded by the only person I had left. He applauded me for my never-say-die spirit and the way I had scrapped in my dogfight with the big C, and how I had treasured and protected my loved ones. He advocated that I persevere with my meditating and continue going out with the kids as a release from the Madness of "Our House" in the middle of our street. He went on to say that if events took a turn for the worse, he could supply antidepressants. I gave his kind offer the elbow because I had endured a bellyful of toxic chemicals already. He also suggested further weekly appointments, which I gave the two thumbs up to. So, the result was not to be locked up in a nuthouse or given a lobotomy, but to be sent on my not-so-merry way to join the sad crazy people who were roaming free.

The days would be spent on my sick sofa being victimised by the monster wife that I had tied the noose with. There were further fits of rage as she screamed, "Hurry up and die" - or shrieks of Wicked Witchy

Poo laughter as she recounted more tales of sex with her new boyfriend. When my enchantress missus left home to meet her spellbound lover I almost roared, "Don't forget your fucking broomstick." I gritted my fangs as an alternative and took the kids out for the day. We took in Blackpool Zoo (never again, coz I am fully awake with my compassionate eyes wide open and I detest zoos), a walk along Lancaster canal, a stroll in a forest to snap photographs of trees and bluebells and of course, countless visits to the nearby lake to feed the ducks. The ducks instantly recognised us and would rush over in a frantic waddle to take the bread from our hands. My broken heart and mind ensured they never went hungry as I escaped the four walls daily.

On 9th June I drove Jo to Chorlton-cum-Hardy in Manchester to view and take snapshots of the four houses I had lived in during my childhood and youth. Joyous and joyless memories mobbed my mind: my mum, my dad, my brothers, girlfriends, pool games, street football, piss-ups, sneaky joints of weed in the small cemetery and hot nights of lust on cold nights in the meadows and the parks, leaving the tell-tale grass stains on the knees of my faded blue, bell-bottomed hippy jeans.

We scoffed lunch sat outside one of my old haunts, 'The Bowling Green Hotel'. I used to partner my mate Kevin Kennedy (Curly Watts of Coronation Street fame) in the pool doubles team. The regulars in pubs we visited to play our matches were surprised and elated and asked him for autographs, but no one asked for mine. I would have to wait years before anyone would want my autograph when *The Death and Life of Psycho Syd* (book and film) kicked arse around the planet.

As a matter of fact, I am a fibbing rascal because believe it or not I was once swarmed by a group of schoolkids begging for my signature. In the late 90's I consented to give a lecture in a high school located in the middle of nowhere in China. A lonesome wild place seldom visited by white foreign devils. I was on stage answering questions about my life, England, the Queen, pop music, football, my family, food, religion etc. I lived up to the eccentric travelling Englishman as I supplied warm-hearted, off-the-wall, rib-tickling replies which had them shouting and howling with laughter. I even waxed lyrical about my beloved Manchester City, but they had only heard of our arch-enemy, Manchester bloody United. Bet they know about God's own team in the here and now as United are living in our shadow at long last.

After an hour the show was over, and the kids cheered, applauded and left the school hall whooping and chanting hysterically.

I was dumbstruck and checked to ensure that I hadn't been giving the presentation with my zip undone. Lol. That day I was a "Supersonic" "Rock N' Roll Star". I left the building only to be greeted by a wall of more than 600 screaming schoolkids waving notebooks, begging for my autograph. I signed as many as possible as the teachers led me through the frantic out-of-control mob to the safety of my car. Once in the car, faces were pressed against the windows, fists pounding on the vehicle as it struggled to make its escape. I felt like the fifth Beatle; Psycho Syd! A once-in-a-blue-moon experience - or was it? Although a similar future occurrence would more than likely entail selfies in this era of modern technology.

We finished our lunches as I reflected further on the days of my youth, in a futile effort to keep visions of my wife in intimate ecstasy with her lover far away. It was tough keeping a grip on my sanity, but I had to, for little Jo's sake.

I drove back home heartbroken and distraught and reached a cold, soulless empty house and dished up something for Jo to eat. Much later my happy wife entered. She looked up and down my feeble, cancerous skeletal frame with disgust. Then chuckled, before taunting, "You are nothing; absolutely nothing about you can match my new boyfriend." She then danced upstairs to her FFB, leaving me pulverised. Little Jo just stared at me. I reached over to him and gave him a big kiss and a tender warm hug. I felt like crying my eyes out but didn't coz I had to be strong for my kids. It was a crying shame what they were going through too.

Gobbing on Life

The nights were spent on my sick sofa with eyes glued to suicide sites. I was sick to death of living like a moron, physically and emotionally crippled. I was seriously dreaming of topping myself. Should I hang myself or I how about slashing me wrists? Whatever, but it must be quick. I really was sick of living. I wanted to die.

However, I must hold my bony hands up to being a bit of a "Mardy Bum," because I had already tasted more than my fair dollop of pain and therefore, I was searching for painless methods.

Anyway, let's continue this morbid theme with a few facts about suicide: Putting a noose around your neck and hanging yourself is the most popular way of killing yourself. Women attempt suicide more than men but men complete suicide more than women. Famous suicide spots include San Francisco's Golden Gate Bridge, Japan's Aokigahara Forest and Beachy Head in England. In all these spots there are signs urging potential victims to seek help. I heard a sad story about a man who killed himself by jumping off the Golden Gate Bridge. He left behind a note saying: "I'm going to walk to the bridge and if one person smiles at me on the way, I will not jump." Alas, not one person smiled. Among famous figures who committed suicide: Sigmund Freud, Cleopatra, Mark Antony, Brutus, Judas Iscariot, Hannibal, Nero, Virginia Wolf, Adolf Hitler, Ernest Hemmingway, Sylvia Plath, Vincent van Gogh, Jack London, Dylan Thomas, Judy Garland, Rudolph Hess, Pontius Pilate, Socrates, Kurt Cobain, Gary Speed and a hero of mine, Ian Curtis of Joy Division. Remember the song "Love Will Tear us Apart" Well, love has already ripped me to fucking shreds.

The method of choice for the person who wants a reliable, peaceful and painless way to snuff it is Nembutal. Marilyn Munroe is rumoured to have used this drug to end her life. It has been taken off the market because of the ease of accidentally or intentionally overdosing. However, it has been used to euthanise patients in clinics in Europe and is still used by veterinary surgeons to send large animals across the rainbow bridge.

My father was prescribed this barbiturate in the early seventies during a period of illness. As a curious teenager I confess to stealing one and taking it with a few pints of bitter, which left me in a warm, dreamy hypnotic state. I will not get to sample it again because it is almost impossible to get one's *Death Wish* hands on. You must cough up an extortionate sum of dosh on some shady website and even then, there is a high possibility that you will end up with nothing or with a wrap of worthless powder. Alternatively, you must fly to Mexico for a risky attempt to illegally bribe a Mexican vet to sell you a fatal dosage. I'd not got the money to consider either sleazy deal, so another life ending technique had to be discovered.

I couldn't stomach the idea of a prescription drug overdose because they are rarely successful, acutely painful and mess up your internal organs, with the risk of permanent lifelong damage when you more than likely survive. I also couldn't get my head into hanging myself and slashing my wrists didn't cut the final exit tape for me. Of course, burning myself alive, hara-kiri in the belly, cutting my throat, power-drilling my brain or gulping litres of bleach didn't appeal for obvious reasons.

Therefore, I leapt to the conclusion that jumping was the way I would end the nightmare. I had to select a very high place where death was a certainty because I didn't want to survive as a vegetable or be locked away in a loony bin for my failed attempt. Hence, I opted for the infamous high cliffs of Beachy Head where I would jump into the unknown and "Kiss Off" into the air to this desperate life of pain and insanity.

There are an estimated 20 deaths a year at Beachy Head. The Beachy Head Chaplaincy Team conducts regular day and evening patrols of the area in attempts to locate and stop likely jumpers. Employees at the pub and taxi drivers are also on the look-out for people contemplating suicide, and there are posted signs with the telephone number of the Samaritans urging potential jumpers to call them. I constantly daydreamed of the long drive down there and acting in a casual cool manner on my way to the cliff, without being spotted by some goody-two-shoes who would try and talk me out of escaping my living hell.

My morbid obsession with death meant nightly visits to the gloomy pro-suicide sites. They supplied masses of peace in my dark mind, with their seal of approval that it was A-OK to depart this mad world if one's cross was far too much to bear. Naturally I pondered the age-old question: is there life after death? Would there be nothing? Maybe I would be tormented in Hades for eternity? FFS. Out of the frying pan into hellfire. Would the bad karma from taking my own life mean an even worse next existence, such as being born as a poor animal, fated to be cruelly skinned alive for its fur? Would I be a ghost and suffer helplessly in the spirit world as I observed the sorrow and anguish of my poor children?

My kids were the safety net that kept me at arms' length from death. I just wouldn't be able to live with myself if I created any additional hurt, confusion and misery for them. My self-inflicted death would haunt them for the remainder of their lives. They were innocent and didn't deserve that. And I most certainly didn't intend to grant the Wicked Witch's wish and die. It would be gut-wrenching to make her dream come true by handing my death to her on a silver platter. My mind was unhinged, and I surely was a potential suicide case.

Whenever the intense urge to 'do myself in' overwhelmed me I would focus on my kids and say to myself, "End it tomorrow." I even telephoned the Samaritans once and had a heart-to-heart chat with a concerned compassionate bloke, when I was on the edge.

***

The bright sunshine of July was above my cloudy mind as we nourished the eternally greedy ducks. The smashing news was that the dreaded cancer was nowhere to be seen but on the flip side, my missus persisted in being a nasty piece of work. I continued looking after the kids while the wife rendezvoused with her new fella before returning home to ridicule and mess with my mind. On one occasion she waltzed in and boasted, "He spent £100 on a hotel and £12 on a steak." I was gobsmacked at the fucking cheek. I had bought her a house and paid for her parents to build a home, spent thousands on keeping her in luxury and flown her to exotic locations around the sodding world.

Enough was enough. I was a livid madman fighting to control my murderous hidden temper which had secretly been building up for months. She was playing with fire because this red-hot furious rage was ready to erupt and vent a volcanic fury that would destroy her and all in its path. You should be shit scared of people with knives in their backs!

My mate Janet was still supporting me, but I was struggling to cope. I continued to expose my troubled mental thoughts to my shrink once a week and floated to meditate regularly too, but visions of suicide were always on my mind.

Anna, a lovely close friend who we had partied and travelled with in Laos, dropped by on her holiday back home. The missus was out galivanting as per usual. Anna was very sympathetic to my predicament and told me that all my mates back in Laos were concerned and sent their best wishes. She had kindly brought us gifts too. When my wife returned, she rushed upstairs and refused to come down and meet Anna. I felt embarrassed and apologised to our friend.

After Anna had said her farewells the wicked one thundered down the staircase in a demented rage and flung her gift away. Ah-ha, the reason was as plain as the Pinocchio nose on her deceitful face. She just couldn't look anyone in the eye from the past, because they knew the truth of how I had loved her and totally transformed her life. However, it was simple to lie to people who knew nothing about us. Maybe her new man didn't even know she had a husband; or were they both keeping their sly fingers crossed that I would be "Knocking on Heaven's Door" in the very near future!

On a rare occasion we went to kick a football with Jo in a local field. She even took a few not-allowed-on-her-FFB photos of us both together. Later, upon viewing the pics with my self-critical beady eye, I spotted a beautiful sexy girl with an ugly ghostly man near to death. She looked fabulous but I was just a creepy weirdo. I didn't belong here. But I will stay for just one day more.

She was still her nasty and vicious self as I continued to bite back on my anger. One summer afternoon little Jo took her hand and placed it in mine, looked at his mother and pleaded, "Stop being bad to daddy." It was heartbreakingly sad to witness his despair. Before I had time to hug him, she smirked, "I have got you a new handsome daddy when your daddy dies." Poor Jo looked destroyed. He cried, "But I don't want a new daddy."

That was the very moment that the straw broke the camel's back. I decided that it wouldn't just be a case of suicide, because I would murder the Wicked Witch first! I wouldn't cut her into tiny little pieces or torture her as she surely deserved but just cover her mouth and nose with duct tape until she suffocated to death and I would down the 40 sachets of the strong morphine I still had and kiss my God-given arse goodbye, grinning madly, knowing the evil-hearted one would never again breathe another sadistic breath. Things were out of control now.

***

The 11th July was the Wicked Witch's birthday. I didn't kill her or buy her a new broomstick but like a fucking chemo-brain mad idiot gave her money for clothes. I had lost the plot. You must consider that I had

had over 260 hours of mind-bending toxic chemo chemicals pumped into my dying body and had spent over eight months out of my skull on morphine. In my unbalanced state of mind, I did what was necessary to make life easier. But my kindness to the one who was abusing me was slowly eating me up inside, just like the cancer had done.

She had a chocolate hedgehog birthday cake too. That was for all the pricks she had been getting. And talking of pricks, whenever my partner was not out with her new lover, she was demanding a session of sexual action with me. Her sex drive had intensified greatly because of her affair and I was second choice. Yes, I was a "Substitute" for another bloke. Of course, I knew full well that while she was at it with me, she was thinking of him. Painfully, so was I!

Ann, my brother's wife, spotted the concealed rage inside me. She urgently advised that I get rid of my she-devil before something disastrous occurred. I knew she was right. So, I informed my missus that she could go and live with her new boyfriend and visit Jo whenever she liked. She refused point-blank. Why? Was he married? Would she miss victimising me day and night? At times I would find one or two hundred pounds in her coat pocket. Was she a kept woman and paid for her sexual services? Could she be on the game or even working in the Thai massage parlour in Blackpool town centre? I hadn't a clue, but it was obvious she was up to no good.

I continued gritting my teeth and biting back hard on my anger as she spent an age dolling herself up prior to going out to meet her man, before returning home to laugh and taunt. One evening I was upstairs when she danced in from her day of pleasure and laughed, "Hurry up and die you ugly old monster, because I have a young, handsome, fit and healthy dad for Jo." BANG. Krakatoa erupted. One year's raging molten fury exploded. CRASH. She was on her back with my left hand gripping her throat, my right fist above her bulging eyes as my insane grinning face glared in menacing rage. My power shocked, surprised and impressed me. A "Seven Nation Army" couldn't hold me back. The only thing missing was an old cassette playing "Stuck in the Middle with You". I laughed into her startled eyes as I pulled my shaking fist back, ready to smash into her shocked evil face, and continue punching and punching until I reached the very back of her deceitful skull, before singing "Ding Dong the Witch is Dead". WALLOP never happened. Just as I was at the point of screaming hurry up and die, you wicked fucking witch, as I smashed her lights out, a picture of Jo's innocent face jumped into my deranged mind. I leapt off her and stood shaking as the adrenalin raced around my body.

She sprang to her feet and began viciously punching herself in the face as hard as she could. Good Lord it's a miracle. Thank you, sweet Jesus. She is doing my dirty work for me. Jo rushed upstairs and saw her. She ceased her furious onslaught and started snapping photographs of her self-inflicted bruised mug. She smirked as she put me in the picture that this was evidence for the dibble (police) to get me locked up in the monkey house. The obnoxious fucking cow. She had probably been goading me all along in the hope that I would hit her, so she could get me nicked and jailed.

Later that day Jo broke the headline news to my brother, his Uncle Jeff, that his mother was hitting herself and taking photographs. If only she knew how close to death she had been. Jo saved her from murder, just as he had saved me from suicide.

The very next morning I contacted the immigration department and cancelled her right-to-remain visa application before booking flights for next week, the 1st August. It was time for action. I arranged for Eugene to stay with friends at the Buddhist centre. I informed the Wicked Witch that her visa had been refused and that she should get her shit together in case we had to fly. I didn't let the cat out of the bag regarding the date of the flights because I didn't want the evil-hearted one to suddenly do a vanishing act at the last minute. She had to go because we would both end up dead if we remained in this house together.

Luckily, I had just received a lifesaving £3700 from a PPI claim, otherwise I wouldn't have had the dough to do this.

Yippee, in just a matter of days I would be on the other side of the world in the land of look and see. Once again under the "Fat Old Sun" in beautiful tropical Laos. All things were not "Hunky Dory" though, because I was stepping right into the lion's den. I was taking the skyway to the "Danger Zone." I would be in her manor, so god help me because I would have no rights whatsoever there. Would she destroy me? Would she steal Jo and leave him with some distant relative in a remote mud village? She would be signing her own death warrant if she did.

It was a bloody terrifying ordeal to face but I knew full well I couldn't take any more shit here. Looking back, of course I shouldn't have made that psychotic decision under any circumstances, but now I am viewing the dilemma with logical eyeballs.

At least I would get to taste the sights, smells, colours and sounds of my favourite place on the planet before I was either burnt in a temple by the side of the Mekong River or buried in a grave in Blackpool, if I made it back home in one piece.

I was like a pussycat on a hot tin roof as it got within spitting distance of departure time. Would she get on the aircraft? Would she suddenly hold my hand and love me again? Shut up you soft-as-shite "Achy Breaky Heart"; the grey matter is boss now. Understand? Well, this *Neverending Story* is about to return to the Far East where it all began. What the bloody hell will happen next? We will find out soon enough because the flight departs tomorrow.

The Sound of Silence

(August 2013)

The daggers in her eyes knifed me as she glared with malice before swivelling and heading to the bedroom. If looks could murder! I had just divulged the news that we must depart Blighty and that the cabbie would be banging on the front door in three short hours. It took her all of 30 minutes to squash a hand-picked selection of outfits into the large black holdall. My bewitched heart had been a soft touch as the remaining boots, shoes, jeans, tops, coats, belts and dresses could fill a fashion shop for a size 8 female with small feet!

She waltzed downstairs and smirked before revealing that she was going to meet a girl for two hours, before slamming the door and disappearing into the night. You think I'm an idiotic idiot? Do you think I just got off the banana boat? You're such a cheating "Liar." I didn't give a monkey's toss who her final rendezvous was with; I just needed Mrs Wicked Witchy Poo on that shiny silver aeroplane that would soon *Reach for the Sky.*

A couple of hours before I had hugged Eugene in his humble but cosy room at the Buddhist centre. My meat-munching lad would have to pig-out on vegetarian food because wolfing down animal flesh was prohibited. Television was forbidden too, but he would be able to view movies on his laptop because the building had wi-fi. His girlfriend was allowed to pop round and stay so he wouldn't be forced to live the life of a celibate monk after all, would he? Attending meditation classes was free of charge, but I visualised him on the main road scoffing fish n' chips, rather than sitting in the lotus position following the middle path to enlightenment.

I felt heavy-hearted leaving him, but he was well looked after. It was only a 15-minute stroll to school, and he was just around the corner from my brother, his Uncle Jeff. I promised I would telephone him at least twice a day and of course, he could call me if he had a problem. It would only be a matter of weeks before we were reunited again. I deposited wads of dosh in his bank for food and any other stuff he may need. Of course, I would miss him like crazy. After all, I had raised him all alone as a single dad since he was knee high to a grasshopper. From two years of age to the ripe old age of almost 16. From a toddler to virtually an adult. But he was still my baby.

I lingered impatiently waiting for my partner to return from her final hush-hush get together. Would she arrive in time? The suspense was killing me. After two hours there was no sign of the Wicked Witch. Had she performed a vanishing act? My frantic grey matter triggered off pictures of her being a dirty all-night stop out before she eventually arrived at the door with a massive victorious smile disco dancing across her angelic face. I was at my wit's end as I repeatedly called her mobile, which was switched off. I started to panic, curse and swear as I paced the tarmac in front of my humble two-up-two-down. I popped my fraught gaunt head into the pub across the road but no sign of my elusive missus. The bird had flown the nest. Shit! Just 10 minutes until the taxi was due. I was distraught as I phoned one last time. She chirped, "See you in five minutes." She swanned in a few minutes before the cab pulled up outside our door. Phew! A bit too close for comfort, my relieved tree reflected.

I glanced at my sick sofa and sang in my head, "See you Later, Alligator." We all jumped into the spotless private hire car, which was driven by a welcoming Polish bloke. The opening tune he played on the journey to Manchester Airport was 'Shine on you Crazy Diamond." He was an avid Pink Floyd fanatic. The eargasms of Floyd sounds for the one-hour dead-of-night drive to the airport left me all tingly and dreamy, just like a proper trippy-hippy. The psychedelic music was a melodic "Paintbox" in my skull as my eyeballs focused on the distant car headlights on the horizon. I really did feel "Comfortably Numb". I was still floating on "A Pillow of Winds" upon arrival and the cabbie got a smile-inducing tip for his spacy "Magic Carpet Ride" through the night to the airport in plenty of time for our upcoming trip through the black starlit heavens.

With my feet firmly back on terra firma, I propelled the trolley loaded with our bags to stand in the snail's-pace queue for the check-in. We eventually reached the counter and handed over our tickets and bags. We were suddenly informed that myself and Jo would not be permitted to board the aircraft because British passport holders were required to hold return tickets when entering the kingdom of Thailand. Bollocks! We only had single tickets. Was this my guardian angel's helping hand, ensuring we did not venture into the treacherous "Danger Zone" with the Wicked Witch?

Jo also held a Laos passport which was surreptitiously stashed out of sight. It was imperative that he travelled on his British passport in case the evil-hearted one turned nasty. In this worst-case scenario at least, I would be in with a shout of getting him out of the danger zone if we had to "Run Like Hell." But no worries, because it appeared that she would be flying without us. I casually mentioned that we were wed and produced our marriage certificate. The poker-faced official all at once smiled and crooned, "That is fine, enjoy your flight." I was gobsmacked. It looked like I would be "Walking on Thin Ice" in the sweltering tropics after all. Life is an oxymoron and I was a poxy moron for sticking my neck out and foolishly embarking on this jeopardous journey.

Into the departure lounge, where we had a surprising unanticipated meet-up with my niece Helen and her boyfriend Scott, who were off to the States for a holiday. We would all be flying by KLM to Amsterdam to catch our connecting flights. Us to Bangkok, the City of Angels and them to "New York, New York" - the Big Apple. They totally blanked my missus. Her turn for a taste of her own medicine; the silent treatment. They chatted with me and hugged and took photos of little Jo. I felt awkward, but my family refused to have anything to do with her. The Wicked One was unfazed and didn't give a shite. She knew only too well she had all the time in the world to get her revenge on me! The red-faced horned demon makes work for idle hands.

I'm "Leaving on a Jet Plane"; don't know when or if I will be back again. Whatever happens I would be reunited with Eugene, either back in the UK or in Laos, in the very near future. I was missing him and worrying about him constantly. We took to the inky black skies for the short-but-not-so-sweet flight to Holland. And yes, it was my turn for the silent treatment.

We had touch-down in Amsterdam, but it felt more like Coventry. The undesirable pleasure-paralysing four-hour wait for our connecting flight to Bangkok was withstood to the "Sound of Silence". In a restless nightmare I sat with Jo as my nemesis kept us at more than a few dozen arms' lengths away. It seemed like I not only had cancer but the plague too. I dared not provoke the silent one because the last thing I needed was a shouting and screaming match in the airport.

As the invisible teardrops fell, I was tempted to gulp a few beers for a bit of Dutch courage. Woe is me, because I was still sickly and feeble and alcohol stung like buggery when it came into contact with my radiated throat. Therefore, a piss-up on the demon booze was not to be. My mind was entangled in Double Dutch befuddlement. The gobbledygook thoughts created a turbulent agitation inside my skull. I just didn't know what to do next.

The versatile idiomatic phrase 'Double Dutch' can also mean using the pill and a condom at the same time. That may well be, but I couldn't conceive the birth of a happy ending and felt totally fucked. I did consider taking Dutch leave and scarpering out of the airport with Jo and retreating to the UK the very next day. The missus couldn't tag along cos she had no blooming visa. However, it seemed to be written in the stars that I was fated to enter the "Danger Zone" with the Wicked Witch. I lounged in the airport comforting and chatting with Jo while the silence from the missus grew like cancer. I was given the icy cold shoulder from her who was never out of sight, or out of mind.

At long last we were seated on the Airbus for the 12-hour long-haul flight to Thailand. The missus was civil but colder than a witch's tit in a brass bra. I was in high spirits as our aircraft jetted far above the fluffy white clouds. The thrill of yet another adventure was pulsing through my veins, with elation racing in my brain. This was the meaning of life. Soaring high like a "Freebird," with countless unique destinations and wonderful escapades to be experienced to my heart's delight.

Life is far too magical to just be: "Birth, School, Work and Death." Too many people never live their dreams. They are miserable, just plodding on in a gloomy meaningless job they detest, merely to put food on the table and pay off their debts on the 'never-never'. A vision of a lottery win or a two-week holiday in the summer keeps them walking on the treadmill of their grey mundane existence. They are ruled and programmed by the lies slithering out from the television; living in a mindless dream world, unaware that this is not true reality. Then they die never having really lived. What a blinking waste.

There is a handful of obsessed and deranged people who run the world, create wars, control the media and sell us junk food that makes us ill, before cashing in on the pharmaceuticals that keep us alive but rarely cure. Most of the planet's population are living in Plato's cave, only viewing the shadows on the walls but never venturing outside to see the truth. The saddest thing of all is that these people never think of leaving their prison because they know of no better life. Either I am one of the minority that has opened their eyeballs, becoming aware of this contrived unreal life we are indoctrinated into from birth, or I have completely lost the plot.

The dazzling sunrise left me breathless as the vivid hues of orange, red and yellow splashed an abstract masterpiece on a sky-blue background, jogging my memories of daily life in tropical paradise.

A gargantuan contrast to cold, black, grey and white Blackpool. We touched down in the oriental city of Bangkok. The bags were grabbed before strolling through immigration and customs. We stepped out into the sweltering humid heat of exotic Siam. I was in seventh heaven.

We jumped on an air-con bus for an hour's drive through the traffic to Don Muang in northern Bangkok. I was in no fit state to withstand the overnight train ride to Laos, so I opted to stay "One Night in Bangkok" to recuperate before embarking on the final leg of this perilous journey. The wife was as quiet as a church mouse, but I got the bad vibrations that there was a dirty rat seething inside. We got off the bus into the scorching heat of Bangkok and sweated our way to the main road for a taxi to transport us to the hotel. I could feel Lucifer walking next to me. Suddenly, the Wicked Witch lost control and a tirade of hellish abuse was flung my way. Her shouting and screaming had passers-by open-mouthed and startled. In the old nick of time her red-hot satanic fury thawed as the taxi pulled up. A short while later our weary bodies were snoozing deeply in the land of nod inside the air-conditioned hotel room.

We didn't stay "One Night in Bangkok," we lingered for a full five! The world was still my oyster and I was loving it. The only blemish in this lush utopia was the tainted hateful love that was dished out by the Wicked Witch. In all truthfulness I must hold my shaky hands up to the fact that I was dawdling as I delayed the risky ghost train ride into the "Danger Zone." I shuddered as I pondered what kind of shit she would throw at me once she was queen on her own turf. God help me because I would be at her mercy.

I telephoned Eugene each day and was mucho relieved to discover all was "Hunky-Dory" and he had settled in well at his new spiritual abode. His girlfriend would call round and they would cook veggie meals together. Maybe he'd see the light and become vegan one day. "Little by Little."

The lion's share of the time was comprised of chilling in our super-cool den; the air-con hotel room. I would venture out into the blazing heat to buy food and drinks before returning dripping in sweat, with an English mad-dog look about me. "Some like it Hot" but I like it hot-hot-hot. I scoffed my vegan nosh while my missus ate meat, fish, rice and noodles spiced up with a fornication of Red-Hot Chili Peppers. Jo had a mishmash of everything except the chili. We washed it down with slurps of ice-cold water. Jo would then sleep it off and the heat was on once more as me and my partner would get down to a session of hot lust. A crying shame it wasn't "Hot Love". She was quite friendly but without even the tiniest drop of love or affection. It was either loveless lust or nothing.

I met my beautiful daughter and we enjoyed a lovely time together. I congratulated her on winning Miss Universe and told her how extremely proud I was of her. She was saddened by my illness and my piteous physical condition, but also deeply comforting. She even offered to pay for Botox treatment for my crow's feet! My laughter lines chuckled in amusement as I replied, "No thanks, love; it would need a full head transplant to make a difference and they only do those in weird sci-fi movies." I hugged her and told her how much I loved her and that I would see her soon. Then it was to the market, shopping for food and drinks for the wife and Jo, before another bout of loveless lust.

***

I took the opportunity to visit an old friend, David, and his Thai wife Bomb, who lived nearby. Bomb would have been the perfect name for my explosive partner, rather than David's amiable, easy-going better half.

I first bumped into David at the railway station in the City of Angels in the late '80s. We were both journeying by overnight sleeper train to Butterworth in Malaysia to renew our Thai visas at the embassy in Penang. These iron horses were invariably ridden by several expats embarking on the mandatory three-month visa trip. The restaurant carriage was the place to be in the evening. As the train chugged through tropical southern Thailand, copious quantities of Singha beer were quaffed. Roars of laughter filled the carriage from the politically incorrect jokes that were reeled off and everyone eagerly joined in with a sloshed singsong of tunes such as "Daydream Believer" and "Bohemian Rhapsody" in the bleary party atmosphere. The following morning, we would hand our passports into the Thai Embassy in Penang, for collection the next day.

The night in Georgetown, Penang, traditionally involved a slap-up Indian banquet, flooded with bottle after bottle of Malaysian Anchor beer, leaving us all three sheets to the wind yet again. One time we defaulted from our customary curry and booze and visited the local cinema to watch the classic British comedy *Carry on Screaming* which made a wonderful nostalgic change. On the third day we would collect the passports before boarding the overnight locomotive back to Bangkok for the inevitable piss-up before arriving at the crack of dawn, frazzled and dehydrated, with a painful head-banging drum solo making an almighty din in the brain-damaged skull.

David was a 50-something-year-old chap, neatly dressed in a clean pressed white shirt, black trousers and shiny black shoes. His friendly Thai wife was with him. The thing that snatched my attention though, was the large bottle of Thai beer that was being swigged. We said our hellos and instantly hit it off. I declined his kind offer of a bottle of booze because I stuck rigidly to the rule of never slurping alcohol before 7pm. We had a fabulous trip and David turned out to be a very generous bloke. He paid for an Indian meal and the hotel room for both me and my American colleague, who was also doing the visa run. He even splashed out and bought half a dozen bottles of whisky for the expats to guzzle on the train-ride home. He didn't work but lived off the money from some property he rented out back home in London.

David and Bomb became my very close friends from that moment in time and I frequently visited and stayed overnight at their detached house in the suburbs. David would drink a bottle and a half of whisky and inhale 100 cigarettes a day! He was funny and interesting and usually well pissed by sundown, just as I was opening my first bottle of beer. Bomb would cook me delicious veggie meals. We got on like a house on fire; roaring with laughter.

They were both massive animal lovers and always had at least a dozen rescue dogs, which were allowed a free run of the house and garden. They even had a rescue goose which would attack any visitor. Once the gate was opened, I would sprint like *Billy Whizz*, avoiding the excited hounds with a huge angry white honking goose up my arse as I raced for the safety of the front door. It never caught me but there were a few close calls. Phew! The "Sound of the Suburbs" was a cacophony of yelps, barks, yaps, growls and howls, much to the annoyance of the nearby neighbours. Sadly, the last time I visited about 3 years ago, David was quite poorly and had had to quit the cigarettes but was still hitting the bottle.

On the corner of every soi (street) was a motorcycle gang of smiling men and women wearing brightly coloured bibs; each with their personal number on the back. These motorcycle taxi drivers would pass you a helmet and zip you through the traffic to your destination for a nominal fee. I handed over my 20 baht note (35p), donned my crash hat and five minutes later was on my feet in front of the large white sliding gates of David's residence. I rang the bell, which was the signal for the canine chorus to begin. This is the "Sound of the Suburbs"; woof-woof-woof. Bomb walked through the yapping hounds to the gate and looked at me without recognition. This unexpected reaction was something I would have to live with. The bastard cancer had utterly transformed my appearance. I was a new man; old-looking, thin and gaunt.

Bomb suddenly froze in the midday heat and stood open-mouthed and wide-eyed. "Syd, is that you?" she whispered. I nodded and grinned. "My God, what has happened? Come inside and let me know." I didn't have a wild goose chase to get to the front door because the pitiful thing was now over the rainbow bridge in heaven. In all likelihood flapping its massive wings in hot pursuit of any unfortunate soul who had unwisely stepped onto its cloud as it honked, "Get Off my Cloud"

I sat on the sofa and was instantly smothered by a pack of hounds who were all in need of a fuss and a belly rub. There was no jovial David with his large glass of whisky in his hand. Bomb informed me he had died just a couple of weeks ago and she had recently lost her mother too. It was my turn to freeze and stare in shock as my heart sank. Poor Bomb, I felt so sorry for her. Life appears to be mostly comprised of suffering and pain, with all too few moments of happiness and bliss.

I gave her my commiserations during this very sad time in her life and described my tragic tale too. She was aghast. She had met my partner on a previous visit and revealed that when she'd looked into my partner's eyes, she only saw raw selfishness, with not a single drop of love for me. She advised me to put her on the train to Laos and forget about her. Every single inch of me knew that she was 100% correct, but the pig-headed nincompoop inside my batty brain compelled me to enter Laos to put this heart-breaking dilemma to bed once and for all.

Bomb did kindly offer me the opportunity to reside at her house and begin a new life in Thailand upon my return from Laos. Her thoughtfulness touched my soul but there was no way on planet Earth that I could impose my critical health situation, my broken mind and two kids on a good friend in such deep, sorrowful grief. We bid each other farewell and resumed our solitary journeys of sadness and pain.

Danger Zone

And on the 6th day God created Adam and the Ants and all the other animals and on the 6th day in Bangkok I brought into being tickets for the overnight express to Nong Khai. Nong Khai is a sleepy town by the side of the mighty Mekong River, where the Friendship Bridge leads travellers into the People's Democratic Republic of Laos. My beautiful daughter met us at the station the evening we were departing. She informed me she had changed her first name to Panvilas. Kids will be kids! We hugged, chatted and took photographs before saying our goodbyes.

We climbed into the second-class air-con carriage containing about 30 sleeper beds. I had the lower and my missus and Jo took the upper. After dumping our bags, we went to the restaurant car for food and a drink before retiring to our ready-made beds. I lay back questioning what the hell I was doing as the train headed towards "Danger Danger High Voltage" with my shockingly deadly other half close at hand. And I felt a proper loser on the bottom bunk as the winner was high above me. I took deep, deep breaths as I reflected that the Wicked Witch had me by the spherical spheres. Literally too, because later that night I felt a devil sliding next to me. She blew my mind before the fallen angel climbed back to the upper bunk. Heartbreak will be my epitaph. The express train continued, taking me nearer and nearer the danger zone. Would I survive?

Early the next morning we were promptly stamped into Laos. As a rule, I would be sparkling with twenty-four carat elation as I stepped into wonderland once again. This was the place where I wanted to die. Be careful what you wish for, Psycho! On this dicey trip the euphoric buzz was contaminated with apprehension because lovely Laos was now unsafe. I felt so sad.

We captured a taxi and half an hour later we were home on the land I had shed blood, sweat and tears for just a few years back. Warm welcomes from her family. They were delighted to see us all again. Even the missus was amiable and smiling. The calm before the storm?

After her family discovered the sadistic, inhumane behaviour of my wife in the UK they were stunned, appalled and deeply sympathetic. They could only say, "We are sorry, and we really pity you." Sadly, there was absolutely nothing they could do because in the land of the piss-poor, the one with the house, land and a spellbound Caucasian husband is queen and rules the roost.

I was still dwelling in the territory of the past. Sweet memories of tender romantic love and happiness were like honey in my lovestruck mind as the painful betrayal was brushed aside and swept under the carpet. Like all broken-hearted lovers I longed for life to be like it used to be, all lovey-dovey, full of kisses and goo-goo eyes.

I went day after day to a major transport company to observe operations with the purpose of securing a long-term full-time position. In my bewitched dreamy mind, I had pie-in-the-sky visions of a sparkling new beginning with the missus; then flying Eugene here and living happily ever after in perfect harmony, as if the betrayal had never occurred. I persisted with this pipedream, oblivious to the fact that pigs were never going to fly. I had lost all sense of logic because I failed to consider my serious health issues and that it takes two to tango. And as you already know, we did tango every day but sadly the wife was never going to allow me to quickstep back into her heart too. I had better get used to "Dancing With Myself."

***

One bright, "Good Day Sunshine" morning, I swerved my Yamaha scooter to avoid a stupid girl who was riding her motorbike directly at me on the wrong side of a back road. Before I could scream, "You fucking idiot," I threw my wheels onto the side and agonisingly slid along the gravel in my short sleeve shirt and thin cotton trousers. Ouch and treble ouch! Blood was oozing from my left forearm, elbow and knee, rapidly colouring my shredded shirt and pants.

In Laos hardly anyone has a license or insurance and if I dared to file a complaint I would be found at fault and fined for being a rich foreigner. I stared at her in disbelief, held my tongue and returned home. I endured the next hour stinging in the shower, gingerly dabbing off the blood and picking small bits of black stone from my wounds with tweezers. The Wicked Witch just sneered with disgust. Not a drop of sympathy.

I did come in useful though, because I dipped my hand in my pocket for the food and paid the bills. I coughed up £300 for house tax and gave her younger brother the £100 he needed for college, even though he had flogged Eugene's computer for a pittance because he didn't think we would ever return.

As I scribble this, I am aghast at how blind I was. She was my heroin and I was addicted. I would allow any abuse as long as I got my next fix. She would repeatedly let me know that without her I would be alone forever and die a lonely old man, because the cancer had made me so ugly that no one else would be seen dead with me. And yet she was still sexually intimate with me daily! Why? Was this another form of entrapment to keep me hooked? Probably not, because I just think she liked sex in all honesty. It brought to mind women who are physically and emotionally abused by their partners yet without fail, repeatedly return back to their abusive other halves. They must have diddly-squat self-esteem, just like me.

August waved bye-bye without even a speck of headway having been made. Will someone please give me a slap and wake me up when or before September ends. I was overall ignored but thank goodness there wasn't the screaming angry abuse anymore. We visited Udorn Thani in Thailand a couple of times for a spot of shopping and a night away. It painfully brought back recollections of hand-holding romantic trips in the past, long before the bastard big C reared its vile head.

On 7th September we ambled along the banks of the Mekong River. Again, Jo put his mother's hand in mine. She smiled and left it there for a few seconds before taking it away. She went out a couple of times with her friends but of course, the ugly one wasn't permitted to join in. I despised myself for allowing her to shit on me in this way. I don't wanna be your dog. Playing the part of the victim isn't much fun. I struggled with an awareness of my oppression, confused by nostalgic love and unable to open my eyes to how it was me, not her who was writing the script and only I could liberate myself, by changing the storyline.

In Blackpool I would escape with Jo to feed the ducks. Here I would take him for a ramble through huge ferns and trees on the wild land opposite our house. We would search for and observe the numerous spectacular tropical insects, which fascinated both of us.

You knew damn well it was bound to happen and, so did I. One balmy evening just as the sun was going to sleep, the barmy Wicked Witch threw a wobbler and went berserk, yelling "Get out of my house and off my land and go back to England." The cheeky bleeding cow. I had grafted for years to buy that land and she had never lifted a finger or done a day's work since the day she had mesmerised me. She considered herself to be the bee's knees, lazily sprawling on the sofa while the maid was busy doing the chores. Her oh-so-hard life included painting her nails, brushing her hair and shopping for the up-to-the-minute fashions. The deranged bastard then twisted her furious face to little Jo and screamed, "And you go with him too." We rapidly stuffed the backpack, jumped on the scooter and got the hell out of there. An hour later she rang and said, "You can come back now." And like a "Puppet on a String" I gladly went there, rather than pissing off and sunbathing on some *Sandy Shore* in Thailand.

Happy Birthday to me, Happy Birthday to me, Happy Birthday Dear Psycho, Happy Birthday to me. I had no option but to howl it to myself because the trouble and strife (wife) purposely forgot my birthday. Yes, the 22nd September and I was 57 years old. The previous 12 months had been a living hell. I was still alive but felt dead inside. On the outside I had the look of a death-warmed-up skeleton breathing in and out.

Fifty-seven years ago, to the day, Manchester United defeated Manchester City 2-0. As luck would have it, today was Derby Day too. As I had not been wished Happy Birthday, handed a card or been given a surprise gift by anyone, I decided to supply myself with a smashing present; I arranged to meet two ex-colleagues at the Highland Bar to watch this year's game live; City v United. The bar was on an outside wooden terrace with several TV screens. It was romantically located on the banks of the massive Mekong River and was owned by a Rangers-mad Scotsman named Andy.

I took my seat with my mates and stared in awe at the wild Mekong sprinting in brown muddy torrents towards Cambodia, before finally spilling itself into the South China Sea in Vietnam. My sky-blue eyeballs peered into the far distance at the village of tiny lights twinkling on the opposite bank. Would I prefer to be watching in a dreary pub in Blackpool? Would I heckers like!

My two football loving pals were the perfect companions to view such a tense passionate match with. Wobbley Bob, a Liverpool supporter and Odd Bjok, a United fan. They were shocked by my ghostly look of death and even more horrified at the treatment dished out by my missus. Unlike the folk in England, they had witnessed my devotion and how I had comprehensively transformed her life. My sky-blue heart beat quickly as I waited for the game to kick-off.

The bar started to fill as more patrons arrived to watch the big match. I spotted a few of my friends but they walked on by without recognition. A second later they were halted in their tracks as a bell rang in their heads. They gawked at me in horror before stammering something like, "My God, is that you, Syd?" By far the best comment was, "Fucking Hell, Syd, I thought you were dead." The news of my illness had spread like cancer amongst the expat community. They were all aghast at my ghostly appearance and even more appalled by my wife's betrayal just when I needed her most.

The place was buzzing with an atmosphere of excited anticipation. Just before the teams came out the lights dimmed, and a birthday cake arrived from behind the bar. My turn to be gobsmacked. Everyone joined in with Happy Birthday as I sat stunned, with a lump in my throat. I was "Holding Back the Tears." And Manchester City beat United 4-1 which was the icing on the cake. I was over the "Blue Moon," but poor Odd was as sick as a parrot as his Simply Red Devils were struck down by God's own team.

I did ponder the fact that we'd played United and lost on the day of my birth in 1956, and it had been 57 years before the derby was next contested on my birthday, and City had been victorious. Was this a sign from the universe that this would be my last birthday on planet Earth? If it was, well, thank God that I was given sweet victory as a final sending-off present.

I rode my orange and white scooter with its Manchester City stickers back home in jubilation at the happy ending to my birthday. I sang the fans' anthem "Blue Moon" all the way home. I didn't know whether to laugh or cry as I sang about being alone, without a dream in my heart and a love of my own. Oh, the irony.

The following morning, I stood perfectly still in my wild tropical garden in deep contemplation. Where was my wife when I needed her most? Gone away. I instantly put a halt to my insane plan of seeking employment because I was in no fit condition to work. I was battling for my life with the Grim Reaper and the odds were still in his favour. It was madness travelling all this way with my very critical health problems in the first place.

It had also become crystal-clear that I was pissing in the gale force wind waiting for a new beginning with the wife. It just wasn't going to happen; she didn't want me. I needed to heal and feel like I was "Somewhere I belonged." My brain screamed, 'Get the hell out of here now', but my besotted heart pleaded for just one more day. If I could fly back in a time machine, I would wear a pair of hobnail boots and give my wishy-washy arse a hard kick and scream, "Get the fuck out of there as of now."

I should have known that things were going to take a turn for the worse when the missus got her younger brother to copy all the pictures and videos of us from my external hard drive.

 October arrived with daily strolls in the woods with Jo. We observed nature and collected different leaves and played hide and seek. It was tragic that Jo had had to experience all this confusion and pain so early in his life. I had continually kept in contact with Eugene and he was fine, but I was missing him so much.

One night the Wicked Witch exploded in a terrible fit of rage. We were in bed with Jo when she completely lost it. Her anger was directed at poor Jo. Not physically but emotionally. She screamed at him, "I hate you; I am not your mother." He was shocked and afraid. I held him next to me as her abuse continued. "Leave him alone," I yelled, "he has done nothing to you." This made her anger boil over. In a terrifyingly evil deep voice, she threatened, "Jo, go to the kitchen and take some medicine and die because if you don't, I will cut your throat." What the fuck was I hearing? I just couldn't believe it! I shit you not; that is what she said. If this book ever kicks off and I am challenged I would willingly go on some TV programme such as *The Jeremy Kyle Show* and for sure, would be proved to be telling the truth. But she wouldn't dare challenge me cos she'd know full well it was the whole truth, the full truth and nothing but the truth! Jo was shaking and sobbing in my arms.

My wife's teenage brother, who was sleeping next door, entered the room and asked Jo if he would like to sleep in his room. Jo just wanted to stay next to me. I was livid and shaking with deep, deadly anger. How could a mother do this to her own son? Was her purpose to incite me to hit her? At that moment I would have gladly knocked her out but that would have been the end for me and Jo. The village chief would have been called and I would have been arrested and Jo would have been left with his vile mother. I just lay there controlling my fury, holding Jo next to me. I knew there and then it was time for me and Jo to flee the "Danger Zone."

I awoke the following bright morning with brand new eyes. The Wicked Witch's sickening treatment of her son had broken the dreamlike spell I had been living under for years. I shook my head a few times as I became aware that the world looked very different today. What the fuck was I doing here? How come I was still with a woman who had been unfaithful, cruel and vicious to both me and my son? I couldn't believe how I had allowed another person to treat me like garbage. Why on earth had I married a woman so much younger than myself? Shit! I was just another gullible old western male who had foolishly fallen for a young Asian girl and was now reaping the bad karma for my crazy short-sightedness. The law of cause and effect had come back to bite me on my arse. However, Jo was innocent, and it was essential to get us both out and far away as soon as possible.

Easier said than done though. If she got the slightest whiff that her Mr Moneybags was going to flee, she would put a stop to that little scheme by any method she could dream up in her black heart. How could I possibly get my backpack, my computer and Jo onto the scooter without raising any suspicions? If it came to the crunch, I would just slyly pocket the passports and external hard drive and casually mention that I was taking Jo out for lunch. Then we'd make a mad half-hour dash for the border. I had to be as cool as a cucumber at this very critical time. I had to continue acting like the pitiful bewitched clown, not letting her see that the spell had been broken.

As lady luck would have it, the wicked one played right into my bony hands. She must have got up on the wrong side of the bed as her fury continued unabated, with double the ferocity of the night before. Thankfully, it was my turn to be the target of her wild screaming insults and vicious taunts. I was relieved little Jo was left alone. No child should ever hear those words from his mother. Unforgivable. She was losing control and I was delighted with the abuse. There is a first for everything, they say. Keep it coming, darling.

I was biding my time, getting ready to pounce if an opportune moment came along. Then I would swiftly grab my stuff and Jo and get out of there without giving her the slightest inkling that I had the 'get out of the danger zone card' secretly stashed up my sleeve. I didn't react to her vile threats or goading, which just enraged her all the more. She eventually exploded and started hurling everything she could lay her hands on at me. Perfect. Thank you my precious. I grabbed my backpack and computer at the same time as dodging and blocking cups, books, glasses and even a DVD player, which hit and cut my arm. Next, I snatched a shocked and frightened Jo and jumped on the scooter and got us the hell out of there. She made no attempt to stop us leaving because she didn't know the spell was broken. Of course, she would be cocksure that I would return in an hour or two, with my tail between my legs. So that gave us about 120 minutes to escape before she began to panic and get suspicious.

We rode to the centre of Vientiane and dumped the scooter with a friend plus £200, so she had enough food to keep her cauldron going for a while. I am not as foolish as it first appears because I had to keep the Wicked Witch blind to the fact that we were scarpering back to England. The last thing I needed was a crazy screaming demon creating uproar at Bangkok airport in an attempt to stop us boarding our flight to safety.

I decided that I would contact her once we were out of Laos and give the impression that we were taking a much-needed break in Thailand. I had always been completely honest and upfront with my wife but now it was time to play her at her own deceitful game. It wasn't easy though, because I was a raw novice and she was a highly experienced five-star expert.

We jumped into a tuk-tuk for the 30-minute tuk-tuk-tuk-tuk journey to the border. I sat down with a monster smile from ear to ear as I held Jo close and breathed easily. Ding-dong, we had outfoxed the Wicked Witch. "Not long now," I assured him, as my smarmy face smirked with deep satisfaction. Suddenly out of the sky an almighty bolt of evil from a black magic wand zapped my mind. She'd been a devious clever cow, I reflected, and there wasn't a black widow in hell's chance that she would allow us to flee her venomous web of pain and torture so easily. She would surely have supplied immigration with our details at some point during the last few weeks in case we decided to make a run for it. Shit!

Why the hell hadn't I woken up from the spell and opened my eyes long before I stepped into the danger zone. I had visions of being arrested for kidnap or some other trumped-up charge and locked up in a tiny concrete cell, while Jo was returned to his cruel mother. Well, that wiped the smile off my cocky face. God forbid that Lucifer had yet another devilish twist of fate lined up for me on this cruel never-ending story.

My claret was pulsating all around my twiggy frame as the old ticker pounded beneath the ribs. All the potential border control scenarios were taking control of my mind as the grey matter hurriedly contemplated each unfavourable possibility. My remaining brain cells then proposed the response that would give the highest chance of success to each imaginable obstacle.

We pulled up less than 100 metres from passport control. I paid the smiling driver, grabbed my black and yellow backpack, held Jo's tiny hand and made my way towards escape. Why was everyone looking at us? I was obviously paranoid. I forced myself not to fidget or appear panicky as I joined the short queue to exit this hazardous land. I acted with an air of bored nonchalance but felt as if I had GUILTY daubed in scarlet capital letters across my sweaty forehead. As we were stood just second in line I mused, *Thank fuck I haven't got a couple of kilograms of heroin shoved up my arse.* The stern-faced immigration official looked me right in the eyes and said, "Next."

I held Jo's hand but wobbled slightly as we took the three short steps to the small cubicle to meet the serious-looking official's relentless steely stare.

Fox on the Run

(October 2013)

I smiled with confidence as I handed over our passports to the hard-nosed official in the kiosk. He studied mine very carefully before looking up with piercing eyes and scrutinising my cheerful face for a relentless ten seconds. My blood ran cold, although I didn't feel chilled as the sweat raced down my cheeks. He stared at the passport once again before shouting, "This looks nothing like you." Shite! It had totally slipped my frantic mind that the bloody cancer had completely altered the shape of my face. Bollocks! I had a vision of him radioing for a couple of Green Flies to cart me off. The police in Laos are called Green Flies in slang because of their green uniforms and for the fact that they always seem to be hanging around shit!

My photograph had a look of life and vigour but in reality, I looked like death; thin, gaunt and very suspicious. I gave the image of a convict in real life but not on my passport photo, which made an amusing change.

I laughed and responded, "Yes, I know, I have stage four head and neck cancer and have recently undergone chemotherapy and radiotherapy as well as losing over half my body weight. I will have to get a new photo and apply for a fresh passport at the British Embassy." He looked shocked. Was it the heart-breaking story or was it my fluency in the Lao language?

"Where are you going?" he inquired.

"We are spending a night or two in nearby Udorn Thani. We will do a bit of shopping and I will nip into the private hospital for a quick check-up to make sure that my condition hasn't worsened," I explained.

His hard face softened with sympathy as he enthusiastically stamped our passports.

He smiled warmly. "Enjoy your visit and good luck." Thank goodness I was fluent in the lingo; it made problematic situations such as this just fade away.

We were still not footloose and fancy free and out of the Witch-Queen of Old Vientiane's wicked web yet. Better shake a leg before my voodoo doll puts a spell on me. We were in no man's land and needed to dash like busy blue-arsed flies across the bridge to arrive at the Thai border control on the other side of the river before we could finally spread our wings. Only halfway there and "Livin on a Prayer" This time my gift of the gab in the Thai language ensured our escape went as smooth as Thai silk. We were now out of the Wicked Witch's territory and in the land of smiles. And yes, I had a massive smile of relief on my mush.

We didn't pick up a 'get out of jail card' or £200 but we were now ready, steady, go as far as rolling the dice and monopolising our new-found carte blanche.

Nevertheless, only when we had our bums on the economy-class seats of the big bird in the sky and were flying back to merry old England, would we be able to breathe a pterodactyl-sized sigh of relief. It was paramount that I was vigilant and on the lookout for any sly tricks my foxy ex-partner might try to pull. The last thing I needed was to fall under her bewitching spell once again. This was not the time or place for being chicken-hearted; it was vital that I was as brave as a lion and as cunning as a Sweet "Fox on the Run."

We jumped into a comfy taxi for the 45-minute drive to Udorn Thani, North-Eastern Thailand. I hugged Jo and grinned. Jo seemed happy and calm. No shouting or bad moods when he was with his father; just love and affection. We scored a room in the British-run Irish Clock.

This Irish Clock is the quintessential Irish pub overseas, with Guinness and Kilkenny Bitter on tap, a pool table, live sports and a tasty mix of western and Asian meals on the menu. The accommodation upstairs was comprised of clean spacious rooms, each with a massive king size bed and a brilliant power shower too. The building was conveniently located in the city centre, close to the shopping mall, the outdoor market and just a condom's throw away from the "Whatever you Want, Whatever you Like" nightlife. It was my home from home.

It was my 'Yabba-dabba-doo' man-cave prior to bumping into my future wife to be. I would break out from sleepy Vientiane for wild alcohol fuelled "It's a Sin" weekends away with an Aussie mate. Dressed to the nines in my glad rags, ready to paint the town every colour of the rainbow on the 'what happens in Udorn stays in Udorn' little jollies away.

Next it became the "Temple of Love" for my "I'm a Family Man" perfect days and nights away with the ones I worshipped. We would take walks in the park, eat in cafes and restaurants and I would splash out on toys and clothes for the ones I lived for. Being close to and treating my family was my idea of a blissful weekend.

And now it was "She Sells Sanctuary" for me and my 4-year-old lad. Yes, I was now a loving single dad focusing on the safety, happiness and needs of my 4-year-old son. Everything "Changes." I had to turn and face the truth; nothing lasts forever.

Now it was time to break the news to my missus that we had pulled a fast one and had outfoxed her. What would her reaction be to the fact that we were no longer possessed and under her spell in the danger zone? Would she explode with wild burning fury when it became apparent that she had been bamboozled and that we had made a monkey out of her? I wondered if there was any chance of her being worried to death about her little "Runaway's" ultra-serious health situation or would she be mega-concerned about the well-being of her son?

I called her up and smoothly announced that we had split the People's Democratic Republic of Laos and were now sitting pretty in the land of smiles. Silence was golden for a full ten seconds until she hollered "What am I gonna do for money?" Well, at least I had my answer. I want "Money." What a surprise; well at least I know what she wants. Sadly, not my kind, faithful heart. She was obviously distraught when she got the picture that she had lost her crying, talking, sleeping, walking, living ATM card. "Little by Little" I had given her everything she had asked for, so now she must be feeling helpless and at a loss as her Mr "Money For Nothing" was on the road to somewhere. I calmed her fears by coolly illuminating that she could collect the scooter from my friend and that I had left her some lovely "Money Makes the World go Around" too. There was no Violent Femme outburst of anger as it must have become abruptly apparent that it was now me sitting comfortably in the driver's seat.

I justified that because of her latest fits of temper, Jo and I urgently required a bit of breathing space to chill out. I assured her that I would give her a call tomorrow. She responded with "Ok". I wasn't gloating or laughing loudest because revenge wasn't in my heart. I was far too sick and emotionally shell-shocked to take delight in this minor victory. Nonetheless, there was a feeling of relief that Jo and I were safely out of range of one of her frenzied violent outbursts. In my lamentable state of body and mind, love, support and compassion were required, not hatred, abuse and heartache.

We ordered some food and sat at a small wooden table on the patio at the front of the pub. Sitting in the corner watching all the girls go by! Plenty more oysters in the sea, I chuckled. I am going to bite my tongue and not reveal what part of the female anatomy oyster refers to in Thai slang, but I am sure you can guess. Don't worry, I was not "Hungry Like the Wolf" on the hunt for another girl, thank you very much. Until I pull a girl who won't stab me in the back, I'll be a "Solitary Man". I managed to slowly eat some chips and baked beans and Jo had some too. I even grabbed a cheeky pint of Kilkenny bitter, which I sipped unhurriedly.

A middle-aged European bloke joined us at our table. We nattered away, and I recounted my traumatic tale of cancer, marriage break-up and our audacious bolt across the border. He looked shocked and was full of sympathy. We continued with our chit-chat and then he left me flabbergasted by asking, "Could you give me your wife's Facebook details?"

I was speechless and glared at him with malice as I thought, *You obnoxious hard-faced twat; "You're Unbelievable"*. I was aghast and through gritted teeth slowly snarled, "No fucking way." He sloped off sheepishly. The narcissistic, self-centred slimy bastard. My entire life had fallen apart, and this out-for-number-one scumbag tries to take advantage in the hope of a possible leg-over. FFS! It would be like me consoling a poor grief-stricken woman whose husband had just passed away. Then in the middle of the heart-to-heart talk, suddenly bursting out with, "He didn't have a snooker cue by any chance, did he?" Just not the done thing, is it? Well out of order! On second thoughts, maybe I should have supplied him with her details, so he could get a taste of being abused, cheated, used and lied to. However, I wouldn't wish that on my own worst enemy, never mind some irrelevant desperate piece of shite I was unfortunate enough to meet.

We woke up fully refreshed the next morning after a well-deserved comfortable deep sleep. We had a super-duper power shower before scoffing breakfast in the sunshine. Jo was happy and smiling. I had not heard even the faintest murmur from little Jo's lips with regards to his mum. He hadn't mentioned her from the time we had left her throwing a fit and everything else she could get her angry little mitts on, right up to the here and now. That was just "Yesterday", but now my trouble and strife seemed so far away.

Chirpy Chirpy Cheep Cheep

(October 2013)

We fastened our seatbelts for the one hour hop to the City of Angels. We took to the wild sky-blue yonder once again, rapidly putting space between us and that cruel fallen angel, the Wicked Witch. "Up in the Sky" I felt as free as a bird. The floaty clouds, the mighty mountain ranges, the majestic jungles, the tiny villages, the silver snaking rivers and the shiny green rice fields all left me breathless as the intrepid part of my mind was in seventh heaven. I took a moment to kiss the sky before being brought back down to earth as the aircraft suddenly plummeted from cloud nine to land at Don Muang Airport in northern Bangkok.

We caught a cab to the awe-inspiring We Train Guesthouse just a ten-minute drive away. I love this place to bits. It is a secluded oasis tucked away from the mad distractions of shops, cars, buses, motorbikes and swarms of busy programmed people. It is perfectly located on an enchanting, peaceful slice of greenery, with romantic trees encircling a fairy-tale lily-covered lake.

Its spotless, air-conditioned en-suite rooms are dirt-free and dirt-cheap. A coffee, tea or snack can be scored in the small café and they serve breakfast, lunch and dinner in the dining hall, with an abundance of vegan options too. There is a gym for the health fanatics and a whopping outdoor swimming pool for the "I'm Too Sexy for my Shirt" types. Wi-fi for your FFB and satellite TV for the buzz of live football, the excitement of a movie or the *Cartoon Network*, to keep the kids out of your hair for an hour or two.

On my first visit way back in the early nineties I relaxed beneath a large leafy tree on the edge of the charming lake as the sun rose in its leisurely way to traverse across the sky-blue heavens. An aura of spiritual vibrations flooded my heart as I sat at one with the universe. In this otherworldly atmosphere I focused on the ever-changing shades of red, orange and yellow sunshine reflected on the glasslike surface. My equanimity wasn't disturbed if a fish suddenly leapt out of the stillness before noisily splashing back in; I just observed the ripples as I continued diving deep into my soul. A dawn chorus of delightful birdsong added to the Nirvanaesque tranquillity. I felt omnipotent in this trancelike meditative state, fully believing that nothing external could disturb my calm inner peace of mind.

The sensation of having made significant progress along the sacred middle path was about to be put to the test. As I sat in this blissful state of rapture a massive monitor lizard, about five feet in length, casually walked up to me and gazed deep into my eyes. It was now my turn to leap, causing the lizard to jump, and twist in mid-air before scampering off as fast as lightning. A split second later it vanished underground in a hole near the guesthouse. Wow, that was a little bit frightening! My stunned mind later reflected that I still had a very long distance to travel before I reached the promised land of enlightenment.

A while later the receptionist opened my eyes to the fact that a lounge of monitor lizards lived wildly and freely on the grounds, but said I shouldn't be alarmed, because they were harmless and afraid of humans.

The collective name for a group of lizards is a lounge; I know that because I googled it. If you already knew without having to look it up, then go and take a running jump into the nearest lake, because nobody likes a smart arse!

I realise that I wax lyrical with respect to this locality, primarily on the grounds that when I lived and worked nearby it supplied a cherished refuge from the day-to-day chaos of life. It probably wouldn't be everyone's cup of tea due to its out-of-the-way location; there are no shops or facilities in the area and the staff don't speak English, either. Anyhow, it was perfect for an adventurous, clever-arsed, multi-lingual dreamboat like me.

In addition, all the proceeds go to supporting abused women and ex-prostitutes, and training them in new skills, such as hairdressing. This helping hand gives them a newfound independence, with prospects of employment; a fresh start in life. The staff are women who have made a new beginning. I love it; therefore, I get my goody-two-shoes God-given arse down there whenever I am visiting the City of Angels

***

That evening I sat on the balcony with Jo, observing hundreds of small geckos on the walls, pursuing and gobbling up mosquitoes. We were hypnotised by these fascinating reptiles as they raced for their next 'mossie' meal. In Thai this small lizard is known as 'jingjok'.

My chilled mind floated back to my early 'English as a Foreign Language' teaching days in an adult education centre in central Bangkok. I was an enthusiastic instructor and absolutely loved the job. I would meticulously plan the classes covering grammar and vocabulary, also utilising pair and group work activities to reinforce what had been taught. However, I would always end the lesson with 20 minutes of madness to "Pump up the Volume." This could be a song, a quiz, tongue twisters or even something obscure such as Cockney rhyming slang. More often than not it would be a game such as: hangman, charades or English Art where a student would draw a picture on the whiteboard and the other members of class would have to guess what it was in English The students eagerly awaited this part of the lesson, with each scholar actively involved, which created a lively, not to say raucous classroom. Their competitive nature meant that they were in it to win it!

On one memorable occasion it was the class versus the teacher at hangman. I created an 'on the edge of your seat' electric atmosphere as I announced, "This is the 1998 World Cup football final between England and Thailand". I could see they were well up for this. I accidentally on purpose ensured that the final score was 2-2 by the choice of words selected. The nail-biting excitement sky-rocketed as I professionally commentated, "We now enter extra time to see who the champions of the world will be; Thailand or England." I then put - - - - - - - on the whiteboard. It was squeaky-bum time! They were frantic as they tried to guess the word. They got some letters but failed as they were eventually hanged. I proudly smiled and loudly announced "England are world champions 1998." It was met with a chorus of deafening boos.

I then instructed, "Thank you students, see you tomorrow and don't forget to do your past perfect tense exercises for homework".

They screamed, "Mr Syd, what is the word?" I sheepishly smiled as I wrote JINGJOK on the whiteboard. As a mass they yelled, "Boo, referee, cheat, foul. It isn't even English." We all left the classroom in high spirits and smiling, as they knew it was all just fun.

The following day we finished off with the 2002 World Cup Final between Thailand and England. I looked distraught and crestfallen at the end of the game as I declared, "Thailand are world champions 2002," to a wildly cheering group of students. We left the classroom that day with my ecstatic class chanting, "Thailand, Thailand, Thailand," much to the confusion of other teachers and students!

My nostalgic dreamy reminiscences had to be put on hold as it was time to telephone the missus. She was friendly and calm and informed me that she had already collected the scooter and her 'root of all evil' stash of cash. I let her know that Jo and I were happy and alive and vowed to telephone tomorrow. I had to call my ex-bird daily because each time I heard her sing her "Chirpy Chirpy Cheep Cheep" tune, I breathed a sigh of relief, because I knew that she was still far, far away!

Well, I woke up the following morning and didn't see my ex-love wanting to torment me." I said, "Wow I'm "Really Free." Jo got out of the right side of bed and was in good spirits, with a splendid contented smile. It was tearfully amazing to witness his little face relaxed and joyous after all the cruel shit he had been through over the last year or so. At that very instant I made the split-second decision to make his face light up even more by declaring that today would be 'Jo Barnes Day'! His eyes opened wide with wonder. Love is the answer!

Once upon a time we grabbed a motorcycle taxi for a breezy dash through the maze of sunshine-lit back streets to the centre of Don Muang. To kickstart 'Jo Barnes Day' the name of the game was to fuel-up, to guarantee that we acquired a chock-a-block toybox amount of energy for this Brothers Grimm trip into childhood wonderland.

For starters, we stuffed our cakeholes with a super-colossal hodgepodge of mouth-watering goodies at our Hansel and Gretelc cottage café, with a vegan breakfast. I had to let my psychedelic imagination run wild to make Jo's day unforgettable. As I was gobbling up tasty morsels, I beamed with satisfaction that the wicked Cruella de Vil wasn't here to cast a dark spell by throwing a childish tantrum and putting the mockers on Jo's fairy-tale day.

"What shall we do next on our day of adventure?" I smiled at Jo.

"Play computer games," he responded.

I waved my invisible magic wand and in a strange mysterious wizardly voice proclaimed, "Whooooosh, your wish is my command." He whooped with glee.

We spent the morning side by side in a tiny internet shop entertaining ourselves with games. I got absorbed in deathly combat, sitting in a bunker mowing down rapidly advancing soldiers with a machine gun, blasting tanks to smithereens with a bazooka and blowing enemy planes to oblivion with missiles.

Somehow, it didn't sit quite right in my peace-loving spiritual hippy tree to be delighting in this online bloodbath. Therefore, I justified my menacing violence by fantasising that I was a courageous animal activist defending the voiceless from an evil army of flesh-eating monsters who wanted to hunt, scoff, experiment on and use the poor animals' furs and skins for clothing.

I was right in the zone now, with renewed energy slaughtering the bastards with a vengeance. The advancing carnivores stood no chance as I defended the innocent creatures who just wanted to live and be happy like me. It is all in the mind, my friend!

I sat breathless and victorious, with a massive Mancunian grin covering my mug, as the game came to an end. "Hey, it isn't half bad being a big kid after all," I chuckled. "Why the heck did I grow up? Fall head over heels in love, get married, and end up alone and broken-hearted so flipping soon? "I Don't Wanna Grow Up!"

"Jo, what would you like for lunch?" I continued.

"Pizza please, dad," he laughed. With a wave of the hand I said the magic word, "Abracadabra."

My one-track mind zipped back to times when I would try to mesmerise the fairer sex. Trust me! With a twinkle in my eye I would wave my magic wand and say the magic words, "Open Sesame." It always worked. I am laughing on the other side of my cocky gaunt face now, because in my grim skeletal state no pretty maiden on planet Earth would be seen dead with me!

Jo must have thought all his birthdays had come at once as he sat wide-eyed in Pizza Hut facing a margherita pizza, french fries, garlic bread and a large glass of coke. Not healthy, I know, but it was his day, remember. He was in heaven and so was I! After lunch we strolled leisurely around the outdoor market. I informed Jo that he could select any toy he desired. He opted for a set of plastic golf clubs and balls. Wow, from Steven Seagal to Tiger Woods. Today he can be anyone he wants in this make-believe land!

We zipped back to our guest house by motorbike for a round of golf on the grass adjacent to the lovely lake. I dug a small hole with a twig and we competed in the initial make-believe land golf tournament. Of course, Jo won; it was his day, don't forget! I presented him with a bag of gold coins I had secretly purchased earlier. He jumped for joy.

Next, I joined him on the slide and finally we went monitor lizard hunting. We managed to track down a couple of these shy creatures and shot them; with a camera, of course. I had always taught Jo that all life is sacred and that we should be compassionate to all living beings and never cause them any harm.

Before dinner we sat by the lake watching the fish. A delicious vegan dinner in the dining hall was scoffed prior to retiring upstairs for a well-earned rest. Half an hour was idled away watching the geckos before Jo ended his perfect day with an hour of *Cartoon Network*. Then I gave him a shower, cleaned his teeth, and tucked him in bed with a kiss and a hug. And last but not least, his favourite bedtime story: *The Three Little Pigs*. Lights out!

As I lay on my bed that night I thought, "I Don't Wanna Grow Up." I was happy but knackered. My body was reminding me that I was still critically ill. This trip to a childlike wonderland had done wonders for my mind but exhausted my feeble frame. It was a day of fun and laughter, totally free of anger and cruel mind games, which was a much-needed change. As my heavy eyelids began to droop, I vowed that I would never lose my teenage sight from this day on. "I Don't Wanna Grow Up."

I opened my teenage eyeballs to yet another bright and beautiful morning. After all, it was just "Another Day in Paradise." Jo begged to make me a tropical fruit juice. I had purchased a slow gear-masticating juicer when I arrived in Bangkok at the beginning of August. It had been put into daily use ever since. It was crucial that I persevered with my vigilant life-or-death fight against the Grim Reaper even when I was on the other side of the globe. I must admit that it had been a burden humping the heavy bugger around in my backpack.

I sliced the dragon fruit, jackfruit and lychees I had purchased yesterday at the market into small pieces and Jo eagerly pushed them into the machine, collecting the liquid in a plastic container. He then presented me with a large glass of delicious tropical fruit juice. "For you, dad," he smiled. I was deeply touched, and it wasn't easy gulping it with the massive lump in my throat. I wiped a tear out of my eye as I gazed out of the window at the lake. I even have a tear in my eye now as I am writing. Just a big bloody softie me, you know.

I pondered, "This must be his way of saying thank you for yesterday." Then I laughed as I mused, "Today must be 'Dad's Day'." Whoop and whoop again. Just the two of us now. A crippled old man fighting cancer and an innocent four-year-old child. We must look out for each other.

In fact, I thought, today should be Bomb's Day! Poor Bomb, losing her mother and her husband within a matter of weeks. Her grief and misery must be utterly devastating. At times a cruel twist of fate can shatter one's dreams mercilessly, leaving a person overwhelmed and on the edge. I can vouch for that and so can you! We have all been there, haven't we?

We would have to visit her to offer what comfort we could as well as say farewell, before we flew back to the safety zone. In my heart of hearts, I knew it was very unlikely that we would ever see each other again.

The harsh reality slapped me across the kisser. I was still at war with terminal cancer and the odds of survival were just like me; very slim. And now I had little Jo to consider too. It appeared that the Wicked Witch didn't want either of us, because we were a stumbling block to her lust for a single life. She had got the house, land, scooter, an overflowing wardrobe full of fashion, seen the world, and been taught English. We had served our purpose and had therefore been ruthlessly discarded. She was ready to take her next step up the ladder while I was clinging to the bottom rung, hanging on for dear life. My full attention had to be focused on Jo, Eugene and my fight for existence from now on.

I sat on the balcony overlooking the lovely lake as Jo was getting his morning fix of the *Cartoon Network*. I was deeply saddened by the fact that I wouldn't be seeing David's smiling face and listening to his off-the-wall drunken humour.

I was entranced once again by this magical lake as my mind floated back to my very first night out with David and Bomb, way back when. It was about 7pm when a half-pissed David steered his old BMW to an outdoor watering hole in the middle of nowhere. The venue was located on the edge of: you've guessed it; a small lake.

A sturdy wooden platform had been constructed over the dreamy water. The lantern-lit tables dished up an idyllic romantic night out under the moonlit heavens for the 'look at how the stars shine for us' lovers and the 'just one for the frog and toad' (road) pissheads too! Gazing at the stars in the night sky or the reflections of the tiny multi-coloured fairy lights in the jet-black water had an otherworldly hypnotic effect. A proper picture book location. I recall the noise of thousands of frogs croaking away in the darkness. Not to the *Beverley Hills Cop* theme song, thank goodness! The bar had a small stage with a smartly dressed middle-aged man playing an electronic keyboard. About half a dozen young girls dressed in elegant flowing costumes would take turns to sing pop and country tunes.

The waitress came over and beers were placed next to our flickering lantern. It was time to order food. David left me astonished when he slurred to the young girl, *Kaow Phat Moi* (pubic hair fried rice). His wife blushed as she admonished him with, "Stop being stupid, David." She ordered *Kaow Phat Gai* (chicken fried rice) for the two of them. I didn't try to go one better than David by ordering *Kaow Phat Kee Ma* (dog shit fried rice) because I don't think it is very big, clever or sensible to take the piss out of people who will serve up the food you will put in your mouth. You just might get what you asked for. I politely ordered *Kaow Phat Pad* (vegetable fried rice). The waitress thanked us and left. Did I just catch a wicked smile on her face out of the corner of my eye as she looked at David? And finally, *Kaow Phat*, pronounced Cow Pat in English, means fried rice in Thai, so in a way we were all eating shit. Lol.

Well, the ale flowed, and a boozy night of jokes and laughter was had. I did inspect my food carefully but didn't find any hairs or anything untoward, although it wasn't me taking the piss, was it? David was a lovely kind-hearted bloke who just enjoyed getting sloshed and having fun. He had a massive soft heart and would do anything for anyone and his compassion for stray animals proved the point. I do miss his quirky humour.

I looked at Jo and he was happily immersed in watching a *Horrid Henry* cartoon. I decided not to gaze into that bewitching lake any more, otherwise we would never fly to Manchester. Maybe this magical stretch of lily-covered liquid was under the control of the Wicked Witch in an evil attempt to keep us entrapped.

We visited Bomb in doggy heaven. She stated that she was fine, but the torture and disbelief were unmistakably evident in her grief-stricken eyes. She kindly made us a vegetarian lunch and I did my utmost to offer some form of comfort with my kind words. She suddenly advised, "Get back to the UK for a while and sort your life out, Syd."

What other alternative did I have? Zilch; absolute zero. To begin with I was still seriously ill and there was categorically no way I was fit enough to be able to cope with any form of employment. I was struggling just to walk, eat, sleep and take care of Jo. It was also imperative that I got back to the consultant at my hospital to check that my condition hadn't taken a turn for the worse. And my cash was starting to run low. It was time to get our arses back to Blackpool.

Yes, back to Eugene, who I was missing like mad. I phoned him every day and he was happy and doing well but it wasn't the same as living with his old man, for sure. And little Jo needed to get back to school too. So, it was back to my two-up two-down on Benefits Street in Blackpool. There was no other way. I was now a single dad and my kids needed me more than ever. I would not let this bastard cancer beat me; for their sakes. Jo's school and the benefits people had consented to the trip overseas in my straw-clutching attempt to solve the impossible. So, there'd be no red-tape shit to tie me up once home.

I sold my wedding ring at a gold shop for about £400. This was my way of facing the truth; the honeymoon was over, baby. My missus had been trying to get her greedy hands on my band of gold for the last six months, but I would never reveal where I had stashed 'my precious.' If you are reading this now, my ex-darling, it was hidden in the secret inside pocket of my red and grey Regatta 3-in-1 mountain coat.

Talking of the devil, I gave her a ring (lol) and let her know we were both safe and well. She complained that her money was running out. What a surprise! I told her that I had transferred £100 by Western Union and she could collect it in Vientiane. I didn't tell her that I had bought the plane tickets for the trip back to England. We would be flying high in the sky leaving our witch of trouble behind in just two days' time.

A wonderful time was enjoyed with my beautiful daughter Panvilas on the final day. This included a trip to the local registry office to switch her surname back to Barnes. It is a long-drawn-out tale but the long and short of it is that her mother had changed her surname years ago. It took a couple of hours, but she left the office with a happy smile as she had now returned to the Barnes clan. Welcome home!

I gave her a monster hug, expressing how much I loved her, vowing to keep in touch and promising to visit her after I had kicked the cancer into touch. She left with a big smile and waved bye-bye. I stood there with tears in my eyes because the truth was plain to see; I would never meet her again.

On the lucky-for-some 13th October we boarded the huge antiseptically-clean Norwegian Airlines "Silver Machine" for a ride to the other side of the sky. Oslo was the destination, where we would connect with a smaller aircraft for the short hop to Manchester. I clasped Jo's hand as I sat relieved but very heavy-hearted. It was always a downer flying out of tropical paradise to gloomy Northern England. At least I had the consolation of being free of the Wicked Witch's cruel claws.

Or so I thought!

The Leaving of Liverpool

(October to December 2013)

The steel Baby Bird touched down on the gunpowder-grey runway in soggy Manchester. "Oh, my God" I am thousands of miles away from home. My psychedelic head had long ago determined that wherever I lay my hippie hat, that was my home. My tit for tat (hat) had been comprehensively super-glued to the kaleidoscopic land of tropical sunshine in the Far East many equatorial moons back. Now the bloody cancer had exiled me to live out the rest of my days on the depressing drizzly coast of gloomy Blackpool. And the key to paradise had been chucked way out of reach.

"Don't let me be Misunderstood". I was eternally thankful for the National Health Service and the benefits system because without them I would have been stuck up shit creek without a blinking paddle. And let's not turn a 'snug as a bug in a rug' blind eye to the shocking truth that in far too many locations around the globe there is no safety net for the wretched and needy who are living in poverty. If you are sick and have no dosh; tough shit, you remain ill or bite the dust. If you are unemployed without a roof over your skull; hard-lines - you must beg or steal. It may well have been just "Aanother day in Paradise" for me during my travels but for many other poor sods, it was simply one more desperate day in hell.

Well, I'm a "Lucky Man," with my British citizenship entitling me and my two British children to be supported in our hour of need. Admittedly, stretches of my life have been spent living overseas but when employed in the UK I always coughed up my taxes and national insurance. My dear mum and dad paid their dues and both my grandfathers fought in the second world war. Therefore, I felt justified grabbing what I regarded as rightfully mine with both my feeble hands while I was helpless and at "Rock Bottom." I had no other option really, did I?

I pictured myself as a "Working-Class Hero" who had struggled to break out from a drab existence in northern England to snatch a taste of freedom and adventure in exotic locations. Although I have no doubt that the folks on the hill still viewed a scruffy council estate Mancunian scallywag like me as an effing peasant.

In my heart of hearts, the tropics was still my home. Perhaps I had spent a past life in lush wonderland and was eternally being drawn back.

However, I imagine that it was the razorblade-sharp contrast between shivering in a mind-numbing drudge in the gloomy cold and grey, compared to strolling on by in the colourful, live-for-today, sunshine lands of blue skies and warm seas that perpetually pulled me eastwards.

Yep, paradise wins hands down every single time. I visualised my hippie hat basking under a clear blue sky on a far-flung white sandy beach of a secluded tropical island awaiting my return. "When Will I see you Again". Some sunny day?

We jumped into a pre-ordered cab for the hour and twenty-minute drive back to bloody Blackpool. The very second we reached our home from home, we ditched the heavy backpack and collected Eugene and his possessions from his Buddhist shelter with our ever-faithful red Fiat Punto. He was as right as Blackpool rain and overjoyed to see us. He dashed straight up to his room and there he would make camp, unless he fancied a bite to eat or required dad's taxi to run him about. Typical teenager! It was comforting to be with him again.

***

Life was a different kettle of fish now. I was an awfully unwell man; just me, myself and my shadow battling tooth and nail with my lethal enemy, the death-dealing Grim Reaper. The mega-strict iron-fisted dictatorship of herbs, supplements and organic fruit and vegetable juices was religiously obeyed. Sugar, animal products and processed food were taboo. It was imperative that I put in a lock, stock and barrel endeavour to guarantee that my immune system had the bullets to at least give me a fighting chance of outgunning this pernicious disease, for my children's sakes.

As well as fighting to rebuild and rejuvenate my damaged body, I zealously devoted all my remaining strength and power to the wellbeing of Eugene and Jo, who right here, right now were entirely dependent upon me. My paternal instinct was fully wired. I was ready and willing to destroy anyone or anything that threatened my children's welfare and future happiness. You better prick up your lugholes, Mr Big C!

Mornings in our nuthouse by the sea were a frantic hour-long high tide of outright madness. "Eugene, Jo; wakey, wakey, rise and shine, it is time for school," I would holler. This was greeted with not even a fly-speck of activity. They were still miles away in the land of nod. I had to rouse sleepyhead Jo in the shower, brush his teeth, get him dressed, then dish up breakfast prior to chauffeuring him and Eugene to their schools.

The remainder of the day would be used up cleaning the dishes, washing clothes, making the beds and dealing with the never-ending housework before collecting Jo at 3pm. Eugene would cook dinner for himself and Jo, which was a godsend. Later, Jo would reluctantly get stuck into his homework, so he could grab his reward of a spell of computer games prior to a bedtime story and lights out.

At long last my ready-to-drop-dead carcass would flee the bleak real world and hide as a lonesome single man under the double duvet of the double bed. I felt washed-out as I drowned in hopeless despair. My life was a nightmare I had each and every day.

Jo proudly returned home from his first day back at school flamboyantly scoffing a lump of bread he had baked. Eugene was in his final GCSE year. Exams in June. He got stuck into computer games and dodged the troublesome homework. That's my boy!

At the weekends, the kids were yanked off computer games to swing, slide and twirl in playgrounds. From time to time, we took a nippy bracing saunter along the local beach flinging pebbles into the cold, battleship-grey Irish Sea. Of course, we had to feed the eternally hungry ducks at the local lake too.

The dreaded superstore visits for the weekly groceries had to be undertaken and I flipping hate shopping. Jo's mouth would be watering at the displays of doughnuts, sweets, fizzy drinks, chocolate and biscuits, as he was led into temptation whichever way he turned. Even worse, Eugene would feast his eyeballs on eggs, pork, chicken and beef, much to my horror. I made sure that we had mountains of fruit and vegetables to go with the shite the kids demanded. Eugene was not the tiniest bit interested in joining me on a healthy vegan diet, but I was making steady progress with Jo.

Jo resumed his swimming lessons for thirty minutes each week at the local pool. I had been taking him since January and he was slowly improving. He couldn't swim but at least he could put his head under water at long last. His mother had never joined us because she wouldn't be seen dead with her ghoulish husband. Poor Jo, not having his mother to observe and cheer his achievements at the pool was heart-breaking. And poor me too!

On top of the endless housework, the lonesomeness of this solitary confinement was starting to do my head in. I felt like a lonely Freddie Mercury as I vacuumed the carpert and sang, "I Want to Break Free." I wasn't wearing a pink tank top and a black satin mini-skirt though. Maybe next time; anything to brighten this grey miserable life up. And

Freddie was right when he sang about how shit it was, "Living on my Own." I really was down in the dumps; in need of a little friendship and a spot of adult company.

Slaving over a hot stove ad infinitum and wrestling with the daily chores ad nauseum was making me sick. I had never had to do it before coz my mum, girlfriends and wives had always performed those easy tasks while I did some real work to bring home the vegan bacon! Well, "Instant Karma" bit me on my cheeky backside, coz now it was my turn to discover what a thankless soul-destroying job housework was. Although the Wicked Witch had had it easy coz she always had maids to cook, clean, babysit and do the shopping while she brushed her hair and painted her fingernails.

I was a colourful tropical songbird singing sad songs of freedom to my sorrowful caged self. Dreaming of escape and spreading my wings as I flew back to the land of lush green trees, exotic fruit and clear blue skies. My dreamy head was always floating in tropical clouds above idyllic islands reliving past adventures hand in hand with my so-called perfect partner. "Where did you go to my Lovely?". It certainly wasn't easy-peasy, living on my blinking own.

Thus, out of desperation to flee the dreary lonely hours of a dull day, I subscribed to an online rambling club. You could chat to like-minded enthusiasts and sign up to participate in hikes that the members regularly arranged. The fact that I could barely stumble 100 metres, never mind scramble up a hill, didn't deter my intrepid spirit. I chatted to a few walkers online, which relieved the aloneness just a dab.

The endoscopy at Victoria hospital was a doddle. I was becoming accustomed to the eye-watering tube shoved up my nostril and down my throat. I didn't flinch but was relieved when it was done and dusted. I was double-relieved when the oncologist informed me that there was still no sign of the cancer. Blinking heck; I was a walking miracle! I mustn't get all gung-ho though because I wasn't out of the brown and nasty just yet. It was vital not to get complacent. I had to continue with my healthy lifestyle, ensuring that my body and immune system were strong enough to thwart the cancer in its attempt at making an unwelcome return.

On 18th October, it was Eugene's 16th Birthday. We scored him a large cake and sang "Happy Birthday." Wow, how time flies. It seemed just like yesterday when I was singing Happy Birthday to him in a pub in Cheng Du, China. He was 3 years old then. Thirteen years gone in the blink of an eye.

***

I had been chatting to a woman from near Liverpool on the walking site. I was my usual cheeky/flirty northern monkey self and we had a good laugh. She loved doing cryptic crosswords and I would send her a clue every morning. Here are five of my favourites for you to have a bash at; answers at the end of the chapter.

Gegs (9,4)

HIJKLMNO (5)

Take notice of aural sex. (5,2,4,4)

O (8,6)

(3,3,3,1,4)

They are rather tricky and before you ask, the final clue intentionally has just the number of letters in each word. If you can get any of them give yourself a pat on the back because you are as Radio Rental (mental) as Psycho Syd. However, don't drive yourself nuts and get your Primark knickers in a twist coz you can always cheat and have a sly peep at the answers, can't you?

Now, my madcap mind wasn't half bad at filling in cryptic crossword puzzles. After a while I found it a doddle to finish *The Daily Telegraph* puzzle so moved up to the daddy of broadsheet crossie puzzles; *The Times*. I usually managed to finish between half and threequarters of this mind-boggling puzzle and I even completed it once, but it took three flipping days. I recollect an amusing incident back in the early eighties when I was stood in a queue at a corner chippy. I was with two mates waiting to order my chips, cheese and onion pie and mushy peas.

We were all a bit worse for wear after guzzling a few pints of beer. As per usual I was dressed like a bloody tramp in ripped jeans and a tatty old coat. While we were stood in line, I noticed a man in a suit with *The Daily Telegraph* newspaper in his pocket. I slurred to my mates, "Look, *The Telegraph*, I sometimes do the crossword."

The smart middle-aged man turned around and laughed, "More like *The Sun*." His two smartly dressed friends laughed too!

Well, the gauntlet had been thrown down, so I shot back, "Have you finished it?"

He was taken aback by my flippancy and pulled the paper out of his pocket and bragged, "Almost half done, this is a cryptic crossword and it takes time. Not simple straight-forward clues. A lot of brain-work I'll have you know."

I nodded smugly before suggesting that if he handed me the paper, I would finish it off while we waited for our chip suppers. He looked flabbergasted and laughed out loud as he passed me the paper and a biro. Everyone in the queue smiled as their eyes focused on the drunken fool, waiting for the moment I fell flat on my drunken council-estate mush. I soon wiped the smirks off their faces after completing the unfinished half in less than five minutes before handing it back to the open-mouthed well-dressed man. He couldn't believe it and apologised for his ignorance in judging me by my appearance. We shook hands and he left with his friends.

As we walked back, eating our food out of plastic trays, one of my mates said, "For fuck's sake Syd, how the hell did you do that?"

I swallowed a mouthful of the pie and chips and grinned. "I'll let you into a little secret. I did that crossword this morning, so I knew all the answers already, but I wasn't going to tell that effing smarty-pants that, was I?"

They laughed out loud and said, "You are a blinking legend mate. I bet that bloke in the chippy is still confused. He will be telling his mates about the time he met a scruffy nobody who completed half a cryptic crossword in less than five minutes." Our drunken laughter continued as us 'mad for it' Mancs made our way through a posh private estate of large detached houses to our tiny council estate of terraced two-up two-downs

Well, the last thing on my normally one-tracked mind was a romantic date for starters, a bit of slap and tickle for the main course, followed by a peck on the cheek and goodbye for dessert. However, I was buzzing at the prospect of having a bit of banter and a laugh with this scouse crossword fanatic. Although, I had not got a clue whether I would pluck up the courage to meet her in the flesh.

I eventually grew a pair of spherics and boldly agreed to come together with this "Long-Haired Lover From Liverpool" for a pub lunch and a short and sweet saunter along the beach. I was only too aware that "The female of the species is more deadly than the male" but the reckless daredevil in me provided the spunky bravado to escape my four walls and make contact with this potential black widow.

We arranged to rub eyeballs one Saturday afternoon after Eugene had kindly volunteered to take care of Jo. I looked almost presentable in my faded black jeans, black tee-shirt, trainers and olive-green army jacket. I didn't have a bunch of flowers, a packet of ribbed condoms or a victory V (Viagra), because love and lust were the last things on my broken-hearted mind. I had no time for any monkey business. I was still yelping from the Wicked One's abuse, so no fair maiden was permitted anywhere near my heart or any other bits of my anatomy, thank you very much. "I Should be so Lucky". Although you never know; some girls might have a fetish for death-warmed-up monsters!

My bag of bones wasn't a bag of nerves as I cruised to the Wirral near Liverpool for this mysterious rendezvous. I sang along to tunes by Merseyside bands such as: The La's, Echo and the Bunnymen, the Zutons and the Teardrop Explodes. I was a cool beatnik full of pep as I drove up to the meeting place to eyeball my blind date. Bet she will be wishing she was blind once she takes just one peep at my unsightly look of death, I thought.

When we laid eyes on each other it was instant attraction; love and lust at first ogle. The chemistry was pure Goldilocks; just right! Time to experiment! Well, the red horny devil smiled in triumph at the conquered white celibate angel. Shit, I should have brought the flowers and condoms after all. We held hands and ambled to her small terraced house just five minutes away for a cup of coffee and a cigarette. "Are Friends Electric?"

While I was sipping the caffeine and inhaling the nicotine, my lusty libido was burning with the hots! "The Heat is On".and my "Sex is on Fire" I gazed into her smoky eyes and speculated, "Will she or won't she? Would she or wouldn't she? May she or might she"? I didn't have long to ponder because her "Lips Like Sugar" soon pressed against my eager mouth. She clutched my hot-blooded hand and escorted me upstairs as my craving eyes were focused on her sexy derrière in skin-tight blue jeans. Wow, "There She Goes"! I licked my sugar-coated northern monkey lips as I eagerly followed, ready and willing to accept my "Reward" I am not going into the full graphic details to supply you all the 'ins and outs' of this passionate encounter but I am sure you can close your eyes and imagine. No naughty self-pleasing though, coz you have this book to finish.

"To Cut a Long Story Short", we entered her clean cosy boudoir and made passionate lust for 30 minutes. Afterwards she gazed into my sleepy eyes and smiled softly, adding, "That was amazing Syd."

I winked cockily and bragged, "Believe it or not, I am even better the second time around."

Her eyes widened with hero worship as she gleefully squealed, "Really?"

I grinned and replied, "Yes but I need a 20-minute nap first and while I am having 40 winks you must hold onto my naughty bits and never let go. Is that OK?"

She seemed puzzled but happily agreed. After the short snooze, I was revived and up for the repeat performance to conclude the double-whammy. When the encore came to an end, she purred, "That was magnificent. Even better than the first time. One thing confuses me though; why did you ask me to hold your private parts while you were sleeping?"

I smiled as I informed her, "Oh, that is because the last time I slept with a Liverpool girl she stole my wallet."

Hahaha. I bet I had you going, there, didn't I? It is just one of my off-the-wall jokes. I apologise for being a naughty fibber. Merely my warped sense of humour. I blame it on the chemotherapy. I better let the pussy out of the bag and give you the low-down on what really took place that cloudy day in Merseyside before you fling the book in the rubbish bin.

This is the honest to God's truth. Cross my heart and hope to die. I parked my car and saw her standing there. Shock, shock, horror, horror, shock, shock. What in tarnation? I wasn't expecting movie stars and swimming pools, but she was a dead ringer for Grandma out of *The Beverley Hillbillies*. But really, no more fooling around, she was younger than me and just a normal slender woman in her forties. The naked truth was that my *Peter Pan* lifestyle in south-east Asia, being eternally surrounded by beautiful young Tinkerbells and Wendy Darlings (not kids but girls in their late 20s and early 30s), had distorted reality. Welcome back to the real-world, Psycho Syd.

Viewing the event from her perspective, her grey matter must have screamed, "Good Lord! It is *The Visitor From the Grave* straight out of *Tales from the Crypt!* In any case, love and lust weren't on my list of tasks to accomplish today and I was certain that they weren't on hers either. I was here to escape the daily grind!

We popped into a local pub and plopped our bums down on a wooden bench in the empty beer garden as we regurgitated tales of heartbreak, betrayal and loss, blow by blow. Her ex was a cheating pisshead and mine was a cheating fucking bitch as you already know. I slurped a vegan soup as she masticated on a hot dog. A short while later we dilly-dallied along the beach, chirping away like two broken-hearted lovebirds. We gulped breaths of fresh and healthy salty sea air between the drags of filthy, unhealthy tar and nicotine.

We then diddle-daddled to her humble abode and dawdled in her backyard, choking on cancer sticks as we nattered away. Out of the sky-blue her mouth ejaculated, "Syd, one thing I do miss is sex." My jolted eyeballs almost jumped out of their sockets and I nearly shat myself too! I simply nodded and responded, "Me too." Could it be that this liver bird had kinkiness about "Scary Monsters," my unscrewed head sweated? I was scared stiff! Be that as it may, I was not up for a portion of "Monster Mash" in this black widow's boudoir. Under the circumstances, I made my excuses in a shot and got my busy blue-arse fly's body out of her web and flew to the safety of my car with my tail between my legs. Thank goodness, the wheels were still on my car; well, Liverpool does have a reputation you know. I put the pedal to the metal and burnt rubber back to my four walls.

On reflection, a satisfying time was had, and it was gratifyingly enjoyable partaking in a spot of friendly chit-chat with this lovely lady. In all fairness, her unforeseen jaw-dropping remark regarding sex may well have been just that; a comment and not a flirtatious nudge for me to drop my ball-hugging black jeans for a period of "Wham Bam Thank You Mam." Perhaps my once-bitten twice-shy state of mind is making me paranoid!

Three weeks later a letter arrived regarding that day in Mickey Mouse (Scouse) land. It wasn't a love letter but a document putting me in the picture that a speed camera had snapped me driving over the speed limit in Liverpool. I had my naughty arse smacked as karma whipped up a bored-shitless day at a speed awareness course.

Answers to Crossword Clues

1. scrambled eggs
2. water
3. prick up your ears
4. circular letter
5. has not got a clue

Lucky Man

(October to December 2013)

Welcome back to the grim reality of life as a "Solitary Man" and the Groundhog days of unrelenting mind-numbing housework. I once had my dream girl but suddenly I was all alone in a nightmare with no one to call my own. I was a broken "Lonely Man."

On 28th October I took my miserable self to the lonely blustery beach and gazed at the chilly Irish Sea through waterlogged eyes. I was standing all on my own again. It most certainly wasn't a "Wonderful life". My thoughts were 24-carat black and my "Heart of Gold" was shattered into "Bits and Pieces" I was weak, sickly, was rapidly losing weight and had severe diarrhoea too. I was shitting myself in case the dreaded cancer had returned.

I was growing feebler and sicker by the hour. I blotted out my alarm from the kids with a loving smile before and after the school run. Throughout the day, I toiled to keep on top of the housework. I was at my wit's end, convinced that the terminal disease had returned. My frail body was a puny blob of soreness, not aided by the nonstop trotting upstairs screaming, "Shit, not again." Very scary times indeed.

There were still occasional phone calls with the Wicked Witch, just sorting things out. There was no love lost as she delighted in painting bright pictures of her brand-new happy lifestyle. It did me no good to talk with her; it just prolonged the hurt. From my perspective, I was helpless and snowed under in despair, after the unanticipated avalanche of new nightmares had knocked me arse over tit, burying me in pain and sorrow. This sudden onset of illness had taken me right down again.

Piteous I know, but the tears of this broken-hearted clown stung with the realisation that death was just around the corner, coz the dreaded Mr Big C was back. I was so needy of a bit of tenderness and a few words of love and support. Deep down in my shattered heart I understood that the Wicked One would never supply a shoulder to cry on because she just wanted me to die.

If my foggy chemo brain recalls correctly, it was Halloween when I blabbed that I was terribly unwell, had the shits and was losing weight rapidly. I held the phone waiting for the whooping and cheering before the evil scream of, "Yippee, hurry up and die." I was left astonished when she burst into tears and began sobbing uncontrollably. She blubbered, "I want to come back and take care of you." That was the first time in about a year that she had shown any compassionate warm-heartedness towards me. I was startled, and the floodgates opened as my salty tears saturated my cheeks before splashing onto the brown carpet between my trembling feet. My choked-up voice stuttered, "I w-w-will c-c-call y-you tom-m-morrow."

It can't be true; I just froze. What should I do? Could she be sincere, and would I get some love before I died?

I didn't get a wink of sleep that brainstorming night as my perplexed tree unceasingly played 'she loves me, she loves me not' over and over. I was "Dancing With Tears in my Eyes" as my heart jumped for joy, proclaiming that her sobbing was out of love and compassion. A moment later, there were "Tears on my Pillow" as my head warned, *Don't believe her, she is shedding big fat crocodile droplets.* I was really tempted to agree to her request because I was so desperate for some love and support. On the other hand, after the hell she had dragged me and Jo through, my gut reaction was, "No bloody way."

The next day my bleary eyes and frazzled mind eventually crashed on the sofa downstairs for some much-needed zeds. I was jolted out of my deep slumber by the phone. My missus tearfully wept, "I need to know that you are ok and I want to return to take care of you and Jo." Heavens above, this was the loving tongue of the girl I once knew and yearned for. I pinched my half-asleep self to make sure it wasn't a dream. I rubbed my sleepy eyes and contemplated; she sounded wholeheartedly genuine, but I was also deeply suspicious and who could blame me. She loves me. She loves me not.

I interrogated, "You're not itching to return because you are pining for your boyfriend, are you?"

"No, I am not interested in him at all, "I Only Want to be With You" and Jo," she emphasised.

I roused my drowsy visage with a damp face-cloth before gravely notifying her: "It will take everything I have to get you back here. I will have to bear the cost of the flights and the visa as well as transferring enough money for you to live on while your return is being arranged."

I continued in earnest, "The only money I have left to use is the last of the cash my mum left me after she died. So, "I'm Begging You" not to make this request unless you are telling the truth."

She pleaded, "Please take me back. I need to be with you and promise to be nice and take care of you and the children. So, don't worry

Syd, I will be good."

I finally believed her, so I agreed, "Ok, I will fly you back."

She replied, "Thank you so much."

***

My heart and soul were bewitched once again. I was in a state of blissful intoxication, counting down the days to this loving reunion. Holding hands, soft kisses, comforting hugs and kind words of support would be mine, all mine, in just a few dreamy weeks.

I was dying for some affection before I ultimately kicked the bucket and broke on through to the other side. I elbowed the niggling doubt that it was all a pack of beastly lies right to the very back of my cranium. I floated on cloud nine with a peaceful smile on my face, oblivious to any possibility of an unfavourable outcome. Because if this was yet another spiteful sleight of hand trick of hers, then I would just curl up and die. I was in dreamland as I sang, "Oh, what a "Lucky Man" I am."

As I scrawl this, I really can't believe that I agreed to it and you are probably ripping your hair out in utter frustration. You must be raging, "The bloody idiot; if he flies her back, he deserves everything he gets." But hold onto your top hats, cloth caps and pretty bonnets for a moment and grab a view of things from my beanie-covered head. I was extremely poorly, just skin and bones, convinced the cancer had returned. I should have been in bed fighting this hideous illness instead of struggling with the housework and taking care of my kids. Plus, the dreadful fear of what would happen to my children if I was suddenly whisked off to hospital, was constantly stabbing my mind. So, in all fairness I had no option but to take an almighty risk and pray to the supreme being above that she wasn't speaking with forked tongue.

I started to feel a little better but made an emergency appointment to visit my oncologist, who informed me there was still no sign of the cancer. Yippee. Maybe it was just the stress of being alone and swamped with housework that made me sick! It looked like I would still be alive to enjoy the family Christmas in a few weeks' time.

The month of November continued just like October, being taken up with the day-to-day running of the house and looking after my kids. With a difference though, because this time there was a spring in my step. I sang and danced to heaps of *Madchester* tunes as I mopped the floor, cleaned the plates or hung up the washing. I was full of vegan beans and felt like I was gonna "Live Forever." I was completely mesmerised wearing my rose-coloured specs, dreaming of the "One love" I would be getting very soon.

Obtaining a United Kingdom visa for my ex-devil was not a piece of angel cake though. She was unemployed, and I was disabled. However, it would go in her favour that she had previously visited the UK. And it was advantageous that she owned land and property in Laos: the blinking house I had sweated for years to buy that she had kicked me and Jo out of a few wicked times. With that thought in mind, I looked to the universe and voiced, "I'm Begging You" that my "Wonderwall" wife won't turn out to be "Fool's Gold", otherwise I will be crying my heart out with a "Waterfall" of tears." I put this daft song-title wordplay madness down to the chemo too!

I concluded that the best plan of action would be to apply for a Visitor's Visa, so she could stay with her husband and son over the Christmas and New Year period. If the application was a success we would once again be playing happy families before needing to apply for an Exceptional Circumstances Visa, so that she could remain with her sick husband once her Visitor's Visa had expired.

I provided her with as much documentation as humanly possible to support her application. Firstly, I wrote a letter explaining why it was important that we were together for Christmas. Next, I included a report from my psychiatrist stating that it would be a tremendous boost for my mental wellbeing to be reunited with my wife over the festive season. There was an offer of employment upon my recovery from a school in Laos. This was to emphasise that our intention was to resume our life in Vientiane, highlighting that she wasn't scheming to remain in the UK once she got her twinkle toes on British soil. Documents from the hospital as evidence of the seriousness of my medical condition were enclosed. And last, but not least, a copy of my bank statement as proof that I possessed enough funds to support her visit. My loyal friend Janet had kind-heartedly lent me the sum of £800 to make the statement appear a bit healthier. I splashed the cash for the application and booked her an appointment at the British consulate in Vientiane. It was now in the hands of the gods. All I could do was pray, fret and pace the shit-coloured carpet in the living room.

My friends and family were unsurprisingly extremely uneasy with regards to the rash resolution to allow my lovebird to fly back. Janet cautioned, "I am happy to loan you the money but don't agree with your decision because I have a sneaking suspicion, she will be just her same evil self. A leopard doesn't change its spots."

Ann, my sister-in-law warned: "It is up to you but be very careful because I don't think you would be able to cope this time if it all went wrong."

We spoke and skyped daily. She was just like her old young self, with words of love, support and kindness. I smiled self-assuredly as I satisfyingly mused, "You made the right decision, Syd."

The Gods had heard my desperate pleas and her visa was granted. I was now floating in heaven too. I was such a lucky man, yes, I was.

In an omnipotent flash the return tickets were booked; Turkish Airlines - Bangkok to Manchester. In just one week's time I would be standing hand in hand with my beautiful wife. *'Til death us do part*, she would be by my side as I fought this bastard cancer. Her silky touch and tender voice would make the loneliness vanish into thin air. Subsequently, I secured flights from Udorn Thani (an hour across the border) to Bangkok. I had also been transferring cash to her every week since I agreed to her return, so she had enough wonga to live on. It was money well spent because now I was safe and secure, alive in her heart. I broke the good news that the travel was sorted, and she warmly thanked me.

During the days leading up to her departure there was an unmistakable U-turn in her attitude. The warmth in her voice had noticeably cooled; she seemed distant and off-hand. Suddenly, her computer was on the blink meaning no skype sessions, and her mobile battery was malfunctioning, so phone calls were limited too. Mission control, we have a problem. I was spaced out with apprehension and began having second thoughts about my chop-chop decision to give the nod to her undoubtedly sincere, heart-wrenching pleas. But it was a bit like closing the stable door after the horse had bolted because she possessed the visa and tickets already. Or was I just being paranoid?

An additional occurrence stoked up the sneaking suspicions bouncing around my brainbox. A close pal of mine sent a text message spilling the beans that he had just caught a glimpse of my missus in the pub. It was entirely up to her, of course, and I had absolutely no issue with that until I telephoned her and inquired, "Where are you?"

She sweetly replied, "At home."

I responded, "Bullshit, a friend of mine has just seen you in the Samlo Pub."

Initially, she was incensed at being caught red-handed before explaining, "I just wanted to see my friends before I return to England." Fully understandable, but why the slimy deceit?

Another incident which banged niggling doubts into my mind was the time I proposed to switch her flight to Bangkok from Udorn Thani, to depart from Vientiane. This would save her the inconvenience of having to cross the Thai border. She put her angry foot down and refused point-blank. "No way, I have arranged everything already," she insisted. "My brother will drive me," she said.

I retorted, "How can your brother possibly take you when he only has a police car, which won't be permitted to cross the border?"

She hit the flaming roof and screamed, "Don't worry, he will find a way."

Something smelled very fishy. So, I quizzed, "You haven't found a boyfriend in Laos, have you?"

Her tone of voice softened as she responded so sweetly and convincingly, "Don't be silly, I only have you." This left me feeling secure and reassured once more. Could it possibly be that I was way out of order for not trusting her and was just behaving like a sad green-eyed monster? Nonetheless, with all the mucky stains on her blemished track record, no one could point a finger at me for having doubts?

***

On 4th December, I toddled off to delight in watching Jo play a shepherd in the school nativity play. It was a pity his mum wasn't here to share this festive event but at least she would be there full of joy and good tidings for Christmas. And his 5th birthday next week, too.

On the morning she was due to fly she phoned to say she was on her way. She notified me that she would switch her phone off but send me a text from Bangkok. A friend of hers phoned and informed me that a woman who purchased garments in Thailand to sell in Laos was giving her a lift. What the hell happened to her brother?

I was getting frostbitten feet and had a shuddersome feeling of impending doom. The writing was on the wall. I sent her a message stating: "Something isn't right, don't bother coming."

Her reply was a selfie and a text from Bangkok airport "See you soon." Would she still love me tomorrow?"

I had a fretful sleepless night before driving to Manchester airport. I parked my car in the ultra-expensive car park before awaiting the arrival of my loved one.

I was a very unlucky man this red-letter day of reunification because there was a seven-hour delay, due to a sodding problem with air traffic control. Just my luck! This was going to cost me an arm and a leg at the car park, but it would be the best dosh ever flung away, I figured, when I was eventually hand in hand with my wife once more. My mind flipped back to the time when she arrived in April 2012 with hugs, love and kisses. Calm down, Syd. Only six more hours to go.

I beamed with joy as I observed reunited couples laughing, hugging and kissing when they met after a time apart. Their faces were illuminated with pure magical love. I was delighted for them, without even a speck of envy, because my bewitched mind knew it would be my turn very soon.

And then I saw her. I raced over to her with a love-struck smile as my lovelight dazzled all in the arrivals area. I opened my arms and cried, "Welcome home." She stared at me, looked at the ground and marched straight past me.

To say I was devastated was a massive understatement. I wasn't just crushed; I was pulverised. The world stood still as I stood there "Alone Again, Naturally." I whispered to the floor, "Please swallow me up."

My heart sank, and my mind screamed, "Oh no, what the fuck have I done?"

I'm a stupid gullible man, yes, I am!

Wicked Game

(December 2013)

I froze in silent self-loathing for falling hook, line and sinker and grabbing with both eager hands, the tempting bait the Evil One had so sweetly presented before my love-struck eyeballs. She had knocked me out cold with a sly underhand sucker-punch. When I arrived home, I would send my bank details to Barrister Thomas Carruthers in Nigeria in reply to his email kindly offering to transfer $8,000,000 into my account. He wouldn't be a happy-chappy though, because the con-woman extraordinaire had already scammed everything I bloody had.

I was wishing I was sitting in the departure lounge with a single ticket to Timbuktu, Mogadishu or even the moon, clenched securely in my sweaty mitts. I longed to get my Mancunian arse far away as my gullible tree shuddered at the significance of the dangerous dumb blunder I had committed. Sadly, I couldn't do a runner from the scene of her crime, because my children needed me more than ever, now that the Wicked Witch had returned. I finished kicking the shit out of myself before my chilled-to-the-bone mind and body trailed through the crowded lonely airport after the black-hearted one to the car park.

As I gave my sleeping beauty a ride back to Blackpool, I was in a fury with myself for allowing the sneaky one to take me for the biggest ride of my life. I glanced at her snoozing away in the passenger seat and thought, now was not the time to put her through the mangle and give her the third degree; better to let sleeping dogs LIE.

Was it feasible that her aloof polar mood was down to being jet-lagged and exhausted after 12 hours of flying and a seven-hour wait in Istanbul airport? Utter bollocks! "Anyone who had a Heart" would have greeted a missed loved one with a smile, hug and a kiss, however knackered they were. Well, this northern arctic monkey wasn't feeling any romantic warmth. So, stop spouting mumbo jumbo, Syd, and open your bloody bewitched eyes! Once home I was out like a light.

I slept like a log but didn't wake up in the fireplace. I was aroused from my slumber on the sofa with my partner making love to me. She was happy, friendly and full of smiles. I thought I had lost my love, but maybe she did love me after all! No wonder my mind was messed up.

Later that evening, I spotted her using my laptop to chat to a man on her FFB page. I quizzed, "Who is that?"

"Just a friend," She smiled innocently.

For some reason, I had a gut reaction that my dirty rat was not coming clean. Probably, it was the way she had begun to manoeuvre the screen beyond range of my curious eagle eyes. Plus, the fact, that she evaded my questioning peepers. You can't hide your "Lyin Eyes" It did not add up. Something was not kosher.

When my Black Widow at long last crawled off, dragging her drowsy eyeballs to slumber land, it was zero hour for my sleepy head to unravel the web of venomous lies she had been spinning. I prayed with to the Lord above that I was wrong but deep down I knew that my devilish darling had forsaken me once more. At high midnight, I morphed into a hush-hush "Secret Agent Man" once again, in readiness to do my duty and muckrake this filthy case. Time to get to the shitty bottom of yet another dirty whodunit using the undercover spyware tool which I had installed on my computer when her betrayal began many months back.

The moment of truth was realised before you could hiss, "You sly slimy sleazy slutty scumbag." And this ace master sleuth was knocked senseless by the poisonous double-dealings detected. I unearthed that a Hungarian bloke and my wife had been swapping shit loads of mushy messages of love as well as arranging to meet up on umpteen occasions. There were also sickening photographs of the slushy couple attending events together!

My clandestine assignment cracking this mucky enigma had left me disembowelled; powerless and having to stomach the caustic certainty that I had beyond any stinking shadow of a doubt been comprehensively shat on. By putting one and one together I had fathomed the belly-knotting solution to this putrid mystery and the nauseating answer was him and her! My psychedelic life immediately flashed before my shaken and stirred eyes.

I got the picture in my broken heart of hearts that she had been 'at it' with this bloke, as visions of their sexual activities sliced up my mind. I would be pissing in the stormy wind if I challenged her eyeball to eyeball demanding answers, coz she would sweetly cop-out by lying through her teeth. There was no alternative but to elicit the distasteful front-page news straight from the Hungarian horse's gob.

I dived into the distressing burden of gathering intelligence by anxiously scrutinising each message sent back and forth between the darling love vultures. Were they impatiently circling above, flying in wait for me to collapse and pop my Lancashire clogs? That morbid vision sent spooky shivers down my spine.

Sending him a message from her FFB page was a non-starter coz my 'up to no good' missus would spot it in the morning and forewarn the hungry-for-love-n'-lust geezer to keep his goulash gob shut and say nowt. If I forwarded one from my FB page, he would probably not respond and alert his wicked partner in crime. Persuading the Hungarian to yakkety-yak and make a clean breast of things by ratting on his fellow rodent was going to be far easier said than done.

I painstakingly hunted for the tell-tale clue that would reveal the blueprint for my rat-trap. Eureka! At long last I dug up his mobile number from the painful piles of syrupy texts to my two-timing hurtful arsehole of a wife. My one and only shot at accomplishing a bitter sweet victory would be to make an exceedingly awkward phone call. I would have to be on tip-top form to trap him into revealing the naked truth and expose the double-crossing Wicked Witch. I was up for it though, because risky business is part and parcel of being a "Secret Agent Man."

I wasn't on the warpath with him because he didn't know me from Adam. On the other raging hand, if it had been one of my so-called close pals who had been yapping with forked tongue while shagging my missus behind my stabbed back, I would have lost it and turned murderously berserk. The comfortably-sitting bullshitting bastard would not be sitting pretty very soon coz just one look at my manic Manc psychotic grin would have had him smiling on the other side of his two-faced mush.

Firstly, there'd be an impromptu war-dance, wailing "Wig-Wam-Bam" around the coffee table at home as my cries of whoop whoop, whoop ricocheted off the four walls. Then, I'd be flying back and arrowing in on the running bare-faced liar. He would tremble on wounded knee begging for mercy upon meeting a furious warpainted apache warrior in the shadows of the tropical night. This would be followed by a scream of "Geronimo" as "Bang Bang" Psycho's silver tomahawk came down upon his head before I scalped the deceitful twat alive. Then I'd carry the gruesome memento home to use as a macabre litter tray for my brother's black cats. Once a shithead always a shithead.

Well, get off your horse and drink your plant- based milk, so you too can become a compassionate vegan like me!

So, fortunately for this Hungarian József Bloggs, there were no bloodthirsty savage images of vengeance drumming in my deranged lawless skull. I just pictured him as a run-of-the-mill bloke who took the opportunity to 'get his end away' when it was offered to him on a platter by the dishy Wicked Witch.

The maniacal blind rage that was running amok in my bloody brain was aimed and focused on the treacherous target who I could see smiling innocently in the cross hairs of my make-believe sniper gun. It appears the cheating fallen angel had betrayed me yet again. Jesus Christ! This morning's passionate encounter on the sofa was nothing but a sloppy Judas kiss.

Back to risky business. I elected to call him at 4 am, which would be 11 am in Laos. That would grant me just four short hours to meticulously plot my strategy. The game plan had to be engineered to perfection and my cunning approach, flawless. It was imperative that I kept my turbulent emotions under control and gave my undivided concentration to the business of securing the crucial confession. I had to be calm and friendly and catch him off-guard by giving the impression that my missus had blurted out all the sordid details by blowing the whistle already, to have even a sliver of a chance of success.

At 4am I hit the road and apprehensively tramped off beneath the bitter black wintery sky, grabbing deep breaths of icy air as I plucked up the courage to trigger this bone-chilling call. Was I ready and willing to face up to and withstand the insufferable truth? My blood ran cold as I stood still like a solitary ice carving in a desolate open space and dialled the secret number.

To the best of my memory the conversation went as follows;

Hungarian bloke = HB

Psycho Syd = PS

HB - Hello, who is this?

PS - Hi, we have met a few times in the Samlo Pub and my name is Syd.

HB - Hi, what can I do for you?

PS - Do you know ****?

HB - Yes.

PS – Well, this is difficult for me to say but I need to hear your side of the story, so I can make my decision on what to do next. I am her husband and she has just returned to the UK and informed me that she has been having an affair with you. It's obviously distressing for me, but I must deal with it. Can you help me? On top of this I have stage 4 cancer and a prognosis of just 12 months to live so I would be grateful if we can finish this painful saga because stress is the last thing I need.

HB - I am really sorry about your illness and honestly didn't know she had a husband. She informed me she was going to see her child who was living there. We met for dinner a few times.

PS - Thank you for your honesty. She has shown me all the messages that you sent to each other, probably to clear her guilt. If you would just answer one more difficult question, I would be grateful, and it would enable me to resolve my problems here. Did you sleep with her?

HB - Yes, I did. I am so sorry, I really didn't know. It was just a fling; nothing serious. I had no intention of forming a long-term relationship because I already have a girlfriend. I apologise once more and hope you manage to sort things out.

PS - Thank you for being so truthful. Take care and goodbye.

HB – Goodbye.

My dying body stood still in the dead of night and silently cried. I felt like I was spinning out of control. I tried to focus but everything was twisted. Flying the Wicked Witch back in the expectation that she would be a candy-coated sugar plum fairy, magically healing my broken tick-tocker and damaged body, was a catastrophic cockeyed blunder. It felt like a right kick to the teeth.

She had returned as an acid-smeared, tart crab apple goblin bent on tossing me off into the pitch-black dungeon of terror and torture with just a flick of her wrist. Goblins are reputed to be outright evil and greedy, especially for gold and jewellery. Yep, that was my girl down to a tee! Her fiendish objective was surely to exterminate me and smirk in glee, without even a droplet of guilt or a few warm salty tears of empathy as I slowly snuffed it.

"Exterminate, exterminate!" Good Lord, my missus is a blinking Dalek. Chop-chop *Doctor Who*, shake your Timelord leg and get Uranus here pronto. I desperately need to sit my God-given bum in your TARDIS and do "The Time Warp" to another galaxy far, far away from this evil Venus fly trap.

If she was having such a ball or two of a time in Vientiane, hell-bent on revelling in her newfound freedom, why in heaven's name did she Sham 69 me by begging to be reunited and lie side by side with her sick husband? Lie being the operative word!

I was mortified with the realisation that I had been soft-soaped by the dirty brainwashing scrubber. I had been taken to the cleaners as my bank account was spotless of cash! The way she had sparkled as a squeaky-clean loyal partner as she polished off the money I transferred weekly, left me feeling sterile. As she was gobbling up my last bit of cash, she was also noshing on the food supplied by some bloke who was only interested in 'a bit on the side' while his loved one was out of sight, out of mind. My ailing body and my finances were both down to bare bones. I had cracked the dirty puzzle but was sickened with the filthy muck she had attempted to sweep under the seemingly speckless carpet.

Break on Through (To the Other Side)

(December 2013)

I was filled with self-loathing for being so *Dumb and Dumber* while at the same time ablaze with a burning rage at my heartless unfaithful spouse. I fumed home in a fiery fury ready for a hot-headed pow-wow with my two-faced squaw. I hoped and prayed she didn't get an early warning by spotting the smoke signals blasting out of my ears.

Upon setting foot inside my imaginary tepee, I was thunderstruck as I caught sight of the callus cow blissfully caterwauling, "Hey, yay, ha, ha, hey, yay, ha, ha," as she circled the coffee table. I put on a brave face as I roared, "How!" which put an immediate stop to her jolly little jig. "How, how dare you," I hollered. I stiffened with rage as I bent her over the said coffee table and whipped out my totem pole and gave her a proper little big horn, which made her hair stand on end like a startled Mohican. After the punishment came to an end, I demanded, "Who is the big chief?" "You are," she meekly replied. "Another feather in my headband," I proudly smirked with satisfaction.

Of course, I just made that up. So, "Please Forgive Me" for yet another psychedelic journey to the centre of my screwed-up mind. Regressing back and re-experiencing such a distressing stage of my life once more, to write this, is emotionally exhausting. I delve deep into buried films, photographs and notes from that dreadful time, which is like picking a raw nerve. Therefore, when my feelings are galloping unmanageably wild and my tormenting recollections start to cut just a bit too deep, I grant my sensitive soul a much-needed breather. It flees the agonising reality by creating a fictional madcap paragraph. "All Apologies." Hope you understand.

The enraged Apache Indian gently faded, to be substituted by the bona fide me; Nosferatu, that is. I glowered at the ceiling in a floored daze, stupefied by the words uttered by our man in Vientiane. In this otherworldly trancelike dimension, I contemplated what nightmare the next episode of this eternal tragic saga would hurl at me.

I silently crept upstairs on tippy-toes and quietly roused my wife. I whispered, "Sorry for waking you but you must come downstairs now because I have something very important to tell you."

She rubbed her snoozy eyes and followed me downstairs and sat on the armchair facing my sofa. For just a moment, two pairs of confused eyeballs stared deeply into each other. You could have heard a pinhead drop. "Did you have a boyfriend while you were in Laos?" I softly quizzed.

"No, I didn't," she responded innocently.

I continued with my friendly talk. "What about that Hungarian man that you were chatting to?"

"Only a friend, I have already told you," she replied sincerely.

She must have had an inkling that something was amiss because she ought to have hit the flaming roof after being shaken from her beauty sleep at such an unearthly hour to be interrogated for something she hadn't done. And rightly so.

Time for "Enola Gay" to drop the humongous bombshell. I glared icily into her darting eyes before exploding the earthshattering news. I spat, "You dirty fucking liar. I have just telephoned him, and he has apologised to me for sleeping with you because you never told him you were married. He just said it was for sex because he already has a girlfriend. Why the hell have you done this to me?"

She froze like a rabbit caught in the beam of a car's headlights *At the Midnight Hour*. The shock and utter disbelief on her astonished face was startling.

"Did he seem angry?" she timidly inquired. Effing hell! Not a piss-drop of remorse or a heartfelt apology for cruelly betraying her dying husband and stealing everything he had left in the world. The inhumane selfish cow's adulterous eyes were crawling with bitter alarm now that her sweeter-than-sweet image had just been shredded into tiny little pieces. She didn't give a stinking dog shit about my shattered dreams but was just panicking about what her Hungarian lover man would be thinking, now that she had been exposed as a filthy deceitful two-timing bitch.

"Was he the person who drove you to the airport in Udorn Thani?" I raged.

"Yes," she admitted.

The backstabbing lying bastard! I glared at her and thought, *How the hell could you do that to your dying husband?*

It was all just a vile pack of sodding lies and I was the joker coz the joke was on me. I wasn't giggling though; I was crying my northern monkey heart out. I agonisingly visualised the weepy pair kissing and hugging as they tearfully cried goodbye. At that very same time, I was jumping for joy in Shangri-La because I would soon be reunited with my beautiful faithful angel. I masochistically recollected the moment when she lovingly vowed, "I only have you and need to be with you and take good care of you." My distraught soul howled in hysterical lunacy as my ripped heart dripped bright globs of shiny scarlet misery.

"Why did you come back here then?" I snarled.

"I wanted to study beauty therapy in college," she unemotionally justified as her empty eyes just passed me by.

I was abruptly walloped by a gargantuan full-force thwack in my distraught Mancunian mush as the nitty-gritty truth clouted me straight between my stunned sky-blue eyes. The acute realisation came that to the evil one, I was just an unavoidable arsewipe; a troublesome necessity to be used and abused in her single-minded endeavour to sit on the throne at the top table. After having served my purpose, I would be shat on before being discarded and unmercifully flushed down the shitter.

The piteous reality that I was terminally ill and on the brink of losing my psychedelic marbles coz of her spiteful, below-zero manipulating behaviour, was of no concern to her sadistic jet-black heart. She was ecstatic when I was on my bended knees. In fact, it was an orgasmic bonus as her devious, vindictive face exploded in "Rapture." She simultaneously licked her sinful lips in delight whilst observing her enslaved captive squirming and suffering, his hands tied, as he shed blood, sweat and tears in his futile bid to unlock the heavy emotional chains she had restrained him in. "Oh, Bondage, Up Yours!"

What a "Wicked Game" she played, allowing my to dream in heaven before plunging me into the blackest, most hideous nightmare of my life. The snide double-dealing she-devil had passed me the death card; the "Ace of Spades." No problem darling, I don't want to live forever. Something suddenly snapped before I experienced my "19th Nervous Breakdown". That was the day Psycho Syd died.

The living room gave birth to a supernatural, eerie stillness before setting in motion a tornado of nauseating gyrations. I was spiralling deeper but couldn't feel any fingers on my throat as I choked. It picked up speed like a whirling dervish on amphetamine sulphate as it spun the life out of me. I was a soft-hearted "Speed King" racing away from my hard-headed woman. I flew across the sky and I saw a strange-looking land. The rotating eventually decelerated until "All Stood Still." My twisted, twirling mind came to a standstill. I sat motionless in deathly silence inside a colourless misty box. How Bizarre!" It was peculiar!

The spooky foggy vapour gradually dispersed, leaving me agog in my very own living room once again. Everything was strangely strange. Shadows began to talk. Colours shimmered in vibrating dazzling hues. Objects came alive as stains and scuffs on the walls and furniture fascinatingly danced before my astonished eyes. It was like the onset of a magic mushroom trip. This was the death of Psycho Syd. My crippled bag of skin and bones was still breathing in and out, but my mind had finally snuffed it.

I heard the silence and I saw the dark as my mind finally fell apart. I was destroyed and my soul was as dead as my wife's black heart.

In a trancelike "Sleepwalk" I floated aboard the Starship Stella Mortem ready to race through the starlit sky and discover the meaning of death. "Mother Universe" had spoken, and I was all ears coz I was "Made of Stars." In this supernova spaced-out frame of mind, I viewed my wife with no malice, envy, jealousy or pain because she was made of stars too. We were one. I gazed through the stardust in my eyes with deep pity, understanding that she was suffering too. We reap what we sow, and karma has no expiry date.

My mind was dead, but my soul was almost as free as a bird, though it couldn't fly, fly away because it was trapped inside a physical mass of dying atoms. I was ready to give up the ghost. Soon I would find myself alone and fade away. I would be free.

Once again, I stress that there was no perception of bitterness directed at my femme fatale, who had picked me up with her promises of love and affection before dropping me to the floor with her lies. That had occurred in the past and the past didn't exist except as pictures in my grey matter that I recalled in the present. The only true reality was this moment in time. Death would only occur in the present because the future was also an unreal vision in my mind. The future didn't exist. Death was as natural as birth. Well, I didn't fear the Reaper any longer. In all honesty, death was the light at the end of the tunnel. For the love of God, where was the Grim Reaper coz I wanted to grab hold of his hand and see if there was life after death…

I stood up and felt like a fairy-tale giant in a tiny room as I strode determinedly into the kitchen. *Fee, fi, fo, fum, I smell the blood of a Manchester man.* I grabbed five sachets of powerful morphine from the remaining 40 and a tall glass of cool, healthy, reverse osmosis filtered water. The buzzing from the refrigerator sounded much louder. I composed myself on my sick sofa and attentively poured out the contents of the first sachet into the glass and following a nifty stir, started to drink.

This wasn't a 'head in hands' suicidal depression, because I was now happy, excited and relaxed. I was deadly serious about the task at hand and buzzing with adrenalin, bent on getting a kick out of my terminal adventure. Or was there life after death, giving me the two thumbs up for countless future intrepid escapades for my itchy feet and crazy mind to relish? Well, I would soon find the answer to that little mystery - or maybe I wouldn't!

It seemed like I was floating in space as I brimmed my glass an additional couple of times, pushing forward with my loony, spaced-out opiated trip to kingdom come. This last journey had a grimy hypnagogic air of foreboding, just like a grainy, shadowy scene from an obscure timeworn black and white foreign film. This was no make-believe, impromptu dramatic play-acting scream for help, in a futile stab at pricking the Wicked Witch's conscience; coz she didn't blooming have one. "When I'm Dead and Gone," she will grieve a river of crocodile tears in public, while pissing herself laughing in secret.

We may have spoken but I fail to recollect any sweet talk or any attempts to dissuade me from my final mission. At least she had the thoughtfulness not to disrupt my concluding couple of hours on planet Earth.

I tottered and very nearly fell flat on my dreamboat face as I zig-zagged to grab the 4th tumbler of council pop. My vision was filmy and my tree soothingly drowsy in my opiated skull. Soaring in tranquilised bliss, being high in Xanadu was heavenly. I was resting in glorious peace and giggled out loud, "Am I Dead or Alive? I ghosted back to my basecamp sofa in readiness for the final ascent. No oxygen necessary! I took a drink of magic potion, glass number four. How did I feel? I felt wonderful.

I gazed at my wicked witch of trouble and saw a hazy pair of them staring back at me. Double vision means double trouble! Were they both giving me the evil eye?

A memory of my wife somersaulted into my fuzzy brain. It was just a few weeks after my dear mother had passed away and I was very poorly on my sick sofa. The harrowingly vivid recollection was of my wife dancing as she sang, "I'm happy your mother is dead." I glanced back at the blurry twins, still aghast at that shocking flashback, which was a whiplash reminder of the wicked cruelty my demon spouse was capable of. My speechless brain concluded, *For heaven's sake go to hell,* before I slurred, "Go to bed and let me rest in peace." Neither of them waved bye-bye or made a sound.

I somehow fetched the fifth sachet of morphine and cascaded it into the glass of water, which I had astonishingly managed to keep almost full to the brim as I swayed back from the kitchen to the sofa. I realised that the subsequent snake to the kitchen and back would have to be the last. This terminal wobbly trip would involve 35 sachets of morphine stashed in my pockets and a large steel pan of chilly Adam's ale in my shaky hands in preparation for the "Final Countdown."

I made spacy headway in this dreamlike hypnotic state, which was becoming more potent by the minute. I supped the fifth glass of my death-dealing elixir, steadying myself for the final stagger to the kitchen. Out of the blue, another mind movie from the past was projected inside my 'high-as-a-kite head.' Once more, the Wicked Witch played the starring role as she taunted, "It would be all my birthdays rolled into one if Eugene, Francesca and your daughter in Thailand died". I was jolted out of my electric dream by this shocking memory but felt no emotion towards the Witch because now my undivided attention was solidly focused on my children. They needed me, and I needed them so today was, after all, not the day to die. My love of my kids pulled me back from the edge once more.

I smiled as my head gently kissed the soft pillow on my sick sofa. The sensation was pleasant. I was deeply in love with my children and the Wicked Witch was irrelevant. My heavy eyelids shut as I passed into another world dreaming and laughing, as I merrily frolicked in my mind with my kids.

Later that day, I blinked my eyeballs open, flashing a 'back from the dead' monster smirk as I savoured the wonder of being wide awake and alive. The joyful sensation of being rejuvenated heart and soul, with renewed hope and new daydreams, had me all tingly inside and out. Remarkably, my physical body felt in tip-top shape too. It was as if last night's delirious mental breakdown had detoxified my body and soul, flushing out the venomous nightmares of the past; leaving me illuminated in the dazzling "Ray of Light" at the end of the scary dark tunnel. It was the first taste of sunshine after so many dark cloudy days. The future was bright; the future was Psycho.

I Believe in Father Christmas

(December 2013)

That very evening, when I was messing about online, I just couldn't abstain from snatching a sneaky peep to see whether the two-timing lovebirds had exchanged messages or not. As sure as night is day, she had dispatched one. She casually spouted, "A man woke me up and questioned me about our relationship last night, but don't worry about it because no one is 100% clean." Yes, she is spotless alright; not a speck of white on her dirty black heart. She had attempted to wipe the smutty slate clean by jumping into bed with the 'cheating scumbags anonymous' mob. It was a bit like the Yorkshire Ripper justifying himself for murder because other sick sadistic killers take lives too.

Even worse, I was referred to as some insignificant man. Not a whisper of the faithful devoted hubby who had depleted his bank account to buy her a house, transformed her life and had just emptied his pockets to fly the deceitful cow back. Our man in Vientiane didn't reply!

The 11th December was Jo's 5th birthday and I was as sure as hell bent on dishing up a memorable super-duper day for him. Prior to Jo returning from school I had dashed about in a batty tizzy, splashing the four living room walls with a rainbow of vibrant colourful pictures and gaudy balloons. I basked in sunny "Instant Karma" as his little face lit up in glee and wonder. He flashed a massive heart-warming smile at me after he laid astonished eyeballs on the brand spanking new shiny Raleigh bicycle I had secretly purchased earlier. Next, a small party and a big cake. He was thrilled to bits as he sang, "Happy Birthday to me," before blowing the candles out. Bless him! He was just a child and it was deplorable that his innocent eyes and mind had been witness to so much spiteful hatred and cruelty over the last year and a bit.

Life persisted in a carbon copy of the previous poisonous conditions. It was as if we had never been apart. The Wicked Witch was still hostile, crabby and aloof while I kept on trucking with a warm, loving smile on my dial for my kids. My exasperation, frustration and apprehension were surreptitiously concealed deep within the dark side of my mind. My gorgeous offspring would view nowt but love, hope and happiness from their doting dad.

Her return ticket was for 7th February, so it was a case of keeping everything crossed that she got her unfaithful arse on that big metal bird for a tearful reunion with Józef Bloggs. I'll bite my lip and bide my time.

I was unwavering in my dogged determination to "Slide Away" from the four-walled prison cell with Jo, because my frightful cancer prognosis meant I was still walking on very thin ice. Little Jo deserved some fun and games with his caring dad, even if the Wicked Witch was part and parcel of each jolly jaunt. Eugene didn't tag along on our days out coz he much preferred hanging around with his girlfriend and his mates. And who could blame him? It was more enjoyable than being within a stone's throw of the adulterous one's scowling mug, I bet.

We drove to Lancaster and munched a pub lunch at a quaint historical pub in the city centre. The Wicked One was ill at ease, seated at the same table as her ill-with-cancer ghoulish partner. She was having nowt to do with me as she gave the impression of never having met such an ugly monstrosity before in her entire life. Thank the Lord almighty for the TV on the far wall, which I could focus on as I chatted with Jo, who was contentedly feasting upon his pizza and garlic bread. And even better, there was a live football match and Manchester City were defeating Arsenal.

An overcast day was treasured in a country park roughly an hour's drive away. This afforded Jo the perfect opportunity to put his riding skills to the test on his good-looking birthday pressie. Despite tumbling over and coming a cropper several times, he loved it. He speedily became adept at steering and braking along the winding paths and the numerous slopes beneath the leafless winter trees. I felt a warm glow inside as I observed him smiling and laughing. There were no smiles from the black thundery Wicked Witch of course, but my focus was on Jo's happiness. I even managed to score some beetroot, apples and carrots at a local farmer's market for my juices.

Four days before Christmas, we ambled near Ribchester. My feeble body pottered very slowly along the riverbank and across a few fields. It was marvellous being out and about in the crisp country air, pointing out sheep, cows, ducks and swans to Jo. My black-hearted beauty stamped her angry foot down and refused point-blank to indulge in a snack and a drink in the village café, because she was too embarrassed to be seen with her ugly beast. It was a crying shame for Jo. And for me too.

"I Believe in Father Christmas" and a massive 'ho, ho, ho' coz my lovely daughter, Francesca, arrived to make merry this festive season. "Good Tidings of Comfort and Joy" galore. The fact that she used the bulk of the time upstairs entertaining herself with computer games alongside Eugene didn't ruffle my psychedelic feathers. I had three of my kids underneath the same roof and I felt good. It was just a pity the shameless 'Oh come, oh ye unfaithful one' wasn't upbeat too. She had a face like a slapped arse. Well, she could French kiss my God-given Manc bum because I was bent on being joyful and triumphant as I celebrated Christmas with my darling children. I sent a loving message to my daughter in Bangkok and wished upon a star that I would see her one last time before pushing up the daisies.

The evening before Christmas we were all squatted on the brown carpet, squashed up in the undersized living room, playing happy families, with the fairy lights twinkling on the jumble of Christmas pressies underneath the tree. I organised 'mad as a hatter' games off the top of my 'as nutty as a fruitcake' bonce. These impromptu capers included balancing a chocolate on the end of your nose for a full minute, singing a song for 30 seconds or hopping to the kitchen and back to the count of ten. The kids loved these madcap shenanigans and even the Wicked Witch became infected with high jinks fever, her sweet smile almost cracking her sour boat race (face). They all toddled off to bed laughing and smiling to dream of Santa Claus while I lay "Lonely This Christmas" on my sick sofa. I was overflowing with emotion this "Silent Night;" rejoicing to be still alive but totally gutted that my partner had pulled the wool over my vegan eyes with her false promises of love and support.

"We Wish you a Merry Christmas," we wish you a merry Christmas, we wish you a merry Christmas and a happy new *Mia*. *Mia* in the Lao language means wife. It would be perfect to be hand-in-hand with a sparkly new faithful wife who loved me from the sexy bottom of her heart, but the likelihood of that miracle manifesting was slimmer than my skeletal frame, given that I resembled the Elephant Man's ugly brother.

I was overjoyed as my kids' faces delightedly tripped the light fantastic with animated fervour, eagerly ripping off the snowman and red-nosed reindeer wrapping paper to get their hands on their pressies. Radiant smiles, gleeful laughter and whoops of euphoric surprise and joyous wonderment danced around our humble room this magical Christmas morning. I drifted back to my childhood with warm recollections of my loving mum and dad blissfully smiling as their three overjoyed children squealed with festive laughter, opening their Yuletide gifts.

I was grinning like the cat who had got the cream as I tore open the neatly wrapped parcels containing my presents. My sky-blue eyeballs were all shiny and sparkly as I hugged and thanked my gorgeous kids. I experienced the eerie sensation of déjà vu once more, there was no present from my wife, just like my last birthday. Jesus Christ! I wasn't expecting gold, frankincense and myrrh; a pair of bloody socks from the pound shop would have done. Yet, she didn't even give me the steam off her piss! She had stolen everything I had and just sat there motionless and emotionless without even wishing me Merry Christmas. Beyond belief!

On the other hand, my hippy psyche is made of different stuff; love, compassion and empathy. There isn't a bad bone in my body; on second thoughts, maybe just one! Notwithstanding the nitty-gritty that she had deceived, cheated, mocked, tormented and plundered well-nigh lock, stock and barrel, it just wasn't in my nature-loving, flower power heart to inhumanely exclude my Venus flytrap from the thrill of unwrapping Christmas presents. I wouldn't do that to my very own worst enemy! In addition, if the pretty one was vacant of her own trove of treasure beneath the tree, she would stick out like a downcast throbbing thumb, which would spawn an uncomfortable thorny ambience. This could give birth to a downer at the high point of Christmas for the kids and absolutely zilch was permitted to tarnish this marvellous moment in time.

I was alive to the sickening reality that the writing could well be on the mortuary wall that I would be inhaling my final lungful of salty Blackpool sea air before Christmas 2014. Consequently, it was imperative that I had joyful mind movies of my kids having fun, to accompany me to the graveyard if I snuffed it before the next "Ding Dong Merrily on High." Now, if it would have been just me and my disloyal partner celebrating Christmas Day together then she would have received exactly what she deserved, and Father Christmas had declared: "Sweet Fanny Adams coz she had been a very naughty girl."

I grudgingly dipped my hand into my not-far-from-destitute blue jeans pocket and scraped together enough dosh for half a dozen bargain-basement gifts for my false-hearted spouse. If my murky chemo brain hits the nail on the head as I write: tights, make-up, shower gel, a hat, chocolate and a belt. I wrapped the six 'bought for a sad song' gifts and placed them under the twinkling tree. Well, it's the thought that counts, isn't it? Eugene and Francesca bought her a small gift each too; so, she did far better than she deserved.

She unwrapped each of her pressies with a sweet smile but the disappointment of not unearthing a 'state-of-the-art' gold watch or an 'up to the minute' iPhone was as plain to see as the Pinocchio hooter on her disgruntled mug.

She was intentionally as blind as a vampire bat to the house, land, vacations overseas and enough in-vogue outfits to last ten fashion-conscious ladies a lifetime or two. She couldn't suck any more blood out of her victim because he had nothing else to give. She had bled him dry. You just couldn't make it up, could you?

I recall her ridiculing me as she flaunted a new leather handbag in my face not many months back. She mocked, "My boyfriend bought me this for over £100; you couldn't afford it." I just shook my head and thought, *You are fucking unbelievable!*

The cupboard was bare this Christmas Day, but Psycho Syd didn't take the Wicked Witch upstairs to give the poor dog a bone because she didn't bloody well deserve it. Therefore, Mr Psychedelic Clever Clogs had the shiny bright idea of driving to the close at hand Lancashire hills to sniff out a country pub with a blazing open fire for a memorable Yuletide scoff.

An hour was spent following the long and winding country roads that would lead to the door of a welcoming village tavern. I felt like the village idiot upon arriving at each hamlet, as the pub was either shut or fully booked. My bright idea was fading rapidly, making me look a proper dimbo! Visions of Joseph and Mary on that starry, starry night in Bethlehem slipped into my frantic skull. Maybe we would end up in a stable too, because we were all hungry enough to eat a horse! Although, just hay for me please, coz I'm a wise vegan man. The missus had a face like a robber's dog, and I was anticipating some Bow Wow Wow earache. The kids were growing impatient too. I would soon have to hold my hands up high and concede that my brainwave was nothing but a fool's errand. We would have no alternative but to retreat home for sugar butties and baked beans on toast for our Crimbo dinner.

Then came a miracle of miracles as the White Hart Inn came to light under a "Twinkle, Twinkle Little Star" in the itsy-bitsy village of Sabden. We were greeted with open arms and escorted to an exclusive private room for a three-course Christmas din-din and a bottle of red plonk. I sat smugly at the head of the table, smirking from ear to ear. I had an upper crust smarmy demeanour about me as I aristocratically declared, "Psycho Syd the council estate kyd does it again." Simultaneously reflecting privately, *You jammy bastard.*

The children were cheerful and even Cruella de Vil had a

bittersweet smile on her normally miserable mush. Sweet because she was starving; bitter due to the detested monster managing to pull victory from the jaws of defeat, meaning that the perfect opportunity to ridicule me was shattered at the very last moment.

Our famished eyes greedily feasted upon the numerous generous portions of food that were adroitly placed on the festive table. Were our eyes bigger than our bellies? We would soon find out as we all piggishly tucked in. There was a harvest of vegan friendly nosh for me too. Laughter and light-hearted banter filled the joyful room as we gobbled up our Christmas banquet. Eventually, we were all satisfyingly satiated and *Abbiocco* (Italian for the drowsy sensation after devouring a massive meal).

I sluggishly sat back and grinned as I realised it was yule-hole time. I imagine you are no doubt assuming that must be Psycho Syd giving the Wicked One a right old doggy-style Xmas stuffing later that yuletide night, but you couldn't be further from the truth. The yule-hole is the hole you must move your belt buckle to after you have eaten an enormous meal; usually at Christmastime.

So, my top tip for today, gentlemen, is after a romantic meal on your very first date with a pretty femme fatale, look deeply into her eyes and whisper, "I think it's yule-hole time, don't you?" The expression on her face will be priceless but more importantly, it will give you a titanic clue as to whether you are going to get your wicked way or be cruelly blown out. Warning: no titanic jokes about going down on her first time out, otherwise you are likely to be sunk to your knees after a sharp icy kick or punch to the cobblers (cobbler's awls; balls).

Once you define the expression she will likely titter, "Goodness gracious me, you are as idiotic as that famous crackpot writer, Psycho Syd."

Please do me a favour and spill the beans on whether she invites you in for a 'nudge, nudge, wink, wink, say no more' coffee or whether she rolls her eyeballs before giving you the elbow!

There wasn't even the tiniest morsel of food left on our 'clean as a whistle' plates. We had scoffed the blooming lot. I couldn't even ask for a doggy-bag so the wicked one could have second helpings tomorrow morning! Meow, meow! She had given me the cold shoulder most of the evening as her focus was pinpointed on posing for seductive selfies; pushing her tits out as she set the booby trap for the five-knuckle shuffle brigade who followed her on Facebook.

Goodbye Kiss

(December 2013 to January 2014)

A few days later I took my wife to buy some oriental fruit and vegetables from a greengrocer in the town centre. Once out of the car she spat, "Keep away from me, I am ashamed to be seen near you. Walk on the other side of the road." I hated myself more than I hated her!

Francesca returned to France to celebrate the New Year with her mother. I hugged her close and affectionately expressed, "I love you and will see you soon." It was always a distressing moment, saying a sorrowful goodbye to my beautiful daughter, because there was every possibility it would be the last.

On the concluding day of the year I battled against the hostile screaming wind and bone-chilling horizontal rain in front of the lawless black and grey waves on the North Shore promenade not far from my house. I glared at the furious sea and just like King Canute, ordered, "Keep the fuck away from me." Its immediate snappy comeback was to crash a riotous monster wave against the breakwater, soaking me to the skin. I was absolutely saturated, looking like a poor drowned rat as I bellowed, "Thanks for such a fitting end to a bastard year." My enraged scream was lost in the cacophony of the screeching wind and the roaring of King Neptune pissing himself laughing. I shivered and escorted my ice-cold sopping-wet body and chattering fangs home before I snuffed it not of cancer, but hypothermia!

On New Year's Day, my wife didn't wish me a Happy New Year, but she surprisingly offered to stick around for 2014 to support me and the kids. However, there was a heavy-duty 'fly in the ointment' stumbling-block to her seemingly humanitarian proposition; the small print which shouted that she could go out whenever she liked and have sex with whoever she liked.

I tossed aside her distressing proposal and refused point-blank to rubber-stamp the sleazy arrangement. I had endured a belly-full of ballyhoo and humiliation already. Enough was enough. I just couldn't stomach any additional shame, self-loathing and embarrassing dishonour.

I glared straight into her smirking eyes and retorted, "Impossible! I am battling for dear life and the torment and stress of any further adulterous behaviour would destroy me. So, the answer is a big fat, no way, José."

She was not my captive slave and had every right to begin a new life and enjoy her freedom but not at my expense. I refused to be a hen-pecked, cuckolded piece of shite for one minute longer. She could slut around to her black heart's content but not while she was living with me.

The following day we took Jo to visit the beach and a park in nearby St Annes-on-Sea. Jo ran wild, wild, wild and wild up the sand dunes; the viper in the grass was glaring at me. The venomous serpent was hostile; hissing with noxious malice because her victim had categorically refused to comply with her 'below the belt' game plan. She was spitting mad at getting the two-fingers up instead of the two-thumbs up.

Without warning the 'nasty piece of work' lashed out as she spat poisonous words of torment and pain. The cruel bitch gloatingly boasted about her enjoyable sex sessions with Jozef Bloggs. For all that, it was like water off a quack quack's back because I had heard it all before and didn't give a Donald Duck (fuck)! I was immune already.

I had a vivid flashback to a shocking incident that occurred a short while after we had become partners. It was a balmy tropical afternoon and we were blissfully snuggling in bed, lolling in the fulfilling afterglow of a sizzle of climatic hot lust. This heavenly euphoria was disturbed by the constant ringing of her bloody mobile phone. I resisted the temptation of flinging it out of the window; instead, like a starry-eyed "Prince Charming," I elected to "Stand and Deliver" it to my fairy-tale princess.

She cut up her heartbroken ex-boyfriend and "To Cut a Long Story Short," she was adamant that it was over as she yelled, "It is finished, you are dumped." "At the Height of the Fighting" she spitefully sniggered, "I am in bed with my new man and we just had amazing sex and I enjoyed it so much." I recall being appalled at how my sweet 'butter wouldn't melt in her mouth' pussycat could transform into an evil sadistic lizard in just the blink of an eye.

She justified her brutal put down by claiming he thoroughly deserved it because he had another girlfriend. I took her word to be gospel because I didn't know back then that she was a lying two-headed bird, did I? In Lao, *Nok Song Hua* means two-headed bird, which translates into English as two-faced. The distraught boy was probably completely innocent and ruthlessly booted into the gutter when something better came along.

Back then I could only visualise a 'they lived happily ever after' ending to this 'once upon a time' new romantic love story. Not in a million light years did I ever imagine that the 'Grimm' day would arrive when it was my turn to face her hateful sadistic side. When that apocalyptic date arrived, I winced as my cold-blooded "Karma Chameleon" kicked me in the balls; just when I needed her most.

I glared directly into her vicious eyes and suggested "Would you like me to fly you back now rather than waiting until 7th February?"

She shrugged her 'couldn't give a shite' shoulders and nonchalantly responded, "If you like." Was she trying to call my bluff?

The very next day I succeeded in switching her flights to 7th January. Rearranging her plane tickets so she could be reunited with her Hungarian bloke a month earlier cost me almost £300. All in all, her false promise of 'I want to love you and take care of you and I have no one else but you' had set me back over two thousand quid, when you consider the money I transferred for her to live on while she was waiting for her visa. Even worse than the loss of the cash was the sickening torment of being knifed in the back once again. She should get her deceitful arse on the plane and fly away pronto before I wrung both of her evil birds fucking necks.

On 6th January, I visited the wild sea on yet another stormy day. The turbulent waves were out of control, just like my life. My wife had constantly taunted, "You will die a lonely old man because you are so ugly that no one will be with you again." The sad thing was that I believed her.

That very night we were intimate. It was a bizarre scenario to the finish of the partnership; it ended as it began, with an erotic coupling of orgasmic frenzy. I endeavoured to visualise that I was making love to the loyal girl I once knew. Sadly, it was nigh-on impossible because my bloody brain kept projecting hurtful porn movies of her infidelity. Eventually we lay side by side, as waves of satisfied pleasure embraced our glowing bodies. Again, my bloody brain tormented me with the cruel realisation that I would never make love to anyone again.

***

Very early the next morning, I drove her to the airport along the virtually vacant pitch-black motorways in a surreally dreamlike frame of mind. There was no resentment or rage; just a deep sensation of melancholy as my mind dexterously turned a blind eye to my wife's latter-day sinful behaviour. In preference, I dreamily floated back to the sentimental days of nostalgia way back down memory lane. I stole a fleeting glimpse of her beautiful face and reflected how we had walked together as lovers.

My soon to be out-of-my-crippled-life-forever partner was touchy-touchy, holding my hand all the way, which was a disorientating turn-up for the books. What in heaven's name was happening inside her skull? Sorrow? Regret? Sympathy? Chicanery? Mmm! I hadn't the foggiest, but I had better stop dreaming and focus on the road, before we both ended up as blood-splattered Crash Test Dummies!

At the airport, I forked over the last bit of cash I had left in the whole wide world so that she could travel from Bangkok to Laos for a tearful reunion with Mr Hungry Hungary. I felt gutted. She vowed to return the dosh, but I wasn't lingering with bated breath on account of her having broken every other bloody promise she had ever made.

She gripped my hand and gazed tenderly into my eyes before declaring that she loved me. What the hell was going on? Was she messing with my mind yet again? As we sipped coffee in the 'nothing to write home about' airport café, she never once released my hand as she stared deeply into my mesmerised sky-blue eyes. Was the bugger hypnotising me? Emergency, call 999. Will my guardian angel please blow out the flame that I am still carrying for this vindictive bastard, who has spent the last 18 months shitting on me?

We stood in silence holding hands near the customs clearance, like two frightened children. We were oblivious to the "Sound of the Crowd" as the manic swarms of programmed homo sapiens vanished into thin air. Time stood still. I felt like a "Spirit in the Material World." On the spur of a magic moment she pulled me close and snogged me passionately for a dreamy lifetime. That was the first time in over a year she had kissed her ghoulish cancer man on the mouth. I almost cried tears of joy and pain but instead softly choked, "Well, are you getting on the plane or not?"

She glanced at the customs clearance, then back into my eyes, the customs once more, returning to my eyes before letting go of my hand and walking away.

That was the last time I would ever see her.

Or so I thought!

I Had Too Much to Dream Last Night

(January to February 2014)

I stared in distress as she nonchalantly evaporated from view and from the bigger picture too; my death-warmed-up life! My stomach was tied up in a hangman's noose as I choked on the knowledge that the relationship was once and for all dead and buried. The asphyxiating heartache cruelly strangled me. I stood still in breathless silence with my head down in helpless desperation. Chirpy, colourful lovebirds flying blissfully high were oblivious to my anguish as they migrated to their cloud-nine destinations for a romantic getaway.

Was I off my psychedelic rocker? Why the hell was I feeling destroyed, because the Wicked Witch just tramped out of my sorry life? I must have been nuts, bananas and a fruitcake, hungering to share sweet love hearts with the inhumane one again. For God's sake, she had treated me like an insignificant, repugnant lump of mongrel shit. I should have been celebrating by tearing off my clothes before joyfully streaking stark bollock naked through the airport chanting, "Ding Dong! the Witch is Dead." Alas, my screwy, self-pitying crushed soul just felt like "Singing the Blues."

I terminated shoegazing and lifted my heavy chin off my chest and motivated myself: "Hold your Head Up" Syd, just hold your head up." I held my head high, also holding back my "Tears of a Clown" as I walked through the swarms of cheery holidaymakers. I sat like a mournful lonely man in my Fiat Punto as I reflected, "No soft and tender caresses for poor old solitary me, on the drive back to emptiness. As quick as a flash I gave my namby-pamby heavy heart a short sharp slap and commanded, "Pull yourself together, you soft as shite bastard, because your children have nobody but you now." With renewed energy and spirit, I screamed at the top of my lungs, "Bring it on."

Just as I slotted my key into the ignition, the phone beeped with a message. And guess who it was from? Yes, the Wicked Witch. And can you guess what it said? I love you and want to be with you! Good Lord give me strength. If I had had any hair, I would have ripped it all out with my bare hands there and then. What the bloody hell was going on? Confusion once again. She sent several similar texts so I replied, "If you really feel that way, I will post photos of us together on your Facebook page." She readily gave the go-ahead, which was an astonishing turn up for the books! I never dreamt in a month of Sundays that she would consent to having pictures of her husband polluting her single and available status!

I drove back to Blackpool along the busy motorways with my thrown off balance tree even busier with flummoxing and frustrating brainwork. Then it all kicked off in my mind; it was World War Three between my wishy-washy heart and my shell-shocked brain.

My brain was beating me up as it mocked, *Why didn't you prevent your soul mate from departing? You should have got down on bended knee declaring everlasting love. It's too late now. You can't close the sodding stable door after the mare has bolted. You don't even have the coin to bring her back, however much she begs and pleads, do you? You are on your arse without even two pennies to rub together coz she has blagged the bloody lot, you weak-kneed simpleton.*

My heart retorted: *Now hold your flipping horses. No point in crying over spilt almond milk. If she loved me as much as she claimed then she would flog the house and sort out the visa and flights. Then we'd have shedloads of wad to start a new romantic life together and live happily ever after; so, put that in your pipe and smoke it.*

Open your gullible eyeballs for goodness' sake. If you think for one split second, she will sell the house, then you are living in a cloud cuckoo land, my tree shot back. *She is a hunter who didn't have a pot to piss in until she spotted her prey and decided to take him for everything he had. She will never part with the house because that is her glorious prize.*

However, be warned because your trophy wife may well be waiting until you finally drop dead. Then she will fix your ghoulish head on a big wooden heart to take pride of place on the living room wall of the house you worked years to buy. That would be the perfect memento for the Wicked Witch to victoriously gloat and cackle over forever. So, dump that in your flaming pipe and puff on it slowly, the brain sneered!

The heart coughed and spluttered before holding its hands high in surrender because it knew beyond any rotten shadow of a doubt that the brain was completely right.

After an hour the war was finally over. The truth mushroomed from the rubble of my bombed-out life. The Wicked Witch had departed victoriously, leaving me defeated, shell-shocked and all alone in the ruins of what once was. There was no love lost on her part, I had served my purpose and she was ready to conquer the next poor victim. I didn't lie down and surrender though, because the Grim Reaper wasn't waving the white flag just yet. And this was a battle I couldn't lose because my kids had nobody in the whole wide world except me.

***

I arrived home and hugged little Jo, holding his tiny hand as I softly explained that his mother had left us again. He didn't appear overly concerned. It was as if he had been expecting it. Eugene knew the score and was more than likely relieved that his dad's bad-tempered missus was finally off the scene.

It was very scary being so ill, living under the dark cloud of a terminal illness, alone with two young children. And the workload of cooking, cleaning and school runs was overwhelming. I should be resting on my sick sofa, recuperating from the debilitating cancer treatment, not working my skinny hands to the bone.

I did post a few photos of us both together on her Facebook page as agreed but she deleted them and commented that someone had hacked her FFB account. And of course she never returned the money as promised. What a surprise!

Over the next four months there were almost as many ups and downs as there were in the passionate relationship with the Wicked Witch. I was in chaos, struggling with the tormenting heartache and the darkest depression known to man. I hid my despair from my children because they had suffered enough already. Escaping the ghost of the wicked one was futile. She haunted each room, shop, film, song and thought. I dreaded spotting the number nine bus which she used to jump on when meeting her lover, because I would fall to pieces and scream inside.

My life was a living nightmare. I only just about coped. When the children went to school, I would vanish under the duvet on my sick sofa in a futile attempt to escape the unrelenting heartache. At 3.15pm I'd collect Jo with a hug and a loving smile before we returned home. I would help him with his homework before cooking up a meal for the kids.

I knew in my broken heart of hearts that I had to fight harder than I had ever done before to have even a smidgen of a chance of outliving this relentless emotional bad dream. "I must flee my four walls and walk," my inner being screamed. Easier said than done when one is critically ill and clinically depressed.

I dropped the kids off at their schools and drove through the harsh winter weather to remote locations in the Lancashire countryside. In the freezing cold, the swirling snow, the biting wind and the teeming rain, I would force 50 painful steps before coming to a shivering standstill. I winced as I gripped the stitch in my side. My icy breath was instantly whisked away by the bone-chilling gusts of wind mother nature was hurling my way. Then 50 steps more. Giving in wasn't an option; I was fighting for my life. After an hour I would struggle back to the car with the icy fingers of madness and despair strangling my broken soul. The heater was banged on full blast during the drive back to the haunted house. Once home, my death warmed-up carcass would lay low under the duvet in a fruitless attempt to evade the ghost of the Wicked Witch. She was always on my mind.

At the weekends, I would drag Eugene and Jo away from computer games for a chilly hour in the middle of nowhere. I focused on each painful step up a hill, through a forest or along a river. The kids shuffled along, twiddling their thumbs deep inside their warm coat pockets as their pitiful dad stubbornly kept on going. Their reward would be a hot meal by a roaring fire in a remote country tavern.

I met up with a handful of different women I had been chatting to on the walking site. They were civil but never asked for seconds and who could blame them! A down in the dumps cripple who took an eternity to limp half a mile, wasn't the ideal hiking companion for an "I Love to go a-Wandering" enthusiast.

I continued taking my herbs and supplements, slurping the fruit and vegetable juices, meditating and visiting my shrink. He was concerned that I might top myself, but I was dead serious when I reassured him that suicide was out of the question, because my children had no one else except their broken old man.

***

A mind-blowing experience occurred at the local meditation centre one nippy Monday evening. I was seated in silence with eyes wide shut as I struggled to focus on the breath entering and leaving my nostrils. A sense of helpless frustration tormented me as the never-ending mind games and mind movies thwarted all attempts to flee the misery.

Then, in the blink of an eye, a 'wakey-wakey, smell the cloud nine organic coffee moment came to pass. I awakened with eyes wide open. The nightmares had disappeared, leaving me wide awake in dreamland. I had been miles away chained to my sorrow but was suddenly right here right now. My unattached soul smiled in pure bliss as my body tingled with warm flowing vibrations. I was tasting perfect reality for the very first time.

The velvety ding-ding-ding of the meditation bell aroused my eyeballs to a shimmering golden Buddha, a radiant orange-robed monk and a brand-new sparkling world. I just glowed in astonished awe as pure love and happiness trance-danced ecstatically in my joyful soul. *Heaven is on earth*, I smiled. *But so is hell,* I smiled once more. It is all in the mind!

In this euphoric state I floated upstairs to the bathroom and gazed in wonder at my gruesome visage in the looking glass. "Mirror, mirror on the wall, who is the ugliest of them all? You are Psycho Syd. Take a bow, you ugly fucking bastard," I chuckled with glee.

I found this realisation highly amusing as well as spiritually enlightening because I fully understood that the ugly fucker smiling back at me wasn't me. It was just trillions of cells; bones, blood, muscles, organs, glands and tendons and it wasn't me. This must be what happens when we die. We wake up from a bad dream suddenly aware of who we really are. And it isn't the rotting corpse that has just given up the ghost!

I swam, flew and soared for an hour in the vibrant land of Nirvana. No regrets, no fears, no worries and no bloody suffering. This is how we are meant to live our lives. Not as brainwashed puppets, conditioned since birth to compete, fret, argue and stress over shit that doesn't really matter.

Unhappily, my overpowering thoughts eventually wrestled back control once more. *Welcome back to your nightmare,* they grinned.

I was back existing as a mindless zombie in the plastic world of plastic people.

Whenever I hit a low point, I would ring the wicked one, clutching at straws for a word of kindness or a droplet of sympathy. All I got was a "Psychotic Reaction" and a manic scream of "Hurry up and die!" I knew only too well that I had to sever all contact for my own sanity.

I did have a sly peep at her FFB page and was appalled when it revealed that she was trying to scam her countless admirers. She was begging for money because her mother had a tumour! What had happened to the hungry-for-love Hungarian geezer? Why didn't he help? Her fans replied with excuse after excuse over why they couldn't transfer any cash. They were either wise to her underhand tricks or just tight-fisted wankers! And I later discovered it was all bullshit. There was nothing wrong with her mum. Surprise, surprise!

In February, my wife made a dramatic return. Not physically but in lucid dreams. Night after night she would be mocking me as once again, she romantically strolled off into the sunset, hand in hand with yet another man. Flaunting gold and new clothes as poor me and the kids were left destitute in a rundown wooden shack. I just couldn't function in the morning because "I Had Too Much to Dream Last Night."

Was there no escape? Seems not, because the dreams have returned with a vengeance as I scribble this chapter. The nightmares of betrayal, humiliation and utter heartbreak have had me waking up in a cold sweat in the middle of the dark night.

However, on a couple of occasions, the dream ended happily. Once, I met a blonde-haired girl with blue eyes on a bus and we just clicked. Another time a lady with black hair on a train. It was instant attraction and love at first sight both times as our passionate bodies were clinging together, our lusty lips moving closer and closer. Before we kissed, I would wake up with a proper morning glory. Sadly, without a blonde or raven-haired nymphomaniac besides me. I had no alternative but to accept the harsh reality that I would be alone until the day I died, just like the Wicked Witch had hatefully foretold.

I inevitably received updates regarding the ex from the various friends who were still appalled that she had abandoned her dying husband and her son. The latest hot-off-the press announcement was that she was sitting pretty in the Samlo pub, messaging on her mobile. Each news flash knifed my heart, but I just couldn't resist being a nosy parker. I had to know.

Jo's caring teacher Miss Haslam recognised that I was struggling to cope and set up a support team to assist. A monthly meeting was arranged at the school where cooking, housework, homework, the children, my health and state of mind were discussed. They were very supportive, even though I found it embarrassing needing help from outside. I had always been my own man. Pauline, a family support worker, would pop round to the house once a week, encouraging me to keep on top of the overwhelming housework.

At half-term on 16th February I grabbed the kids and escaped the haunted house. We stopped at an isolated youth hostel in the Brecon Beacons in South Wales for a couple of nights. Vexed black storm clouds bombarded our mountain shelter with ferocious torrents of bitter rain. We huddled around an open fire playing computer games. Jo delighted in flinging small logs onto the blaze, guaranteeing that the dancing flames kept us toasty as the vicious weather screamed outside.

We took the opportunity for a soggy walk up to the top of a small hill when there was a break in the weather. Twenty minutes later the heavens opened once more, with even greater savagery. Later that day I left the kids toasty warm by the fire and walked alone through the storm. My dreams were tossed and blown far away and I just couldn't visualise the light at the end of the dark tunnel. None of these dark clouds had a silver lining. Half an hour later I arrived back at the shelter sopping wet and jumped into a hot shower before joining the kids by the flames.

That night we went to a pub in the village and sat next to a roaring fire. We had a slap-up meal while watching Barcelona play Manchester City. City lost but I did sup two pints of Dragon Heart, the Welsh real ale. It was my first taste of the taboo demon booze in a long time and I felt as pissed as a broken-hearted rat.

Dizzy

(March to April 2014)

March blew in as I looked high and low for my lost marbles in my very own non-existent padded cell. Dark depressive thoughts tortured me as I climbed the walls in search of an escape. I did manage to flee my despondent black mood briefly on the 2nd March with Manchester City's 3-1 victory over Sunderland in the League Cup final at Wembley before returning back to despair.

In this disconsolate state of mind, I frantically begged the doctor for some anti-depressants. Once home, I gulped one tab of Citalopram and sat eagerly awaiting the peace and calm from a long-lost memory to make a welcome return. "Hell's Bells," I was met with panic and fear as my world fell apart. The kitchen carving knife appeared gigantic and very, very shiny. It was the centre of my attention as it glowed and called, *I am over here waiting for you.* I shuddered and sat trembling in the living room, keeping far away from the glistening blade in the kitchen.

I never popped one of those happy I am a robot pills again. It took five hazy days for the distressing side-effects of just one tablet to wear off. Daytime panic with shaky unease, followed by shocking loud-coloured nightmares each scary night. Fancy supplying medication which causes panic and suicidal thoughts to patients who are deeply depressed. The world is off its head.

Ian, an ex-colleague of mine who was still teaching in Laos, divulged that my ex had started working as a barmaid in a sleazy pub. He said that the evil bunt was flirting with all the new foreigners, who were falling over themselves for her attention. Well, she needed to earn money as she hunted for a new sucker with a big ATM card.

I made a sensible decision for once in my life by deciding to stop struggling like a cripple in the middle of nowhere. I was far too ill to keep up this foolhardy act of bravado. My kids needed me.

***

My dreamboat eyes practically popped out of their head as I ogled a photo of a blue-eyed blonde on the walking site. And she was a dishy vegan too. Perfection. Maybe she was a Manchester City supporter, loved washing dishes, listening to Joy Division, deep meditation and the odd session of physical ecstasy too. By gum, the universe had spoken, so

I sent her a message. She responded in a flash, and we exchanged phone numbers.

Her name was Sandy and she was a City fan. Alas, not God's own team but Stoke City. She was on the payroll of the local council as an office worker. Several health issues, not to mention cheerless depression, were part and parcel of the baggage she came with. Join the club, baby! It was just my rotten luck that an extra item of luggage was a boyfriend. Even though they were going through a rough patch and living apart, all mental pictures of love and lust were swallowed up before you could whisper, "Shall I buy the vegan condoms, or will you?" Having already tasted life as one of *The Walking Dead*, there was no way on earth I would be party to a betrayal. Introducing another poor sod to the "Boulevard of Broken Dreams" just wasn't going to happen. Be that as it may, in no way am I implying that she was the tiniest bit interested in a "Basket Case" like me.

In the evenings we would provide one another with a shoulder to cry on as we sobbed out our anguish, sadness and fear. Our sorrowful heart-to-hearts invariably concluded with heart-warming inspirational dreams, which empowered us into believing that sooner or later there would be a happy ending. Having support from a friend in the same sinking boat was comforting and ace therapy.

The minute we met she fell head over heels in love. Not with me but with little Jo. It was 26th March as we stood under the majestic trees of Delamere Forest. I was overjoyed witnessing Jo squealing with delight as we played hide and seek. Later, we were darting around like medieval heroes in our impromptu Battle of Delamere Forest. Scooping up armfuls of ammo from the forest floor, taking cover behind the mighty trees, before making a frenzied attack. The air beneath the healthy green foliage was awash with screams, whoops and airborne fir-cones. My little soldier was loving it.

The day ended with our new friend mollycoddling and mothering Jo in a nearby pub, where our battle-weary bodies were treated to some hot, tasty grub. This was just what he needed, I reflected. I may well be a doting dad, but Jo needed a woman's touch. Come to think of it, so did I!

***

I received the very welcome two thumbs up from the oncology department as it was announced that the dreaded cancer was still nowhere to be seen. Phew! A bit of good news during these dark gloomy days. I meditated

220

daily and on a handful of occasions ascended to the land of pure bliss for a few minutes before my troublesome thoughts dragged me back down. Pauline, the family support worker, dropped by weekly. She commented that it was a pleasure visiting me because of the devotion and deep love I had for my children, even though my life had fallen apart.

My youngest brother Stephen dropped off an Xbox 360 for Jo. From that moment in time he just couldn't get enough Minecraft. To be perfectly frank, I was relieved because it gave me a bit of peace and quiet.

I remained in wonderment after the astonishing realisation that there was indeed a place of no suffering here on planet Earth. At the close of March, Mister Postman delivered a book I had ordered online: *The Power of Now* by Eckhart Tolle. I was astounded by the truth and wisdom in the book. The main message was that the NOW is the only true reality. Also, that there is no unhappiness when you live in the NOW as suffering only exists in time; the past and the future. It opened my mind and magically transported me to nirvanaesque bliss. This time for a full week! Not in dreamy dreamland but in a crystal-clear reality. The real world was crisp and vibrant when not clouded with my foggy thoughts. Euphoria pulsed through my veins as once again I sparkled with love in my heaven on earth.

I felt like an otherworldly visitor observing the bewildered humans controlled by the meaningless conversations they were having in their minds. Torturing themselves with the past that couldn't be changed and the future that hasn't even happened and will never happen because everything happens NOW. For an entire week I was free from all that madness. The dust had been washed from my eyes and I could see everything just as it really was. I smiled in rapture as I lived in the peaceful space between thoughts.

***

On 6th April we rendezvoused with Sandy once more for a laid-back ramble through some ancient woods close to Frodsham. I was still poorly and unsteady, therefore I happily spent the day observing Jo and his mother-like friend chasing each other. Their laughter bounced off the treetops as they hurled handfuls of leaves into the air. Sadly, our new friend couldn't have children, so Jo was like the son she could never have, and she was like the mother he didn't have. They adored each other.

We had met at the far end of the woods, where we left Sandy's car before cruising in my motor to a pub in Frodsham. The brainwave was to walk from my car at the pub in a leisurely manner through some woods and meadows to her car. Then she would drive us back to the pub for a well-deserved bite to eat. However, the finest plans in the world can always go tits-up when an unforeseen element throws a spanner in the works. And this was just one of those occasions, as you will soon see.

Following an adventurous few hours of fun and games under the trees, we eventually spotted Sandy's car in the distance. It was a sight for sore eyes as our dog-tired bodies longed for a comfy sit-down. Our rumbling tummies were hungering for a mouth-watering feed too. The instant we arrived at the car our vegan chum suddenly cried, "Oh no, I have left my car keys in your car. I am so sorry; what a dizzy blonde I am."

We opted to walk along the road back to my motor rather than traipse back through the woods. Just as we set off, I stuck out my thumb on the off chance of getting a lift. Lo and behold, a van pulled up. A friendly environmental worker smiled and said, "Jump in." He kindly went out of his way to drop us off at the pub where my car was parked. Fantastic. Time for a hot meal and a well-needed rest for our weary bones. Or so I thought!

We were relaxing in the cosy lounge, scrutinising the menu for vegan options when our dizzy friend shouted, "Shit, I have lost my mobile phone." I grinned as I teased, "You really are a dizzy blonde, aren't you?" I called her number, which was answered by a cyclist who had picked it up off the side of the road. We arranged to meet him at a pub about three miles away.

I drove Sandy to her automobile before we both went to meet and thank the cyclist. Finally, we were sitting pretty in a quaint country pub with plates of delicious vegan food in front of us. Sandy was as happy as Larry with her phone and keys safely back in her possession. And you'll never guess what I was supping. A pint of Dizzy Blonde! Yes, you heard correctly. I chuckled with delight when I laid eyes on the draft beer this pub had on tap. Dizzy Blonde - a real ale by the Robinsons brewery. You just couldn't make it up. It was as if the universe was having a laugh. I just had to have one and ordered a pint for the cyclist too. I was grinning like a Cheshire cat as I put my lips to the Dizzy Blonde and drank. I love coincidences like that, and I bet you do too.

Janet and her lovely sister Jacqueline paid us a visit with surprise, surprise Easter Eggs for the kids. Janet had been an angel, standing by me from the moment my very sick body limped into the UK. Supporting me through the terrifying cancer treatment, being there as I screamed in despair, while my wife betrayed me, and always lending an ear as I battled depression and loneliness. It took a few months to return the money I had borrowed to bring the Wicked Witch back, but she never complained. A loyal friend indeed. Janet, my brother Jeff, his wife Ann, as well as a few friends back in Laos helped me survive the nightmare. I would never have made it without them and am eternally grateful.

Funds were tight as you can well imagine, but we managed to get a day out during the school break. Nothing pricy, just a windy walk up a crag in Yorkshire. I did have to splash out £30 in petrol and a few bob for a pub lunch but it was well worth it to be out and about with my kids.

 The solitude was strangling me, as my vacant heart beat with aspirations of rubbing eyeballs with 'the one'. It was another lonely day with no one here, except me sitting silently, nursing my broken heart. Consequently, I grew a pair and joined all the needy souls in the heartless world of online dating. Well, the sphericals would come in useful if I pulled my dream lover, wouldn't they? I scribbled a friendly yet inspiring description of myself, uploaded a recent pic and chopped a few cheeky years off my age. Ridiculous really, coz the bloody cancer had added about twenty! I lounged back in anticipation, looking forward to the messages of love and desire that would soon be flooding into my inbox.

It was a total wash-out because no one responded. This was the day of the cougar, where females in their fifties were hunting for a 20 or 30-year-old partner. Bloody hell, what chance have I got. Who the hell is seeking a fifty-something-year-old monster? Maybe a 95-year-old grandma searching for a 55-year-old toy-boy for a bit of 'slap n tickle.' Instant bloody karma.

I had been spoilt rotten living amongst the birds of paradise in the Far East and having my pick of young nurses, teachers and secretaries. Now I was on the frigging scrap heap, being blown out by old boilers that only needed maintaining once a year. Sexist Syd, I hear you shout. And you are completely right, of course. However, I wasn't in the same league as the unfairer sex of the species on this site. They were sexist superstars. Plain Janes would demand that their prospective dates be good-looking, fit, have their own hair and teeth and sorry, no fatties. Bloody hell, a ghoul like me hadn't got a shout in hell. "What about my sparkling mind and warm heart," I screamed, as karma bit my arse again.

"Serves you right for marrying a girl half your age," I hear you mutter under your breath. I understand where you are coming from but in my defence, I plead innocence because the mitigating circumstances clearly reveal that the bitch was 140 years old in doggie years. That's my pathetic excuse. Woof woof.

One day I contacted a fit maths teacher from nearby Darwen, who was a good-looking slender blonde and not yet a grandmother. We exchanged a few messages before swapping phone numbers. We even enjoyed a chummy chat one evening. Woe is me, coz that potential soulmate vanished before I could declare, "I don't have my own hair and all my fangs, but I am kind and passionate."

A few days later a flirting match kicked off with an attractive European lady from Preston. Would I score this time, or be ruthlessly booted into touch? She prick-teasingly divulged that she would only reveal her nationality if we ever met in the flesh. Bloody hell, she was giving me a hard time already! I was man of the match as I charmed her with my tender heart, turned her on with my naughty innuendos and brought tears to her eyes with my romantic dreams.

My Mancunian banter seemed to have had the desired effect because she let the pussy out of the bag by revealing that she had fallen head over heels for me, which caused me to fall arse over tit in surprise. She passionately declared that I made her feel like a teenager for the first time in years. Looks like I'm gonna score, doesn't it? If we ever meet, I will have to show off my ball skills with a skilful display of keepy-uppy!

She proclaimed that she couldn't linger any longer and insisted on a date. I may be a whizz-kid keyboard chatter-upper but was worried stiff that once she grabbed a flash of my hardened features in real life her jaw would drop before crying foul play. For that very reason I was hesitant. I emphasised that I wasn't God's gift, in fact more like Lucifer's revenge after the bashing the big C had cruelly dished out. She purred, "I don't care about that. We must meet each other."

The match would kick off at 11am on neutral ground; the white windmill in Lytham St. Anne's. Maybe she was Dutch? I drove along the coastal road with a bunch of fragrant flowers I had scored at Marks and Sparks. No vegan condoms or victory V's cos I wasn't counting my chicks just yet.

I was five minutes late as I parked my tiny red Fiat. I snatched a quick peek at an attractive blonde standing by the windmill in the distance. That must be her. Swedish maybe? I took a deep breath and started walking towards happiness or sadness. Love is a funny old game.

It can mend your heart or break it in two.

The seagulls squawked as they floated above the nervy speculation jittering about in my head. I sucked in the slightly salty sea-air as a bitter breeze lashed the tiny bit of flesh I dared to display. I was covered with faded blue jeans, a green anorak, with a dark beanie hat and jet-black shades. Only the lower half of my face was on show. My self-belief was non-existent after being mocked and dumped by my ex. There was no cocky Mancunian swagger as I approached this European femme fatale; just one casual step after another. I ultimately arrived at my goal and uttered, "Hello."

She smiled, and whispered, "Take off your sunglasses."

I calmly removed my shades and then she kissed me full on the lips. Bloody hell, she must be French, I mused. Although she didn't sound French. I heard the crowd in the imaginary stadium cheering as they chanted, "You're gonna get your fucking end away."

We strolled along the shingle beach hand-in-hand. I gazed at the horizon, my heart beating in wonder as the waves gently kissed the shiny pebbles. Every 30 seconds we would stop for a romantic slow-motion mouth-to-mouth. It was just like an action replay each time a goal was scored. This was a dream that I didn't want to wake up from. I looked deep into her dazzling eyes and shot, "You are German." She laughed and nodded. We kissed once more then continued along the beach; heart in heart. I recalled the Wicked Witch taunting that I would be alone forever because no woman would ever love an ugly monster like me again. I felt unreal and smiled to myself that she was wrong. Somebody does love me. Whoop. Whoop.

At the far end of the beach Fraulein Deutschland turned to me and smooched me once more for a long, long, time. I was in seventh heaven. She stared into my mesmerised eyes and purred, "Syd, you are the most amazing, wonderful person I have ever met." *Wunderbar*. I wanted to don some vegan lederhosen, drink a litre of German lager and dance to some Joy Division. Not "Love Will Tear Us Apart", though.

Miss Germany continued, "However, I am very sorry to say that I cannot accept the way the cancer treatment has damaged the lower part of your face. I am really sorry Syd, but us Germans are straight to the point, you know."

I stood in shock as I awoke from my dream to the nightmare. Smiling softly, I said, "It is fine, I fully understand." Then I quipped, "I could always get a face-lift if you like." We sat close together in a

Victorian storm shelter for a while, still holding hands. I laughed and joked as I hid my pain, then escorted my lady to her motor. We kissed another few times before she waved a red card and sent me off.

I walked slowly back to my car with my hat pulled down and the sunglasses covering my face as I hid myself away. I was proud that I had reacted politely and warmly to her crushing admission that I was too ugly for her. I didn't even taunt, "Two world wars and one world cup."

To be honest, I had bucket loads of sympathy for her. Visualise that you are going on a date to meet your dream lover and the creature from the crypt turns up. She must have felt crushed too! The deep connection we had built up online must have triggered the kissing automatically but all the time she must have been fighting against the repulsion of snogging with the living dead. In the final minute the winning goal was scored by Beauty is only "Skin Deep" United against "Owner of Lonely Heart" City.

I drove steadily back along the coastal "Autobahn" and screamed, "*Nein, nein, nein*; emergency, call The Police." I would have more hope of finding my true love by flinging a "Message in a Bottle" into the cold Irish Sea than pissing around with this heartless online dating lark.

I crept into the haunted house and hid under the duvet. I am sure I heard the ghost of the Wicked Witch cackling in *Schadenfreude* ecstasy. "Yes, my dear, you are right. No one will ever love me. I am far too ugly and will die a sad and lonely old man."

I collected Jo from school with a big smile and assisted him with his reading homework, before slaving over the stove cooking something up for the kids. When I tucked Jo into bed, he held my hand and softly pleaded, "Daddy, will you find me a new mum that doesn't hurt me." I smiled as I promised that I would try to find one for him, then kissed him goodnight.

At long last I dragged my knackered body into the large double bed and wept tears of sorrow. Not for me but for Jo. He had suffered so much. I didn't seem to have a prayer of chancing upon a loving partner. Which fair maiden in her right mind was going to be giving the come-on to a penniless crippled skeleton like me, for goodness sake.

The moment before my heavy eyelids shut tight, I grinned. Tomorrow was a new day. No surrender. Bring it on.

River Deep, Mountain High

(May to June 2014)

I experienced the sensation of being a lump of cast-off garbage bobbing up and down as I floated along the river of mangled dreams. I was drowning in self-pity and sorrow, with zilch control over my destination as the current carried me forward to "Tomorrow Never Knows". There were heart-racing turbulent moments desperately clinging onto anyone or anything as I screamed down the rapids. Sluggish lonesome periods of sadness in the doldrums, followed by dark depression when the watercourse took a spiteful turn for the worse, by leading into the venomous jaws of a scary pitch-black cavern. A daunting subterranean nightmare of madness and gloom was endured as I struggled to subdue my hysteria.

In the panic I yearned for a folkloric emerald-green genie to magically materialise and grant me not three wishes but just one. Whoosh, I was back upstream sitting pretty in the paradise I once knew. Sadly, that time and place was nothing but a flashback in my demented mind. The tough-to-swallow truth was that my utopian lifestyle had vanished in a puff of black smoke many full moons ago. It no longer existed, yet here I was desperate to return to a place that was no longer there. The cruel insanity of a broken heart.

The torrents carried me onward as life flowed on, within me and without me. It was either sink or swim as I faced each new challenge head on.

"Is that the hairdresser's?" a lady enquired.

"Sorry, it isn't. This is an out-of-work single dad, so I probably won't be able to help," I chuckled.

"I don't know about that, perhaps you can," the mysterious female replied cryptically.

To snip a long story short, it was the maths teacher from Darwen who I had fleetingly chatted with last month. And now, she had just called my number in error!

We chuckled about her blonde moment and arranged to meet at an off-the-beaten-track country café on Sunday, 11 May. Thoughts of a quick blow-dry and a hot hair-curling love affair were not at the front, or even the short, back and sides of my usually lusty mind. The confidence-shattering sudden kick to the goolies by the German lass had put an immediate halt to any aspirations of love and lust. A bit of useless information is that the word gooly (singular), meaning testicle, originates from the Indian word goli, which translates as ball.

Focusing on the well-being of my children was the solitary factor keeping my drowning head above water. Eugene was either in his room playing computer games or out and about with his girlfriend. He would only give us the pleasure of his company when he decided to join us for dinner or needed dad's taxi. Typical teenager! I would take Jo to playgrounds, a park or the beach after school and at the weekends we would "Run to the Hills" for a breath of fresh air and the treat of a pub lunch at a village tavern.

***

I was up for a busy weekend for a change. On Saturday 10th May I would be meeting Sandy, the dizzy blonde at Leeds Vegan Festival and on Sunday I had a date on the moors with the maths teacher. I had never been to a vegan festival so that was exciting, and the date was an unexpected bonus I suppose.

On the Saturday, Jo and I joined Sandy at the Queen's Hotel where the vegan festival was being held. She was accompanied by her best friend, 'Big Ted'. Puzzlingly, Big Ted was neither tall nor big. In truth, just a typical slim fellow in his forties. If my foggy chemo-brain recollects accurately, he was nicknamed Big Ted because he reminded Sandy of a large cuddly teddy bear. He made ends meet as a website designer in Manchester. I liked him instantly and got the vibration that Big Ted was one of life's good guys.

I was pleasingly flabbergasted by the masses of vegans fervently snapping up the cruelty-free merchandise on sale. I held Jo's hand tightly as we explored stall after stall of vegan food, soaps, t-shirts, cakes and perfumes. I also did my bit for the voiceless by signing all the petitions presented by the many animal rights groups.

At last I was somewhere I belonged. This was my tribe and we were living the plant-based dream. It made a welcome change from the eye-rolling taunts of, "How do you get your protein?" from the mocking corpse-munchers.

The vegans were a vibrant body of smartly dressed fashionable souls, not the dirty unwashed mob of tree-hugging hippies they are often wrongly portrayed as. I was smitten by the sweet eye-candy in their skin-tight black jeans, fake leather boots and animal rights t-shirts. I was hypnotised by a "Venus" in blue jeans rebelliously wearing a 'Don't eat Animals, eat Pussy' t-shirt. If only I had been sporting a 'Don't eat Animals, eat Cock,' t-shirt. It would have been the perfect ice breaker as I grabbed her attention before smirking, "Tasty t-shirt, love."

I remained goo-goo eyed as these drop-dead gorgeous birds of a feather flocked together. Their eye-snatching vegan tattoos and outlandish face piercings announced that this plant-based, cruelty-free lifestyle was not just a passing fad but here to stay. I'm in with "The In-Crowd"; I eat where the in-crowd eats.

This wasn't the time or place to be at my silver-tongued swashbuckling best, even though vegan females outnumbered vegan males by about three to one! The truth was good, bad and bloody ugly. The good being that most of these compassionate dishy dolls would only date a vegan partner, so the odds were heavily stacked in favour of the rare vegan male. The bad was that they were all a lot younger than me and the ugly was that I was a dead ringer for the creature from the crypt.

Consequently, I wisely dodged making a flirtatious beeline for these delectable vegan honeys. I was still smarting from the savage sting in the tail delivered by my previous Queen Bee. I needed to be a ridiculous old man with a partner half my age like I needed a hole in my head. Been there, done that; lost the t-shirt, lost the house and almost lost my mind. Once love-bitten, twice shy, as the saying goes.

We had a fab time with Sandy and Big Ted. The four of us toddled off to a close-at-hand bohemian cafe to munch a vegan pizza. I even braved a 'naughty but nice' glass of organic vegan beer too. Sandy made a massive fuss of Jo as she mothered him, while Big Ted and I swapped sorrowful memories of smashed hearts and shattered dreams.

I recognised that veganism was destined to be mega as my grey matter commenced brainstorming ideas for a potential vegan venture. Surely there must be something I could do to break free from the mind-numbing world of life on government handouts. My foggy imagination failed to espy the crystal-clear reality that the likely 'end result' would be winding up six feet under in a coffin, rather than flying high as a triumphant entrepreneur sitting pretty in the house on the hill.

***

The following day I met the teacher from Darwen at the remote café on a windswept Lancashire moor. She was a tall and slender blonde bombshell, tastefully presented in a crimson top and slate-grey jeans. I fancied the pants off her. As well as looking the bee's knees, this vegetarian beauty provided me with an unexpected warm-hearted buzz after producing a small bottle of soya milk for my coffee. Her thoughtfulness touched my plant-based heart. She didn't even avert her eyeballs in 'repulsion at first sight' after coming face-to face with my ghoulish visage. Things are looking up, I thought. Although on the downside, she could have thrown up when she popped into the loo, I daresay!

I made none of my off-the-cuff gung-ho flirty remarks because I felt she was way out of my league. In all honesty, after being dumped by the Wicked Witch and rejected by Fraulein Deutschland I sensed I was out of every woman's league. Relegated from the Premier League to the Sunday pub team league in just one season. No longer dining at the top table and not even bin-dipping for scraps. The final score was that I was starving to death.

We had an engaging amble through some romantic shady woods, chirping away about this and that as the birds and the bees energetically made public it was the spring season. Not for me though; it was still winter in my broken heart and not the time to 'go forth and multiply' with this mathematical head-turner. And when all is said and done, things just didn't add up because she was a smart uptown teacher on a decent monthly salary and I was a scruffy downtown nonentity on benefits.

I drove back to Blackpool flying high after a couple of blissful hours with the teacher. Please Miss, if I don't do my calculus homework, will you give me six-of-the-best?

My football team Manchester City were flying high too, sitting pretty at the top of the Premier League. They just needed to defeat West Ham United in the final match of the season to get their hands on the trophy. Liverpool were waiting in the wings for us to do a 'Steven Gerrard' and slip up, therefore victory was vital in this potential banana skin encounter. At 4.55pm I stood in the crowded pub across the road from my humble abode, nervously watching the game on the big screen, before singing "Blue Moon" at the final whistle, as we were victorious and deservedly crowned champions. A perfect ending to a "Perfect Day."

***

Astonishingly, Miss Bombshell was enthusiastic about getting together again. "The Lady and the tramp" rendezvoused on two more occasions that merry month of May. First off, there was a bit of banter and a hot coffee in a cafe before hitting the great outdoors for a leisurely walk in England's green and pleasant land. She was wonderfully patient as my feeble damaged body doddered along, repeatedly halting for a five-minute break to catch my breath. Each meeting, my new ladyfriend supplied me with a bottle of water and a couple of bananas. What more could a cheeky northern monkey like me wish for? And don't send your answers on a postcard please, because I wouldn't know where to put my face, when our post-lady delivers the next package of herbal tonics.

We got on like the proverbial farmhouse on fire. Chattering about anything and everything, slagging off our old flames and causing each other to giggle with our childish jokes and riddles. Swapping anecdotes from the good, sad and mad old days would leave the pair of us either shocked in disbelief, angry at the injustice or pissing ourselves laughing at the absurdity of it all.

She would tutor me in the German language and I provided instructions in Thai. Deep down I was fantasising that we could teach each other how to speak in tongues but I knew full well that those oral language exchanges were just imaginary lip service; empty hollow thoughts.

On a more positive note, it was heart-warming having a friend to phone up for a natter in the evenings, which would be followed by spending time searching for a café and an interesting location for us to visit the next weekend, when Eugene would kindly take care of Jo for the afternoon.

I would often dream that maybe, just maybe, the friendship would develop into something a tad more romantic. To walk hand in hand, perhaps with a tender kiss… I supposed I wanted to have my Angel Cake and eat it.

Out of the sky blue the missus forwarded an image of herself smiling as she posed next to a white aircraft. My beady eyes spotted that she was wearing the Supergirl t-shirt I had bought her when we visited China in 2010. If I had known then what I now knew, I would have got her a Wander Woman (lol) top instead. She explained that she was in Sam Nuea, in the north-east of Laos, visiting some distant relatives. Good for her, but Messenger proclaimed that she was a dirty rotten liar because the image was sent from Luang Prabang airport, which was nowhere near Sam Nuea. She was more than likely having a dirty weekend with the latest western bloke she'd picked up. That was up to her but why was she lying to me and messing with my mind? A leopard never changes its acne, I suppose.

On the 3rd June Jo attended his first Young Carer's Youth Club evening, thanks to Pauline, my family support worker. This weekly get-together was organised to provide young children of severely disabled or terminally ill parents with a refuge to break away from the heartrending set of circumstances they faced at home. Once a week they would meet up for a couple of hours to smile, laugh and have fun with playmates who were enduring a similar tragic homelife. My eyes would well up with tears as I observed these innocent young kids running wild, laughing and playing.

The pitiful truth was that in a very short time they would return home to their seriously sick parent or even worse, a mum or dad who was about to die. I watched my son, Jo, as he painted a picture of the sky. I was alive to the harsh reality that his dad, the only person he had left in the whole wide world, had a death-sentence hanging over him. I smiled warmly at Jo and the other kids as I screamed inside with fury at the steely-cold nightmare that these poor kids were having to live through.

Two weeks later Pauline dropped off a jumbo box of creative toys and games such as jigsaw puzzles, artbooks, board games, paints and building bricks to entice Jo away from his unhealthy addiction to computer games. Each evening after his homework was done and dusted, we would have an hour of dad and lad time, building, painting or participating in a game of snakes and ladders.

He was highly competitive, and it would be anarchy in the living room if he happened to lose. Pure pandemonium as he shouted and stamped his feet in rage, subsequently flinging the game to the floor. I sat him down, explaining that losing was part and parcel of life and that he must accept it with dignity. He should learn from it, then try his best to be victorious in the future. Was I speaking to Jo or myself? His angry outbursts became a thing of the past following the promise of an hour of computer games after dinner if he took defeat on the chin without throwing a tantrum. Problem solved.

The weekend get-togethers with Miss Bombshell were progressing perfectly. It was a bed of roses having my very own agony aunt to share my wacky mind with. She was a single mum with two teenage kids. This gorgeous Penelope Pitstop had put her foot down by pulling the plug on wedlock after discovering that her partner had been doing a Dick Dastardly with some other woman. I suppose that made me an agony uncle, come to think about it. Even so, I wasn't at the races with regards to driving off into the sunset in her compact pussycat. I was no Peter

Perfect by any stretch of the imagination.

Nevertheless, my wishful thinking involved the pipedream that one day before too long, the following hot- off-the-press read all about it headline would appear in the *East Lancashire Telegraph*: 'Agony Aunt and Agony Uncle Fall Head Over Heels in Love on Misty Moor'. "And piggie-wiggies can fly," I chuckled.

On 22nd June, at long last, Jo met Miss Bombshell upstairs in Morgan's café in the small town of Barnoldswick. Barnoldswick is one of the longest place names in the UK without repeating any letters, although the locals refer to it as Barlick. It is also home to Silentnight, the UK's largest bed and mattress manufacturer. Perhaps I would be a future customer if I ever pulled the girl of my dreams, but for the time being I would have to snooze quietly, all alone in my fleapit.

Jo and Miss Bombshell hit it off instantaneously. He held her hand as we sauntered along the Leeds and Liverpool Canal. When we sat down for a drink and a banana he softly kissed her cheek. That peck on the cheek kissed my heart too. It was heart-warming witnessing him getting a drop of motherly love. I did do my best as a single dad, but I suppose it just wasn't the same.

As we resumed our slow walk, Jo startled the pair of us by asking Miss Bombshell to hold daddy's hand. We gawked at each other, shrugged our shoulders before obeying our 'Lord and Master' and walked on hand in hand. A few minutes later he left us open-mouthed when he badgered us to kiss. We refused but his relentless pleading resulted in our lips awkwardly touching for a split second, putting a halt to his constant pestering.

And much to my astonishment, at that very instant I knocked off itching for Miss Bombshell to be a conceivable love-mate but was chuffed to bits that she was a close friend. The chemistry just wasn't there; it wasn't meant to be. I experienced a whopping sensation of relief that cold water had been tossed onto my 'ready and willing' "Achy Breaky Heart" and my rampant one-eyed trouser snake, thus extinguishing all desires for love and lust. I didn't want anything to fuck up this beautiful friendship. I glanced at the Silentnight factory on the other side of the canal and smirked inwardly; *Sorry, you have just lost a customer.*

I did feel shedloads of sympathy for little Jo. The sudden abandonment by his mother at a very young age had unquestionably affected him adversely. He was without doubt determined to replace the mum he had lost but that improbable occurrence was only going to transpire if I came across 'true love' sometime in the future. "You Can't Hurry Love", can you?

***

Ian and I had been ace drinking buddies for many years whilst I was in Laos. He was a stocky, quietly spoken Englishman in his fifties, always ready to laugh. He had a "Heart of Gold". I would portray him as the quintessential ex-pat who enjoyed a beer, watched live football, dated a local girl and taught English as a foreign language. He was living the dream as I lived the nightmare in bloody Blackpool. After my rapid dash back to the UK he had kept in regular contact offering support, as well as supplying me with up-to-the-minute news regarding my little runaway.

He had just returned to the UK for a couple of weeks to visit his mum in Watford. He elected to kill two birds with one stone by popping into his local hospital while he was back home. He explained that he had been feeling a bit out of sorts and had this shuddersome fear that it could be the dreaded motor neurone disease which runs in his family. We didn't meet but I wished him luck.

Eugene hopped over to France to spend a month with his mum and his sister. Upon his return he would be accompanied by my daughter Francesca. I was over the Blue Moon" at the prospect of spending a few weeks with her soon.

I persisted in treading water in the River of Mangled Dreams and without warning I hurtled over a thunderous waterfall, plummeting rapidly into a swirling pool of deep depression. I sensed that I was going under, powerless to escape my intolerable predicament. I really was up shit creek without a paddle.

I was fed up to the back teeth of enduring the dire after-effects of the chemo-radiotherapy. There was pain in my jaw, neck, back and arms as my muscles kept locking tight, causing me to scream out loud. I was unable to swallow solid food and choking up over a cup of yucky phlegm every morning was another ordeal I had to live with. I felt more dead than alive! And to put the cat amongst the pigeons, the tormenting thought that the bastard cancer was more than likely to return was always there.

On top of that, there was the never-ending housework, shopping, cooking, school runs and taking care of the kids. At times I had no energy and was either shivering or burning up with fever. The loneliness was

234

eating me up inside, too. I had no alternative but to struggle on because my children had no one else. I knew full well that I was incredibly fortunate to still be breathing in and out, although most of the time it didn't feel that way. I was sick to death of my life.

There had to be more to life than just clinging on in a dark depression, robbed of any promise of change. A flashback to the jam-packed vegan fair produced the brainwave to form a company; Loving Kindness Limited. I decided to import the rare, high quality 'Lao Mountain coffee' and flog it to restaurants, cafes and at vegan fairs. Initially not for profit, but in the distant future I would be able to escape benefits and lead a normal life, if the business took off. At least it would furnish me with a dream while I washed the pots and slaved over a hot stove.

I approached the coffee supplier in Laos and reached an agreement to be their sole UK distributer. So far so good. The fly in the ointment was that the minimum quantity that could be shipped was an almighty 500 kilograms. To get the business off the ground I would have to splash out approximately six grand for the coffee and its transportation from the mountains in central Laos to my terraced house in Blackpool. With no assets and trapped on benefits, how on earth was I gonna pull this one off. Not to be deterred, I swiftly threw together a business plan and made an appointment with the bank.

I felt a complete and utter cheeky bastard upon entering the bank a few days later to ask for a loan of £7500. Who in their right mind was going to give the two thumbs up to handing over seven thousand notes to a critically ill man who didn't have two pennies to rub together? It was going to be a painful experience, just like visiting the dentist; but it was too late now.

A dumbfounded, dazed and ecstatic Psycho Syd floated out of the bank 45 minutes later. The loan application had been approved and the dosh was already in my account. I couldn't bloody believe it. "You lucky bugger," I laughed. It must have been that dog shit I stood in last week. Maybe I should contact a supermodel and ask for a date. If a skint down and out can legally get his grubby mitts on over seven blinking thousand pounds, then anything is possible. I shrewdly decided against lining up any hot dates because business must come first. There was no time for whispering sweet nothings or hot sessions of the 'old ins and outs'. I had 500 kilos of blooming coffee to get rid of.

The lion's share of my unexpected windfall was eaten up before the idea of doing a runner and living on a remote tropical island with my two kids, had had a chance to cross my itchy-footed mind. Once the coffee and the shipping bill had been settled, nine hundred quid remained for printing flyers, booking stalls at vegan fairs and all the other stuff that was bound to crop up.

At some point I grassed myself up to the benefits department. I went into detail concerning my little venture, emphasising that it was all non-profit. They didn't throw the book at me or lock me up in the monkey house, but surprisingly, the bureaucrat interviewing me wished me all the luck in the world. I was told, "We are not chasing a man with terminal cancer alone with two young kids. Therefore, we are 'fine and dandy' with what you are doing but please inform us if you make a profit." Wow, the civil service has a heart. Another piece of good news was that Sandy's friend Big Ted offered to build me a website free of charge.

What I failed to consider was how seriously ill I was.

At the close of June 2014, I was still not clear of the damn cancer and in debt to the bank for the humongous sum of seven and a half bags of sand (grand), plus interest. And in a few short weeks, five hundred kilograms of organic coffee would be on my doorstep. What the hell had I gone and done?

I had better pull my flipping finger out and stop feeling sorry for myself in the river of misery, I reflected. It was time to get out because I now had a very high mountain to climb. Hurry up Psycho, otherwise you won't only be in deep water, but in deep shit too!

If I Had a Hammer

(July-August 2014)

July commenced with me, myself and my shadow popping into the hospital for yet another endoscopy test. I took my place in the chock-a-block waiting room. I was a silent "Solitary Man" studying all the other sorrowful patients with their disfigured faces and burnt scarlet necks. I surreptitiously dabbed a lonesome tear off my cheek upon experiencing an eerie yet fleeting moment of déjà vu. Once again, I was the only unaccompanied cancer fighter in the room.

Before long, my eyes would be flooded with tears because the unpleasant endoscopy test not only evoked a gagging sensation but resulted in my eyes watering like buggery. Eventually, it was my turn to plonk myself down into the comfy cream medical chair in the white examination room. I mused over the only two possible outcomes to this investigation. Either, a 'Thank fuck for that' moment after being notified that the big C was nowhere to be seen. Or an 'Oh shit' occasion if the results screamed that the cancer had made a most unwelcome comeback.

And if the disease had returned, as a rule it would be far more aggressive. And that worst-case scenario would be all my scary nightmares rolled into one as my broken mind and body undertook an agonising journey to death's door. Ashes to ashes, dust to dust.

"Yabba-Dabba-Doo," I triumphantly hollered after the oncologist reported, "All clear Mr Barnes." I wasn't about to make a song and dance about it or blow my own trumpet just yet, though. There were still three more years of intimidating hospital tests to endure. And if I miraculously achieved the impossible by getting the all-clear each time then hallelujah; I would be discharged as a cancer-free homo sapien. That would be the day to sing and dance and hopefully by then I would have a beautiful Wilma on my arm to blow my trumpet for me.

On a more serious note I fully grasped the significance of my "Never say die" mindset in this struggle for survival. A healthy raw vegan diet of organic fruit, vegetables and herbs was the name of the game to stand any chance of winning the war against the bastard cancer.

My mate Ian returned to Laos but didn't manage to visit the hospital during his time in the UK. He commented that he was extremely anxious because he still wasn't feeling himself. I advised him to visit a doctor over there and pronto. The way things were going, it looked like we would be supporting each other from now on.

On the 7th July Jo and I jumped into our tiny red Fiat for a spin down the motorway to visit our dizzy vegan friend Sandy in Newcastle-under-Lyme. Once we stepped foot inside her tidy terraced house, we made ourselves at home. Jo kept an eye on *a Scooby Doo* cartoon on TV, and a hand on Mitzy-Woo Sandy's black and white moggy. Whilst Jo's eyeballs were glued to the goggle box, Sandy and I had a good old natter. She despondently revealed that she was still living apart from her boyfriend. To make matters worse, her 'one and only' was working all the hours God sends as a long-distance van driver, meaning they hardly ever saw each other. She confessed to 'hitting the bottle' each evening in a forlorn attempt to blot out the reality of her burdensome predicament.

I could only offer sympathy and support as well as inspiring her into believing that things would surely get better. It was easy to look into her eyes and utter, "The Future's so Bright You Gotta Wear Shades", because I had been egging myself on with that inspirational phrase for over two bloody years.

During the sunny afternoon we took a trip to "Strawberry Fields Forever." It was a very real fruit farm with a stunning line-up of gooseberries, raspberries, blackberries and countless rows of strawberry plants. Jo was beaming with a massive smile on his happy mug as he attentively selected the largest, juiciest specimens before placing them in his basket. After all, strawberries had been his favourite fruit since he had been knee-high to a grasshopper. We jumped back into the car nibbling on our succulent treasure. Ms S was dropped off back home before the two-hour drive back to Blackpool. By the time we arrived home we had scoffed the blooming lot.

It jogged my memory of a time in the far-flung past when, as a young scallywag, I went scrumping for apples. A dozen were pilfered off a neighbour's tree before I promptly scarpered to the adjacent woods. I proudly lazed in a shady nook by a babbling brook clutching my tasty booty. With a naughty smile and a smattering of self-reproach, I unwisely 'pigged out' on my mouth-watering pickings. In due time I discovered that Hades hath no rage like a bellyful of plundered fruit. I lay on the sofa gripping my painful tummy sobbing, "Never again".

It was a side-splitting first taste of 'never again,' which would be wailed a few years down the road after waking up with a mega *Katzenjammer*, which is German for 'magnificent hangover'. After sneaking into the pub as a naive 16-year-old, I short-sightedly guzzled five pints of cheap man's black velvet; a savage mix of cider and Guinness. My cockeyed act of bravado culminated in a gut-wrenching technicolour yawn as I vomited all over the kitchen wall. My poor mother would be furious and not impressed with the new piece of modern art abstractly splattered over the plain white wallpaper. My vile, foul-smelling concoction of cider, Guinness, mushy peas and carrots would be no masterpiece as far as mum was concerned. I was an artist; a piss-artist.

I rose from the death the following afternoon, feeling as sick as a "Hound Dog", with a thundering headache and eyes like piss-holes in the snow. *Katzenjammer* can be directly translated as cat's misery, but I haven't the foggiest idea why. Although, I did feel a proper pussy for the rest of the day as I pitifully whimpered, "never again". Karma can be a right bastard, can't it?

***

The weekly meet-ups in an 'out in the sticks' café with Ms Bombshell were going amazingly well. Our friendly chinwags inspired me to struggle on. Moreover, the leisurely saunter did my death-warmed-up body and broken mind, the world of good. Jo joined us once but didn't plead with us to smooch or walk hand-in-hand, thank goodness.

I got the painful picture that my broken heart needed a dose of tender loving care, but also understood that this wasn't the time or place for a romantic relationship. I was still in severe shock at being betrayed and abandoned by the woman I had loved and trusted. I just wasn't ready for anyone. I had to heal before I could love and believe again.

I was anxious to say the least when Jo was admitted into the hospital for an operation to have four teeth extracted. I even phoned his mother, informing her that her son was in hospital. She coldly snapped, "I am not interested. It is none of my business." I was shocked to say the least.

I sat fretting in the waiting room as painful mental pictures of my baby undergoing surgery tormented my mind. At long last a nurse notified me that Jo would shortly be regaining consciousness.

She asked, "Would you like to sit next to his bed to comfort him?"

"Yes, of course," I responded.

I was warned that his face would be bloody and that he may be screaming because some children react badly to the anaesthetic. However, not to be alarmed.

I sat next to his bed super-alarmed as my bulging eyeballs focused on my son's blood-spattered face. Suddenly he began crying and pleading, "Dad, help me."

My paternal and maternal instincts instantly kicked in as I held him closely. After all, I was mum and dad, wasn't I? I reassured him, "I am right here, you will be fine, and Daddy loves you."

My heart beat rapidly as floods of tears gushed down my cheeks. I didn't give a fuck who was watching; my baby was hurting and that's all I cared about. I was horrified that my Jo was enduring so much pain and confusion and like any good parent was wishing I could take his place.

Thirty minutes later he was fine. A bit groggy with a sore mouth, but out of the nightmare that I found so unbearable to witness.

He made a swift recovery and a few days later he was 'as right as Blackpool rain'; running around, playing games and laughing his little head off.

My heart went out to all parents whose little ones were suffering in pain as I reflected on the ordeal my son had just suffered. I cried inside at the thought that some mums and dads were living with the horror that their child was terminally ill. And what about innocent kids who were sexually abused by warped monsters or even worse had been kidnapped or vanished without a trace. That pain would be unbearable.

I may well be a peace-loving vegan hippy but if any pervert ever messed with my son, I wouldn't be responsible for my actions if I ever got my hands on them. And I am not joking!

***

On 21st July, Ian sent me a text letting me know that my ex had quit the pub because she had met a man with a lot of cars! Ah, so that is why she didn't give a shit about her son in hospital. She had a new conquest to focus on. Good for her but it still knifed my soul. Why couldn't I just let go and accept that she was nothing to do with me and Jo anymore? She didn't love us or want us. She was ready for a brand-new life far away from us. We had served our purpose and she had moved on. Why couldn't I move on too and start over, instead of crying my eyes out as I lived in the past?

I recalled a few words of wisdom spoken by the monk at the local Buddhist centre: "If someone hits you with a hammer and hurts you, then why do you keep picking up the hammer and hitting yourself after they have gone away?"

I fully understood the truth of his wise words, but I was still humping a ten-ton "Sledgehammer" around and just couldn't put the bloody thing down. Each time I heard a song, visited a shop or gazed longingly at a photo from the time we were together, then "wallop wallop", Psycho's invisible hammer came down upon my head. If I received an update about the Wicked Witch's happy new life, I would clobber myself until I saw stars. I wished I could knock some sense back into my brainless skull and stop beating myself up over someone who wished I was dead.

Ian also informed me that he was now struggling to eat and having problems with his speech. He was terrified that it could be the onset of MND. Once again, I told him to hurry up and see a doctor before he ended up worrying himself to death.

On the 24th July Eugene and Francesca were back from France. My daughter stayed for a wonderful week. One glorious sunny day we went as a family to a picnic site by a beautiful river and took heaps of photos. Another time we got lost in a nearby maze. It was bliss living a second childhood playing with my kids. "I Don't Wanna Grow Up"!

***

At the end of July, the Wicked Witch contacted me asking for a divorce. Where's that sledgehammer? She was quite friendly for once because she wanted something. I just replied, "Give me a few days to think about it."

On the first of August I met a lady who had contacted me by email, asking for a get-together to exchange views on spirituality. The rendezvous spot was a rocky beach near Silverdale, about an hour's drive from Blackpool. She was a tall Czech Goddess clad in pink jeans and a pink top, with a black and white Jack Russell called Bobby. She could have just stepped out of the latest Eastern European fashion magazine. Yours truly had just crept out of the classic 70's horror comic *Uncanny Tales from the Grave*. It was a match made in heaven and hell.

We ambled along the beach discussing meditation, yoga and the meaning of life before having a coffee at a café. I gazed at this heavenly seeker of truth before naming her my Pink Angel. She almost died laughing, wittily responding with, "Syd, you are my Grim Reaper." I would be more than willing to love her to death I suppose!

It was blissful living in the present moment with this gorgeous like-minded being, even if it was only for a couple of hours. Eventually, we said our farewells and vowed to meet up at some point in the future. We went our separate ways, each of us following the middle path to the promised land of Nirvana.

The wife was buddy-buddy once more as she pleaded for a divorce. I clarified that I would be more than happy agreeing to her request providing that she transferred $15,000 to my bank account. She could keep her greedy little paws on the house, land and everything else I had toiled ten sweaty years for. If her new bloke with lots of cars was as filthy rich as I was led to believe, then fifteen thousand greenbacks was mere peanuts to pay off a skint northern monkey like me.

She replied, "No problem. My mother and father have said that it is only right and proper that I send some money to you."

If she kept her word that would be marvellous, meaning I could clear the bank loan and with the surplus treat the kids to a much-needed vacation. I didn't dash to my old laptop to search for a holiday in the sun just yet though. She was as sly as they come and lower than a snake's belly. I knew full well that she would indulge in any dirty deed imaginable to sidestep returning anything that she had pinched from me. And yes, she had stolen it. It wasn't me who committed adultery and abandoned her in her hour of need, was it? As my friend Janet wisely pointed out, 'A leopard never changes its spots'. Therefore, I was agreeing to nowt until the 15 grand was sitting pretty in my bank account and who could blame me? She needed to cough up just a fraction of what was rightfully mine to get this northern monkey off her back.

I lifted the hammer once more upon discovering that my ex had not only been sleeping with the Hungarian bloke and the geezer with many cars but also learnt that she had been 'having it off' with a mate of mine from Sunderland. Bloody hell, once she was single, they are like flies around a lump of shit. In all reality it was me who was the turd because after all, I was the one who was dumped.

I was as chuffed as mint balls when Eugene successfully grabbed heaps of GSCEs He promptly enrolled at Blackpool Sixth Form College to study A levels. I mulled over the fact that he had attended so many different schools around the planet. On some occasions he had spent months off school as we hit the road travelling. What a clever lad, he surely took after his old fella. I was as proud as punch.

A truck arrived with my 500kg of coffee, which took up half the dining room. Shit, what had I done!

A vegan lady from Salisbury had been flirting with me on a spiritual dating site. Her raunchy messages left nothing to the imagination, implying that her idea of a perfect date was a full-blown afternoon of dirty sex. She even enticed me by sending a photo of herself in a red bikini. I licked my lips in anticipation as my libido exploded, thinking, "Wow, she is a knockout". No Viagra needed for this sex bomb. But was I up for it? The last time I'd had a session of the good old 'ins and outs' seemed like ancient history. No need to panic. It must be like riding a bike. Once you have mastered the skill you just jump on and do what comes naturally.

She invited me to meet her in Salisbury. Should I be a daredevil and go? In for a penny, in for a pound, as the saying goes. I burnt rubber down south and chuckled to myself as my one-track mind fantasised that I would soon be burning rubber with the condoms which were stashed in my jeans pocket.

The moment she set eyeballs on me her face dropped to the floor. I instantly realised that there was no chemistry as far as she was concerned, therefore the human biology practical I had so eagerly anticipated would only ever be theory. It didn't ruffle my feathers because rejection was the new norm. It was like water off a duck's back. There wasn't a pussycat in hell's chance that I was going to get Donald Ducked so, I decided to grin and bear it and make the most of this unwelcome turn of events.

I was at ease and chirpy as we politely frittered away a couple of hours chatting. We meandered along the River Avon before having a mosey around the shops. I even splashed out and bought her a couple of bath bombs, so she could clean the sexy body that my dirty mind would never get to explore. Her loss, ha-ha.

As I put pedal to the metal on my journey back to Blackpool I reflected on my previous successes with the opposite sex, from the wine bars and nightclubs in Manchester to the pubs and discos in Bangkok. I was always the one who would pull and get my wicked way. Yet here I was now, not being blown off, but being blown out left, right and centre. Should I fling the contraceptives in the motorway service station rubbish bin or hang onto them before passing them on to Jo in ten years' time? They were of no use to me because it didn't look like I would be getting my 'end away' again during this lifetime. Karma can give you one hell of a painful kick in the balls, can't it?

The friendship with Ms. Bombshell was blossoming, which was the one sparkling light during these dark desperate days. She patiently lent an ear to my fears, regrets and angst-ridden thinking after my life had been obliterated beyond recognition. She was the honeyed spoonful of medicine needed to soothe my despondent mind. It was not all gloom and doom as all our little heart-to-hearts were peppered with off-the-wall jokes, humorous anecdotes and rib-tickling laughter. The significance of this close friendship was nothing to be sneezed at, though. Knowing that Ms Bombshell genuinely cared about my well-being was crucial in psyching me up to continue plodding along the arduous, long and twisting road to recovery.

On the 26th August Ian notified me that he had caught sight of my wife in the pub with a big tall fella in his 40's. "Bang Bang". Ouch my head hurts. I visualised her sitting pretty with a towering, good-looking bloke who had wads of cash and a fleet of flash automobiles. They were holding hands, kissing and so in love. Next, I pictured myself sitting all alone, ugly and without a pot to piss in. Holding my head in my hands, smooching any hope of happiness goodbye as I nursed my broken heart. Life just didn't seem damn fair.

How on earth was it possible that the faithful partner who had worked and given his wife everything he had, was now sitting alone in poverty? Yet, the unfaithful other half who had lied through her back teeth, and had never worked, was now as gleeful as a swine in shite. The dirty rotten two-timing cheat had her thieving hands on everything I had worked for and she even had a brand-new lover to boot. Where was the justice in that?

This shameful one-sided state of affairs is far too commonplace nowadays, with the loyal partner usually getting the shitty end of the stick. I have heard that this idiom is as old as the hills, dating back to the pre-bog-roll and Daily Mail era. During this period a stick was left inside the outside loo to knock the poo off one's bum. Unfortunately, at night without a lantern or if the candle blew out, then on occasions the unlucky sod taking a dump would grab the wrong or shitty end of the stick. Is this the true origin of this idiom or just a load of old crap? I haven't the faintest idea but if curiosity gets the better of you, then you better get your shit together and google it!

Come on karma, hurry up and pull your bloody finger out. How long will I have to linger until she gets her just desserts of a dish best served cold? I want sweet revenge, with my face smirking in *Schadenfreude* ecstasy before screaming, "It serves you fucking right". Don't dilly-dally, karma, coz I am relying on you to ensure that the law of cause and effect comes around and bites the Wicked Witch on her double-crossing arse. And when that day of retribution arrives, I will be pissing myself laughing loudest while the evil one laughs on the other side of her deceitful face. Until that wonderful day I will curl up on my sick sofa, howling in misery with my barking mad thoughts. But remember my love; every dog has his day.

Come to think of it, thoughts are just thoughts. They are not real. It was only my tormenting mind painting pictures that may not be true. He could be fat, bald, ugly and covered in tacky tattoos. His fleet of cars could just be rusty old bangers ready for the scrap heap. They could have had a blazing row. Who knows? The truth was that, whatever he looked like and however much dosh he had, it was none of my bloody business.

Thoughts cause suffering; without them there is no pain. Time to retreat to that warm, peaceful place beneath my mind. Nothing can hurt me there.

I instantly stopped suffocating in self-pity after Ian revealed that he had just been diagnosed with the dreaded motor neurone disease. I gasped in terror at this cruel twist of fate. Lord have mercy! This pernicious illness leads to difficulty in speaking and swallowing as the poor victim's limbs waste away. There is no effective treatment or cure and the average sufferer will only survive for two years after diagnosis.

He was terrified and asked me for help and support as I was the only person he knew who had been given a death sentence too. He continued, "Other people who have never experienced the horror of living with a terminal illness haven't a clue how it feels". That comment hit home as I recalled spotting people crying on Facebook about a headache or diarrhoea. I would fume, "You lucky bastard; if you only knew what it was like screaming in agony with terminal cancer!"

I stressed that I was always here for him and would message daily.

I hid under the duvet that night and sobbed. Not tears of pity for my sorrowful life of pain and loneliness. Or droplets of heartache over the discovery that the woman I loved was as happy as Larry with her new fella. These flowing tears were for my close friend who was scared shitless, numb and confused after being informed that he was going to die.

I was transported back to that shocking day in May 2012 when I was handed the DS1500 form by the clinical nurse. I flashed back to the moment when time stood still, as the words 'TERMINAL ILLNESS - Life expectancy less than six months,' screamed out at me. And right here right now, I was reliving that earthshattering time, once more experiencing the very same hysteria that my friend on the other side of the planet was now tasting.

I gradually recaptured my self-control and joylessly concluded that there was always someone worse off. It was almost two years to the day since the traumatic cancer treatment had thankfully ended. Miraculously, I was still alive. Now it was Ian's turn to walk that mind-numbing "Boulevard of Broken Dreams" Been there, done that (wrote the guidebook).

Once more I drifted back to the evening following my cancer diagnosis, when I endeavoured to look on the bright side of death by grasping that a person paralysed from the neck down was irrefutably in a much worse place than me. That futile attempt at uplifting my terrified spirit only lingered for a few split seconds before my scared-to-death mind shot back to ME and the sharp truth that I was fighting for my life. The vision of the paralysed person vanished without a trace as my survival instinct kicked in. I had no alternative but to focus my undivided attention on me and my struggle, if there was to be any hope of this life or death battle ending victoriously. Dying was not an option back then as my wife and kids needed me!

I have no idea what weird logic incited my madcap mind to unexpectedly navigate back to an episode 14 years earlier. I was squashed on a bus with my three-year-old son Eugene. We were just about to embark on an exceedingly jarring journey from Kunming to Jinghong in south-west China. I knew that this cramped 18-hour overnight trip was a distressingly bumpy, twisty nightmare over half-finished mountainous roads. Eventually, the following afternoon, we would stumble off the boneshaker as frazzled nervous wrecks.

I had endured this appalling bad trip in days gone by, so was savvy to the ordeal which lay ahead. To mollify my anxiety, I imagined a convict locked up in a tiny prison cell. He most certainly was worse off than me. What would he give to be at liberty to travel on this bus? The ride began with me chirping like an uncaged "Freebird. It was all in the mind; I smiled. After just 45 minutes of twisting and shouting "shit", I finally screamed, "Fuck it! I would rather be chained to a slimy wall in a medieval dungeon". I thought to myself, maybe the grass isn't always greener after all!

I arrived the next afternoon dazed and stunned, clutching Eugene's tiny hand. The lucky lad had slept like a baby throughout most of the journey.

***

At midnight on 31st August I lay wide awake contemplating the meaning of life. I gazed into the black atmosphere of my lonely bedroom, speculating whether the monster was under the bed or in my tortured head. On occasions the bedroom would be momentarily illuminated as rays of dazzling light from a car's headlights danced across the walls. Then it was darkness once more. A bit like life; mainly glum black periods with fleeting moments of sparkling joy. Nothing is permanent. Everything changes. Life is the space between two dates on a gravestone. "Birth, School, Work, Death." "Life's What you Make It." So, chop-chop Psycho, pull your flipping socks up and grab your remarkable second chance of life with both hands.

I should be "Dancing in the Street" celebrating that the effing big C hadn't returned as well as cheering hip-hip-hurray and tossing my beanie up to the sky because my kids were happy and healthy. Ian's tragic situation continued to affect me emotionally, but at least I could stand by him in his hour of need by supplying unlimited support and compassion.

My mind floated down to the dining room and the massive boxes of coffee that I needed to flog. I wasn't sure that I was healthy enough to succeed but I would try my damnedest. I also kept everything crossed that my dirty ex would come clean by transferring some of the filthy lucre she had nicked from me. At least that would ease the pressure from my foolhardy brainwave of going into business when I was still half-dead.

I am not certain whether I started talking to myself before my heavy eyelids shut tight, or after I nodded off to sleep.

"Syd, do you really think the grass would be a brighter shade of green on the other side of the world? Would life be rosier if you were back in the arms of the woman who lied, cheated, stole, mocked, abused little Jo, screamed hurry up and die and abandoned you when you needed her most? Syd, my old friend, do you honestly feel you would be happier? Open your mesmerised eyeballs, mate; she has a new lover and she wants you to die."

"And one last thing. Hurry up and fling that bloody hammer and never touch the fucker again. You know it makes sense. Do it now. Zzzzzzzz"

Wake me up when September Ends

(September 2014)

A repulsive potty-mouthed tongue-lashing of hostility blasted off from the Wicked Witch's mobile phone in Laos. It rocketed straight to the shiny Satellite in outer space prior to ricocheting and landing in my dumbfounded lugholes in Northern England. "Fuck you, fuck off," banged on my eardrums. I was rather taken aback because in all the years I had known her, she had never used such profanities.

What specimens of lowlife was she mingling with now? Was her new suitor afflicted with Tourette's or was he just some knuckle-dragging amoeba with shit for brains whose only response to anything would be "Fuck you or fuck off"? None of my business but whoever her new English language instructor was, then he or she should be given a pat on the back for the splendid job in tutoring advanced level *Toilet Talk for Dummies*. The heinous one had passed with flying colours.

Now, 'hold your stallions and mares' before pointing the finger and suggesting that I am the pot calling the kettle black. I am not being hypocritical by paying attention to the speck of dust in her eye while ignoring the log in mine. Nor am I implying that I am an angelic saint and that a four-letter word has never crossed my Mancunian lips. I am not striving to be a smart arse, doing my level best to sway you into believing that I am an innocent goody-two-shoes. I wouldn't have a prayer of pulling the wool over your eyeballs because having read my tale of woe up to this point, you will have become accustomed to my colourful choice of words. I wouldn't get away with it in a zillion years!

I would just like it to be common knowledge that I never ever 'eff and blind' in public. On the other hand, if I was glued to a large-screen TV watching a vital football match with the lads I would be the first to call the referee a blind bastard, but with a group of strangers I would, respectfully, just call him blind.

In all honesty I was flabbergasted and dismayed at my wife's unanticipated barnyard mouth of manure. Yet another one of life's little turn-ups for the book; my 'silly young moo' was suddenly 'swearing like a trooper'. I never swore in front of my wife and kids and of course my wife was free and could use foul language if she liked. I think I was just startled that someone I had known for eight years who had never used bad language was suddenly a foul-mouthed monster.

I presumed it was because I had dug my heels in by refusing to agree to the divorce, she so desperately craved, until she coughed up the $15,000 I had demanded as settlement. There was no alternative but to stand firm because clearly Eugene and Jo deserved something from my ten years of graft in the People's Democratic Republic of Laos. Why should the adulteress be given carte blanche to pinch everything?

When all is said and done, not only had I bought the house, but I had constantly supported her family too. From hospital bills when a relative was ill to school fees for her younger brothers and covering the funeral costs when her grandfather died. I'd even purchased the building materials for her parents' new house. I would happily agree to the divorce, but surely, she must have a speck of decency to go with that speck of dust in her eye.

We both knew that if she could wriggle out of wedlock without handing over what was rightfully mine and the children's then she wouldn't think twice about it. The deceitful one had no scruples or sense of fair play. I was awaiting the feeble excuse that she was keeping the house for Jo. That wouldn't wash in a month of Sundays because she would never allow her ill-gotten gains to leave her slimy thieving hands.

Then she could lead a conscience-free life as Lady Muck, painting the air blue as she swore at the top of her lungs in her new boyfriend's home. At the same time playing the sweet benevolent fairy godmother by granting her relatives permission to live in the house she had stolen from me. Of course, I felt bitter and had every right to as I sat struggling to make ends meet in a rented two-up two-down.

I responded with, "You have been having a wonderful time dating many different men while I am stuck here alone with two young children, fighting for my life. So why in heaven's sake are you so angry with me?"

"Fuck you, I am not a prostitute in Pattaya," she spat.

I tried to clarify that I was not implying anything of the sort but was just highlighting how different our lives were. She refused to listen, boasting that she had been to Singapore and Australia. She gloated as she forwarded two images. The initial one was of a small bungalow her boyfriend had either built, bought or rented, which was nothing much to write home about really. This was followed by a photograph of a glass of orange juice and a massive steak on a table near a sunny beach. The beach looked lovely and the drink was tempting but the steak just disgusted me. Since becoming vegan, I no longer saw a piece of meat; I saw a murdered animal that wanted to live. You don't impress me,

Missus Scumbag. What will it be next? Monkey's brains, bear's paws or stinking pig's trotters?

Well, not a good start to the month; "Wake Me Up When September Ends."

***

My mind floated back to the late 80s when I idled away a few intrepid months backpacking around the Far East. This was before the new-fangled era of Facebook and mobile phones. To contact my dear mother, I had to send a postcard that would arrive about a fortnight later or spend a night's beer money phoning home from a post office. Even then the conversation was never clear and invariably had a time delay, causing confusion. In the 21st century it only took a split-second for the Wicked Witch to give me a loathsome earbashing or forward a vile message. Welcome to the modern world.

Mind you, immediate communication was not always a pain in the arse. On the plus side it enabled me to respond instantaneously to Ian's urgent cries for help. His latest text explained that without supporting his jaw with his hand he would slur. As he was employed as an English language teacher, clarity of speech was paramount. His goal was to continue tutoring until mid-December, which would top up his bank balance, hopefully giving him sufficient cash to see out his final days on planet Earth. He paid a speech therapist $20 an hour to help him achieve that goal.

He mentioned that his arms were terribly weak and before long it would be his legs. His next sad message emphasised that he would progressively waste away until death. All hope was lost because there was no cure or possibility of recovery. He despairingly confessed that 'doing a Robin Williams' was constantly at the front of his mind.

I disclosed that I could identify with where he was at, because not so long ago I had planned to 'throw the towel in' and 'end it all'. And just like Ian, I had been captivated by famous people who had committed suicide; everyone from Ian Curtis to Adolf bloody Hitler. I speculated whether it was a matter-of-course for desperate souls mulling over self-murder to be fixated upon the famous who had carried out the ultimate sin. Did it make the final deed easier and more justifiable, to link oneself with a deceased superstar? Not that I am in any way implying that Hitler was a celebrity, but you know what I mean.

I don't know, but it just goes to show that stardom, bags of money, luxury cars, massive mansions and so called perfect-looking partners cannot guarantee happiness. We all suffer; that's life.

Ian continued with this morbid topic. "Eugene and Jo saved your life because if you would have been alone in Blackpool with cancer, that may well have tipped you over the edge and you would have done yourself in."

I knew he was right!

His friends advised him to return to the UK, but he wasn't convinced that going back was the better option. He rationalised that even though he would receive support, hospital treatment and welfare benefits back home, the truth of the matter was that he would unavoidably end up in a hospice. The thought of slowly wasting away, unable to talk, trapped in a wheelchair with an oxygen bottle in cold boring England, was terrifying. Passing away in colourful Laos under the warm tropical sun felt natural and certainly preferable to 'kicking the bucket' in a hospice cold and grey.

He elaborated that people in the UK hadn't the foggiest idea of what it was like in Laos; living in the moment under the big yellow sun as life slowly flowed by. Being alive inside the bright vivid masterpiece of golden temples, quirky street markets, wandering monks, laughing kids and old wooden shophouses; now that REALLY was living. In comparison, England was a grey scribble of deep-in-debt robots existing in unhappy chaos as they struggled to save for the next must-have gadget they had been programmed to buy.

They appeared happy with their new house, shiny motor, large flat screen TV and state-of-the-art whatchamacallits but take a quick peep into their bewildered glassy eyes and tell me what you see. Yes, that's right; anger, pain, greed, misery, hate, jealousy, confusion and sorrow. And why, you may ask? They have everything that money can buy. But they don't because their brainwashed minds can only focus on the next 'all-the-rage' thingamajig they need for instant gratification.

"I will be happy when I finally get my hands on the new iPhone. Just wait until the Joneses see it," they smirk. And they do feel joyful briefly until their insatiable mind swiftly moves on to the next gizmo, then the next, then the next.

In contrast, the old man cycling along the bank of the mighty Mekong as the first rays of sunlight illuminate the city; now, his eyes sparkle with magic, happiness and pure contentment. And one last thing; the weather in England is shit.

As I visualised the real-life picture Ian had so artistically painted, a tear of sadness fell from my right eye, followed by a droplet of rage from the left. I craved to be alive in that dynamic equatorial landscape and would be back there in a shot if only the woman I had loved and trusted hadn't ruthlessly betrayed me.

Ian recounted a time when he had worked on a house on a shitty decrepit council estate. Its sole occupant was an old man who had once been employed on film sets. The walls were proudly adorned with photographs of him next to famous people he had met, such as Peter Sellers and Roger Moore. He used to have a great life but now he was sad and boring, just living in the past with his memories.

Ian's little anecdote touched a nerve. I closed my eyes and was sitting by a remote temple in Laos, swimming in a tropical sea in Thailand and travelling along a high mountain pass in China. Then I opened them to a pile of unwashed dishes in the sink as the pissing Blackpool rain flung itself against the kitchen window. Now it was my turn to be the sad old sod living in the past.

***

I resumed my meditation practice, both at home and at the local Buddhist centre. I urgently needed to silence the tormenting thoughts of regret as my out-of-control mind flashed up images of me, the pitiful victim. For short-lived periods I managed to conquer my self-critical thoughts by focusing on the breath and remaining totally present. Only I could be my own saviour, by changing my mind.

Fighting the cancer, healing my broken spirit and taking care of the kids was a challenging full-time job, to say the least. And now I had the burdensome task of flogging 500kg of coffee banged onto my already heavy-hearted workload? It would be futile, slamming the stable door because the horse had already done a runner. Welcome to another fine mess, Psycho.

No point in weeping over spilt almond milk, so I promptly pulled my holey socks up and booked a stall at the upcoming Blackpool Vegan Fair. The flyers were designed by a monk in exchange for half a dozen bags of coffee. They were an exquisite blend of gold and brown, oozing with oriental spirituality. Perfect, and let's face it, not everyone can shout from the temple tops that their artwork was created by a Buddhist monk. I hurriedly got them printed along with a large roller banner in readiness for the big day.

When I originally ordered the coffee, I stipulated that 80% should be ground and 20% beans. However, the proprietor persuaded me to import all the coffee as beans and grind them myself as and when I received an order. Convinced that he knew what he was talking about, I agreed and purchased a small coffee grinder from Argos. I soon regretted my decision because grinding the beans was an absolute nightmare. Giving the two thumbs up to his suggestion was one of the worst decisions I had ever made in my life. It took a full hour to grind just six bags.

Firstly, I would carefully slice the top of a bag of beans, then empty the contents into a dish. Next, I would pour a third of the beans into the electric grinder and once finished, I would spoon the powder back into the bag as further beans were being ground. Finally, I would meticulously reseal the bag. Then I would swear my fucking head off as I grabbed the next bag.

A tedious mind-numbing procedure and I needed 180 bags for my stall, which took 30 hours of relentless toil. Had the owner made that recommendation to save himself the bother of grinding or was he really giving his expert opinion? I will never know.

On the 14th September I arrived at my table in the Winter Gardens, Blackpool with about 200 bags of coffee, 500 flyers, two kettles and no end of disposable cups. This out-of-the-ordinary coffee came in three subtle blends; the powerful Elephant Express, the flavoursome Naga and the delicate White Parasol. The coffee was elegantly displayed, while the roller banner announced that an organic mountain coffee was on sale here. I was knackered, and the doors hadn't even opened yet. Luckily, I had Eugene, his girlfriend and little Jo to help.

The doors opened, and the throngs of vegans came in. The Barnes team went into action. Eugene and his girlfriend boiled the water and I handed out cups for passers-by to sample while Jo gave out flyers. The majority bought a bag after just one taste. Ms Sandy our dizzy-blonde mate joined us in the afternoon and babysat Jo, taking him to visit other stalls. The fair was an immense success as most of the coffee was sold.

What I didn't tell anyone was that I was exhausted, and all my muscles kept locking up. It made me realise that I was still very poorly. Had I bitten off more than I could chew?

***

The following day Alfie, a black rescue Staffordshire Bull Terrier, became a fully-fledged member of the Psycho Syd tribe. This two-year old snub-nosed bundle of love wagged his tail in a frenzy of excited glee as he greeted his new family. He had a few invisible flecks of brown fur on his back that would magically appear in the sunlight, a paintbrush of white on his neck and gentle amber eyes.

The kids had been badgering me for over a year to get a pet, but I doggedly turned a deaf ear to their persistent pleas. After all, I was at death's door so what would happen to the poor animal if I gave up the ghost and snuffed it? I finally caved in but insisted that it must be a rescue animal; I would never buy from a breeder because I loathe callous arse-wipes who use this heartless method to get their hands on some filthy lucre so they can buy a new fridge-freezer or pay for a fortnight in sunny Spain. Bastards. And if you buy from a breeder so you can flaunt your expensive pedigree dog then you are no chum of mine either. Open your eyes and realise that these are living beings; not money-making objects to be bought and sold. Rant over.

Eugene and Jo vowed to take him for walks and clean up the poo, but you don't have to be a spaceship scientist to figure out that it was 'muggins' here who ended up doing the dirty work. I handed over £100 and welcomed the new member of the clan to his forever home. Alfie arrived in a cage, but I instructed the rescue people to take it away because no dog of mine lives in a cage. Although, on second thoughts maybe I should have kept it just in case the Wicked Witch made an unexpected return. Once the rescue people left, Alfie made himself comfortable on HIS sofa.

Over the next few weeks we had a ball with our new pet. Each evening after school was frittered away fooling around in fields, in a park or on the beach. Jo would run wild, shouting and laughing as he chucked sticks for his dog to fetch. Alfie also joined our weekly strolls with Ms Bombshell and had a whale of a time exploring and sniffing in the Lancashire countryside. He was a playful non-aggressive creature; great with humans and other dogs. And let's face it, he was living the dream. From a cage to a sofa, plus lots of love, food and walkies. Getting a pet was a wonderful decision.

Alfie became my best friend. I would tell him everything about my broken heart, the cancer, my loneliness and he listened like a good faithful boy!

On the 19th Ian sent word that he saw my ex going into the Samlo Pub and that he almost didn't recognise her. He remarked that she looked fat, jaded and spotty without her make-up on. He spat, "She looked fucking ugly!" She did occasionally have an outbreak of acne, but I never spotted it because love is blind.

On the 20th September Jo and I met a Polish woman who had contacted me through a free dating site. She was in her early 40's and her thirteen-year-old daughter and a son about Jo's age would be joining us. Happy families! We picked them up in Liverpool and cruised to the nearby red squirrel sanctuary. My date couldn't speak a word of English, so her daughter translated our tittle-tattle. It was awkward, but it worked.

The three kids had a fabulous time chasing each other on the vast beach, picking juicy blackberries and observing red squirrels in the forest. Next, a pub lunch. I knew we wouldn't see each other again because she just wasn't my type. She was friendly but far too strait-laced for an oddball like me. Would anybody ever be my type? Possibly a strangely strange spiritual gothic vegan chick with itchy feet and a lust for life. Is there anybody out there?

Nowt gained; nowt lost I dare say. It was a breath of fresh air having an adult to natter with, despite using a translator. And viewing Jo having fun outdoors away from his computer meant the trip was well worth it, even though this lady was not the one for me. We uttered our farewells before I drove back to man's best friend - Alfie.

On the 22 September I had reached the ripe old age of 58. I never thought I would make 56 to be honest. Will I still be knocking about at the big six-zero and will someone still need me and feed me vegan food if I hit 64? We had a small cake and an Indian curry. Alfie got some too!

Lying in bed, I conjured up colourful memories of past birthdays to light up that lonesome "Black Night": initially, warm recollections of an excited toddler eagerly ripping off the shiny wrapping paper concealing his presents. Then beaming with pride at blowing out all five candles in one go as the family cheered, clapped and sang "Happy Birthday". Later, I had fuzzy flashbacks of sloshed blurry nights in my youth, which were viewed as a flop unless I got blind drunk and spewed my guts up over the pavement on the zig-zag home. Finally, there was nostalgic reminiscing over sweet romantic nights with my wife in a beer garden under the starlit heavens. Painfully, the last three birthdays had been a knife-wound of heartache, confusion and sorrow. Yes, it was my birthday, but I felt so damn lonely. However, the good news; it was one year closer to death.

Well, that morose thought went straight for the jugular. I was battling to survive with a *Death Wish*. It was like slashing my wrists because I wanted to live; it just didn't make bloody sense. Well, it was

255

a case of chin up and keep clutching at straws in the hope that the next birthday would be heaven on earth.

On the 23rd September Ian forwarded some rather surprising news. He had contacted his ex-girlfriend for the first time in months. This on-off relationship had been tempestuous to say the least, but under the desperate circumstances, his thirst for a taste of love before he kicked the bucket was understandable. Another poor soul clutching at straws! They agreed to meet outside Nazim's Indian restaurant, just a stone's throw from the Mekong River. The moment she laid eyes on Ian's atrophied frame she burst out crying and begged him to marry her.

Ian accepted her proposal and subsequently, an impromptu Laotian wedding ceremony was thrown together in her village about 40 kilometres outside the capital. Ian coughed up $5000 for the dowry, the party and other incidentals. Would he live to regret his rash decision to tie the knot before he passed away? He planned to teach just one more term at Vientiane College before living and slowly dying in her village.

He snatched my breath away by adding, "I hope she takes loving care of me and doesn't do a ****." Bloody hell, my wife's name was being used to depict the ultimate betrayal a woman can commit. When the "Whispering Grass" divulges her newfound claim to fame, the notorious one will be as proud as Lucifer.

I had received sympathetic and shocked remarks such as 'callous', 'disgusting' and 'inhumane'. A close friend of mine who had been an ex-pat for decades once ventured, "Syd, I have heard some appalling stories of deceit and cheating by Asian wives but yours is by far the worst I have ever witnessed. I am so sorry, mate."

Ian continued, "And if my wife does a **** I will swallow the magic pill and end it all. I am dying anyway. I refuse to spend my last moments with my missus screaming "hurry up and die", with vile taunts about shagging another bloke. I would rather be dead."

I instantaneously screamed back to the nightmare that I had lived and died through. I recalled an instance where I was on the floor in agony with my neck, shoulder and back muscles cramped up. My skin was burnt and blistered, with open wounds seeping pus. My wife sneered at me in disgust. I looked into her eyes and cried, "Where have you gone? Why are you doing this to me? I love you, I love you, I love you."

She stood towering over my pathetic body and sniggered, "My new boyfriend has only told me he loves me once. That is why I love him."

My knee-jerk reaction to Ian's statement was, "If I hadn't had my kids, I would have taken the so-called easy way out, mate. Believe me, being betrayed and mocked by the woman I loved and trusted was a fate worse than death."

Ian revealed that he was still wed to a Japanese woman he had not seen for donkey's years. He pointed out that it would be futile applying for a divorce because the Laotian red tape to make the marriage official and legally binding would take at least a year; and by then he would be dead and buried. So, it made perfect sense to just live 'over the brush' with his new wife until 'death do us part' without having the burdensome task of having to deal with countless interviews and a mountain of paperwork. The village wedding meant that they could live together until the bona fide wedding papers were signed and sealed.

He blurted out, "I have two teenage children who are living with my Japanese wife in Africa. Maybe I should visit them one last time this Christmas."

"You must, mate," I stressed. "It is crucial that you see your kids one last time, letting them know how much you love them. Please fly there while you are still fit and able, for your sake and theirs."

He agreed and told me he would start looking at flights immediately.

Ian's new wife moved into his apartment to lend a helping hand supporting her hubby as he endeavoured to complete his final term at the college. One day they popped into a nearby temple seeking spiritual advice regarding the illness. A monk advocated a beer, chicken and pork free diet. "Thank Buddha he hadn't forbidden sex too," Ian chortled. The holy one then handed over a bag of twigs and leaves with instructions to boil them up, let them steep and drink the herbal tonic. Ian did as was asked and spent an hour sipping the concoction, reporting back that it tasted like shit!

A weighty matter of concern was that Ian was becoming anxious about his appearance. The kilograms were rapidly dropping off his dwindling frame. From a fat bastard to a streak of piss in a matter of weeks. I knew the feeling only too well. Join the club.

Ian quizzed, "How did you feel when you reappeared in Laos as a grim skeletal member of the walking dead? Did you find the stares of shock and the gasps of horror distressing?"

"I didn't give a northern monkey's toss mate, because I wasn't really there. I was living in my head as my mind focused on the painful reality that I had been knifed in the back by my partner; everything else was merely a blur."

He mused for a minute, before replying with, "You are very lucky, no one expected you to pull through."

Speaking of the she-devil, she contacted me threatening to return to the UK and take Jo off me. She gloated that her new partner-in-crime was filthy stinking rich and that he would pay $5,000 or even $10,000 to guarantee success. I saw red. I sensed that this menacing provocation was primarily because I refused to be her lapdog and play ball. There was no way I was going to sit and wag my tail agreeing to the divorce until she handed over a slice of what was rightfully mine and the children's.

The Wicked Witch was playing with fire. I had lost my health, job, house, mother and my wife and the deep love for my kids was all I had left to live for. If in the unlikely event she took Jo, she would not be needing a divorce because she would no longer be in the land of the living. That would be the straw that broke the camel's back.

When a person has lost virtually the whole shebang, and you 'step over the line' by stealing their only remaining reason for living, then you'd better get ready to shit your pants. Death for me would have been a godsend, a welcome escape from the non-stop physical pain and mental torture. I had zero fear of death, pain or prison and unless you'd a similar 'happy to die' mindset, my advice would be to keep your bloody distance because if you took Jo, I would be the 21st Century Witchfinder General. Therefore, Ms Wicked Witch, if you have the brass neck to confront me with your new bloke and a gang of heavies, then believe me I will not be calling your bluff when I vow to massacre the bleeding lot of you, eagerly awaiting the onset of round two in the fires of hell.

I recalled a tale I had heard regarding an extremely 'head the ball" nutter from Blackpool who was challenged by a drunken thug outside a pub. He smiled as he glared into his antagonist's eyes before grabbing a pint glass and pushing it into his own face. With rivers of blood flowing down his manic face he grinned, "If I can do this to me, just imagine what I can do to you!" The thug instantly backed down and fled for dear life. And I have a sneaky feeling that this is not an urban myth but the truth, because I have met this bloke and he is one scary mother.

Not that I wanted to murder the Wicked Witch or anybody else, but if my reason for living was snatched away then I would have been twice as scary as the above bloke. I don't doubt for one second that my wife still had some love for Jo, but it appeared obvious that her love for her son was secondary to her love for herself and her lust for wealth.

The red mist cleared from my eyes and my rage abated. I knew it was just an empty threat, but my mind had overreacted and gone berserk. The likelihood of her carrying out her threat was minimal and even if she did, the chances of a court agreeing to her request would be remote. He was safe here attending school, swimming lessons, seeing his school friends, his aunt and uncle and his dog. The school, my family support worker and many friends would attest to my love and devotion, which could all be proven with photographs and films. No court in the land would remove him from a safe loving environment in England and send him to an unknown future in a developing nation.

I toddled off to bed all peaceful and happy, without any angry visions of murder. I meditated until my heavy eyelids shut tight. I felt someone nudging me and I slowly opened my dreamy eyes. My imaginary friend smiled and whispered, "September is over now."

Thank fuck for that because I had just had a terrible dream!

Apeman

(October 2014)

I love you too lol!" was the mind-boggling text message my drowsy eyes awakened to, on the first day of October. Far more mystifying was the 'I love you' message I had previously forwarded to this young lady, because to the best of my knowledge I hadn't sent one. This romantic folly couldn't have been committed during a lonely drunken stupor because I was no longer a beer-monster. In fact, hardly a drop of alcohol ever passed my now 99.9% teetotal lips. Maybe half a pint of real ale, three or four times a year.

I shuddered upon discovering that each female on my mobile phone contact list was in receipt of an 'I love you' message. My cheeks were scarlet, and my bloody brain was befuddled. What on earth was going on? Was someone taking the piss? I went downstairs for a coffee to clear my mind and find out the answer.

The culprit was little Jo, who had been firing cupid's arrows of love to all my female friends. "For Heaven's sake, why?" I shouted.

He looked up at me with his sad cherubic eyes and softly whispered, "I am sorry Dad, I only wanted to find you a new girlfriend."

My heart melted as I asked, "Why do you want me to have a girlfriend."

"So, I can have a new mam," was his heart-tugging response.

The lump in my throat almost choked me to death as I recalled the dreadful emotional and physical abuse he had suffered from his real mother. The time she had screamed she was not his mother and that she hated him. The numerous occasions she had lost control, hitting and kicking him. And finally, the painful reality of the abandonment which had deeply affected both of us.

I hugged Jo, gently explaining that one day I would have a girlfriend who loved us both, but I had to be careful because she must be the right one. He pleaded with me to find a mam who would love him and not hurt him. He then promised not to send any further texts. I wrapped my arms around him and gave him a massive loving hug before dragging my crushed soul back upstairs and silently crying my eyes out.

Next came the cringeworthy task of convincing each girl that I hadn't sent the message of love, but my son had. Would they believe me, or would they be thinking that I was a sad sod using my cute young boy as a 'fanny magnet' in a desperate attempt to break the ice? I winced at the very thought. They all found it rather amusing and felt sympathetic towards Jo's quest, however, no offers to cook dinner, wash the dishes, keep my bed warm and supply Jo with shedloads of mothering were forthcoming. I wonder why?

***

Life dragged on in a loneliness of never-ending housework. I would flee the humdrum chores by daydreaming of the upcoming weekend jaunt with Miss Bombshell. Having a close friend to share my thoughts with for a couple of hours on a Saturday inspired me to keep plodding on. Eugene was studying at college and largely spent his free time with his girlfriend, like most teenage lads.

Ian explained that he hadn't informed Vientiane College about his illness because he was worried sick that they would dismiss him. The name of the game was to complete the term and build up enough cash to keep him ticking over until the day he finally passed away. He was depressed and angry at the injustice of being shot down in his prime, just when life was going so well. Tell me about it, mate.

On the 18th October Eugene reached the age of 17. We celebrated the occasion with an Indian curry, followed by a small birthday cake in the living room. Eugene then left us and took his girlfriend to the cinema. My little boy was now becoming a man.

The nights were drawing in and visions of another chilly winter in Blackpool prompted me to treat the three of us to warm winter coats. The days of shorts and sleeveless t-shirts under Surya, the Buddhist Sun God, were long lost but not forgotten memories It was time to wrap up because soon it would be icy breath and frozen fingers time in the company of that cold-hearted devil, Jack Frost.

***

Physically, I was nowt but trillions of cells with each cell needing to be nourished. The gastrointestinal tract - the tube from my cheeky 'Manc' gob to my God-given arse - did the job of feeding my hungry cells. Taking in food, digesting it, extracting energy and nutrients, before expelling the waste. My strategy of supplying each of my precious cells with a daily dose of organic fruit and vegetables seemed the logical method of keeping them healthy.

Of equal importance was omitting all processed food. Any food that was kept in a packet or a tin was off-limits. Surely giving the cold shoulder to foods that had been chemically corrupted by additives that completely changed the natural flavours and colours to give them a longer shelf life, was just plain common sense. These convenience foods provided healthy profits for the money-hungry corporations, but unhealthy outcomes for the consumers who scoffed this mass-produced shite containing zero or very little nutritional value.

And as a vegan I wasn't going to ingest animals or their secretions which would be detrimental to my physical well-being. And from a compassionate aspect I couldn't bring myself to be the cause of another sentient being's death. A pig, a dog, a cow or a cat are all living beings; they feel pain and don't want to die. We have been conditioned since birth to feel that it is fine to eat a pig or a cow but wrong to eat a cat or a dog. In my opinion it is wrong to eat any animal. Remember, meat is murder and it is not the food our biological make-up demands and your karma for eating the rotting flesh and secretions of a dead animal will more than likely come back to bite you on the arse with some form of illness.

My brainy grey-matter had no doubt that we are naturally frugivores. Our physiology closely resembles primates that live on diets of primarily, fruit, berries, nuts, seeds, herbs and leaves. Do your research and you'll discover that we are nothing like carnivores, omnivores or herbivores. Check out jaws, digestive systems, teeth, sweat systems, stomachs, skin etc. Get it into your thick, brainwashed skulls that, like it or not, we are frugivores.

Now this was fine and dandy when early man flourished in a tropical paradise, with an abundance of fruits, nuts and seeds. However, once the species began to migrate to colder climes with a scarcity of the perfect food for our biological make-up, then a shift in diet was crucial for survival. Fortunately, our bodies are awesome and can exist on foodstuffs that are less than ideal. So, animal products and starchy vegetables were gobbled up. I strongly believe that the discovery of fire played a significant role in mankind's consumption of animal flesh. Cooking the dead animal tissue, muscle and organs made it far easier to chew and digest.

Now go and have a swift glance in the mirror at your teeth. Study the four incisors and two tiny pointed cuspids. What do you think they were designed for? If your answer is to tear into the skin of fruit, then grab yourself a gold star Little Mr or Ms Clever-Clogs. If you are shortsighted enough to believe that they have any similarity to a carnivorous big cat's massive canines, which have evolved to rip raw flesh, then don the dunce's hat and stand in the corner.

And I am fed up to the back of my fruit-munching molars when I hear knuckle-dragging dinosaurs banging on that cavemen ate animals; therefore, it is fine for us to scoff them too. As I have previously pointed out, our bodies are incredible and will survive for lengthy periods on unsuitable substances. People who drink a bottle of whisky a day, chain smoke, or are addicted to hard drugs don't drop dead instantaneously, unfortunately most of them usually pay the heavy price with an early death or a chronic illness.

Similarly, modern man is consuming processed meat such as bacon that is a class one carcinogen, slimy mucus-forming dairy and heaps of junk food that are making him overweight and sick. The huge corporations that sell and market this unhealthy disease-causing shite only want to get their greedy hands on your money. If I were a conspiracy theorist I would no doubt be implying that these vile peddlers of unwholesome junk food were working hand in glove with the mega-rich drug-pushing pharmaceutical giants. Well, money is the root of all evil!

Therefore, turn a blind eye to my sound advice at your peril. Persist with your gung-ho mindset of 'I will be fine' but, statistics scream, in all probability you will end up as one of the 50% who will be diagnosed with cancer or one of the other poor sods who are struggling with a chronic disease.

Doubtless, many of you will pooh-pooh my egghead ramblings regarding diet and ridicule that I am just a bizarre oddball gushing a pile of old shit. Did you know that medical doctors study nutrition for between 10 and 24 hours during their five or six years in a UK medical school? Well, I have studied diet and nutrition for thousands of hours because my blooming life depended on it. I concluded that by scoffing 90% fruit, 10% green leafy vegetables, with the occasional baked sweet potato plus numerous herbal tonics, I was providing myself with the greatest chance of defeating the cancer and keeping my cells healthy.

As you may well recall, I was handed the dreaded DS1500 document that shouted that my maximum life expectancy was just six months. Yet more than two years later I was still breathing in and out in the land of the living. So, it is as plain as the conk on your face that I must have been doing something right. Maybe this northern monkey isn't as daft as he looks after all!

***

I was still searching for the truth, with two 45-minute sessions of meditation a day. I would focus on my breath entering and leaving my nostrils as I attempted to still my mind. It worked to some extent as I remained present for brief periods of time.

After staring the Grim Reaper slam bang in the eyeballs, I would repeatedly ask myself, Is there life after death? Am I simply an assortment of cells that die, then decay after I snuff it? Are my emotions, thoughts and feelings just chemical reactions and electrical signals? Or do I have a non-physical self such as a spirit, a soul or some form of universal energy that lives on after my physical body bites the dust?

As an angel-faced toddler I religiously attended the weekly Sunday School classes, also saying my prayers nightly. It was uplifting to learn that if I was a good boy then immortality in heaven was mine all mine, once I had stepped through the pearly gates. Although it was an almighty downer discovering that eternal torture in hell awaited if I fell into temptation and sinned. For heaven's sake, how could a God of love inflict everlasting pain on a person he had created in his own image? Good grief, it was like a smart-ass oxymoron dreamt up by a Hell's Angel. It just didn't seem right. Was I missing something?

As I grew up, I went through a period of taking as gospel that immortality was a load of old codswallop. When we popped our clogs then that was it; no sitting on cloud nine playing a harp. Yet, in times of heartbreak I would dip into the Bible, seeking some obscure holy wisdom prior to praying, "God, if you are out there then please help me get through this shit." I guess countless nonbelievers have done the very same. In their misery they clutch at straws, hoping that a benevolent supreme being is listening and with one wave of his all-powerful hand will answer their prayers.

Although, I confess to being spiritual for most of my life. Was it my enlightening journeys to the east or could it possibly have been the 'real me' trying to knock some sense into my thick skull? And who is the real me? Well, it certainly isn't the person you see right in front of you. That person is an imposter who has been created and conditioned with its very own ego and image to live and survive in the world of the plastic people. The real me existed before birth and will continue after death. On a few blissful occasions I have managed to put down my zombified mind and experience the timeless zone of true reality. There is no pain or suffering in that dimension; it is as it is. Anyhow, back to the age-old question: Is there such a thing as eternal life? *Definitely maybe*!

***

The phenomenal Big Ted created a magnificent user-friendly website and online shop. Dazzling gold, yellow and brown pages perfectly highlighted the shiny silver bags of rare mountain coffee on sale. And Big Ted wouldn't accept a penny. This hero certainly deserves much more than a pat on the back and a medal. He will be getting an unexpected treat after my book begins flying off the shelves.

Hey ho, it was ready, steady, go to flog the coffee online, so, I uploaded a link to the website on a post to my Facebook page and waited to see if anyone woke up and smelt the coffee.

On the 24th it was endoscopy time and once more I received the fantastic news that there was no sign of the big C. Getting the two thumbs up was becoming a formality, however it was vital that I continued with my vigilance and didn't get too cocksure. Maintaining my health with a diet of organic fruit, vegetables and herbs was imperative. I am an "Apeman"!

You're Unbelievable

(October 2014)

On the 25th October I grabbed a couple of hundred bags of coffee and drove to the West Midlands Vegan Fair in Wolverhampton. I was accompanied by a man I had bumped into at the Buddhist Meditation Centre. This Liverpudlian fella in his mid-forties offered to tag along and give me a helping hand. He didn't appear to be a devout spiritual Buddhist and later blurted out that he was only at the centre because it was straightforward renting a room there whilst in receipt of benefits. He didn't abide by the centre's strict code of vegetarianism and owned up to sneaking kebabs, burgers and fried chicken into his room whenever he had been out for a night on the lash. We did have one thing in common though; he was also an emotional wreck after the break-up with his ex-partner.

My fellow misfit and I set up the stall and sold most of the coffee. Once again it was hard bloody work handing out samples and reeling off the sales patter. I was fatigued and in pain as my muscles kept cramping up. I treated my pal to a meal and handed him £20 beer-money for his assistance. Obviously not much, but after importing the coffee, paying off the loan instalment, booking a stall and putting fuel in the car I was making Sweet Fanny Adams. The coffee growers in Laos and the bank in good old England were the only ones making a killing.

Mr Liverpool was a friendly chap but there was one thing that really got on my tits. He was a 'Billy Two Sheds'. Whatever I had done he had done better. Anything I owned, then his was a better, more expensive, more modern version of mine. He was obviously insecure, but it did get a tad tedious constantly being reminded of how much better than me this loser was. My compassionate side mused that this was probably his method of rebuilding his self-esteem after losing everything, therefore I merely smiled and nodded at his never-ending bragging whilst biting my tongue.

This aroused a flashback to one rainy afternoon back in the eighties when I was nursing a glass of Robinson's best bitter in a pint-sized pub in central Stockport. A peculiar bloke I judged to be in his mid-twenties was the only other patron in the cosy snug. I puffed on a cigarette as I endeavoured to discover what it was about this chap that had pricked up my ears. Soft Cell's "Tainted Love" was playing in the background as

I surreptitiously studied him. He was wearing an olive-green pullover with sleeves rolled up and dark grey shiny trousers. I was cautious as I discreetly scrutinised him because for all I knew he may have been a psychopathic nutter and suddenly screamed, "What the fuck are you looking at?"

I gazed into my beer as the idiom Curiosity Killed the Cat sprang to mind. Upon taking another sneaky glance I noticed that his eyes were far too close together, his ears were massive, and his nose was bent. Ah, that's the answer. Elementary my dear Psycho. It was his grotesque ugliness that had snatched my attention.

He caught my eye as he proudly flashed his two-remaining tar stained teeth before announcing, "Do you know my girlfriend is a model?"

I didn't spill my beer in surprise but calmly responded with, "Lucky you."

He continued, "And she is going to buy me a Ferrari for my birthday."

"Wow, has she got a sister?" I laughed.

"And yesterday I got a cheque for £5,000," he boasted.

I didn't respond with, "Was that for winning the latest gurning competition or was it for being bullshitter of the year?" Instead, I just smiled and gave him the two thumbs up.

My new-found friend then jabbered, "Any chance of buying me a pint because I have left all my cash at home. Don't worry mate, I'll meet you here tomorrow and pay for all your beer and take you for an Indian meal too, as a thank you."

The idea of spending a drinking session and a curry with him wasn't the slightest bit tempting in the unlikely event that he kept his word, because the truth was that he was an out-and-out liar. However, he would have been the perfect companion for chatting up pairs of females in a nightclub. "Don't like yours mate," I would whisper as he danced with the fat one!

And yes, all you feminists out there are coming across loud and clear as you scream, "Syd, you are a shallow sexist bastard." And of course, you are all correct. And if it is of any consolation, you will be pleased to hear that karma bit me on my cheeky Manc arse as I soon paid the price for wrongly evaluating a girl's dateability purely based on her physical appearance. My wife had left me, explaining that the cancer had made me far too ugly for her. As the saying goes; you can't judge a book by its cover.

Also, once the cancer had left me looking like the elephant man's ugly brother, I was cold-shouldered by the opposite sex. They were blind to my warm heart and zany sense of humour because after just one peep at my uninviting features they'd avoided me like the plague. Jeez, Manchester's cocky ladies' man hadn't had a leg-over since the Wicked Witch departed many full moons ago.

"It isn't fair, beauty isn't skin-deep, you know!"

"It serves you bloody right," you laugh.

"I know that now," I cry.

I bought the poor sod a beer and exited the pub into the drizzle. I stood on the pavement of the busy A6 as cars and lorries splashed by. I pondered that, he knew that he was bullshitting, I knew that he was bullshitting, and he knew that I knew that he was bullshitting. Yet he continued to bullshit. His life must have been so dreary that he had to exist in an imaginary world of models, fast cars and money to feel of any value.

And before you all start mocking this poor Billy Liar, ask yourselves this question. Do you live in the real world or are you living in a dream world too? Are you here in the NOW focusing on the sights, sounds, smells, tastes and touches of this very moment? Or are you living in your own unreal world, fantasising about the Aston Martin you will be driving when you win the lottery: are you sunbathing on the beach of last year's holiday in the sun, or imagining making love to your partner later tonight? (Lucky bastard.) Lift your heavy eyelids and wake up, because very few people live in the real world.

***

The Stockport incident reminded me of a comparable episode that transpired just a few months later in the city of Dublin. I was employed as a truck driver, delivering medical supplies to this fair city. I would drive from Manchester to Holyhead in North Wales before catching the ferry to Dun Laoghaire in Ireland. I would drop off my load in central Dublin, then catch the overnight ferry back.

Alas, on one unfortunate occasion things didn't go exactly to plan. On this fateful day a change in the tax laws meant delays because of the new-fangled paperwork, leaving myself and countless other truckies stranded after missing the ferry. All the B&Bs were full and the only room I could find was in a luxurious country hotel a few miles from the port. I phoned my boss and got permission to rest my weary head there providing I obtained a receipt.

I felt like Lord Muck as I scrubbed the dirt off my grimy body in the massive bath. I was soon brought tumbling back down to earth as I put my oily ripped jeans and dirty t-shirt back on. I didn't have a change of clothes because I hadn't foreseen the unexpected delay.

I was reluctant to visit the plush restaurant dressed like a tramp, having to face the embarrassment of sticking out like a dirty sore thumb. However, my stomach was rumbling, giving me no alternative but to put on a brave face and grin and bear it.

I entered the posh restaurant and felt like a dirty peasant amongst the smart suits and dresses. I imagined the tut-tut-tuts as the hoity-toity snobs thought, "What is the world coming to, letting that in?"

I winced as I scanned the lavish surroundings, seeking a corner to hide away in. Lo and behold, I spotted a vagrant sitting alone at a table slap-bang in the centre. I couldn't believe my bloody eyes. "My goodness, he has got balls," I chuckled. "Thank God there is someone even scruffier than me!" I rapidly made a beeline to his table and politely asked if I could sit with him.

"Go ahead," he smiled.

Abracadabra, my discomfort magically vanished as I sat with my fellow hobo. We were like two specks of dirt on an elegant mirror and I was mega-relieved that I wasn't the only blemish in this ritzy eatery. I bought him beer after beer and a meal too. Sod the expense. As the beer flowed, we chattered away, oblivious to the rich and wealthy nearby. We got on like the proverbial house on fire, discussing Ireland, football, history, music, films and up-to-the minute news, as well as exchanging jokes. We had a wonderful time. After a couple of hours of banter and laughter he thanked me and shook my hand, before leaving me to polish off my final beer alone.

I was well pissed so didn't give a shit about the posh people close by. Although I soon sobered up and started to panic when I thought about paying the bill. Bloody hell, I had spent a blinking fortune. On reflection it had been a great evening and I felt warm inside, having treated someone far less fortunate than me. I hoped and prayed that I had enough dosh to cover the bill.

I nervously called over one of the smart waiters.

"May I help you, Sir?" he enquired politely.

"Can I pay the bill please?"

"The gentleman you were with has already settled the bill, Sir," he disclosed.

I gazed at the waiter in open-mouthed astonishment before stuttering with, "He d-d-didn't look like he had two p-p-pennies to r-r-rub together."

The waiter smiled before informing me that my scruffy drinking pal was not only the owner of the hotel but in fact, owned several hotels, businesses, racehorses, country mansions and was a multimillionaire.

I staggered back to my enormous room in an instant karma daze and sprawled in gobsmacked bliss on my king size bed. Life is sometimes unbelievable. All I needed now to round off this perfect evening would be a knock on the door and a visit from a wealthy drop-dead-gorgeous Irish model.

She would gaze lustily into my startled eyes and sexily purr, "Excuse me Sir, I would just like to inform you that I have a hot fetish for dirty down and outs and would be most grateful for a night of sin. And as a thank you for your services I would be more than happy to buy you a brand-new Ferrari for your next birthday."

I smiled at the thought and fell happily asleep.

However, the 'Billy Two Sheds' bullshitting champion of champions was an Aussie arsehole I had the misfortune of crossing paths with in Vientiane. And to win that prize you had to be a 'Walter Mitty' extraordinaire, believe me! Living in the back of beyond I encountered all sorts of weird and wonderful oddballs. The number of occasions a drunk had slurred, "I shouldn't be telling you this, but I am ex-SAS and can kill a man in 10 seconds," was staggering. I am a gangster, a millionaire, I have five Rolls Royces back home, I am a friend of the US President and the list went on and on. People were just strangers, travellers or misfits who for some reason or other ended up on the other side of the planet. Nobody knew anything about their backgrounds, meaning it was a piece of piss for a nobody to reinvent themselves as a superhero somebody.

Well, back to the Aussie Gobshite. We had both applied for the position of Human Resources Manager at the largest hydropower project in the country. Out of the hundreds of applicants it was down to the final two; me and him. After a final interview I received an email informing me that my application was unsuccessful. Then a couple of days later another email stating that they would like to see me again to review the decision. Wow, things were looking good. Alas, I still didn't get the job.

No problem, I carried on swimming and hitting the gym in the morning and teaching in the evening. Life was great, and I had no sour grapes when I met the successful candidate in the pub one evening and shook his hand, congratulating him on getting the job.

He smiled arrogantly and declared, "Better man won."

What an arsehole. I knew there and then the company had made the wrong decision. I would meet him regularly and found him to be the ultimate "Billy Two Sheds". He was always pissed up and bragging about what he had or what he had done. I once told him that I ran a kilometre in 5 minutes that morning. He smirked, "I can run it in 3 minutes." I blanked the big-headed swine from that moment and carried on enjoying my life in lovely Laos.

Over the next few weeks I would smile knowingly when friends of mine complained that they had just met the most boring, arrogant, drunken arsehole in the world. I chuckled as I said, "Is he a fifty-something-year-old Aussie?" They said, "Yes, you don't know him, do you?"

I responded with, "Yes, unfortunately."

To cut a long story short, the Australian bullshitting braggart was given his marching orders from the job within a few weeks. They must have seen through his web of lies. As fate would have it, I soon ended up being employed by the same company. Another case of "Instant Karma."

Although karma doesn't seem so instant regarding my ex. Will I have to linger until my next life to have the pleasure of seeing her get her just desserts? I would be satisfied to just get a slice of the wonga I was owed from the house and the land in this lifetime. At least I could pay off the loan and me and the kids could escape to the sun for a couple of weeks. So, hurry up, karma; shake a leg and get it sorted. Pretty please.

At the end of October, I received a message from Ian informing me that he had had a massive row with his missus. She had gotten blind drunk, which had led to the almighty argument. He ordered her to leave the flat, but she refused. Eventually she walked out of the door, much to Ian's relief. However, he quickly discovered that his ATM card had left too. He contacted the bank, discovering that an attempted purchase had been made at the market, but fortunately it was declined. Ian cancelled the card and went to sleep.

It was once again Halloween which some folk refer to, as the day of the dead; remarkably, I was still very undead. Halloween: the day to remember the deceased. Would anyone be remembering me next year? Not if I had a say about it because I was resolute in my single-minded mission to triumph over the cancer. So far, so good - and many more All

Hallows' Eves lie in wait for this death-defying ghoul.

Jo got a monster mask and bags of vegan sweets for the trick-or-treaters. I didn't need a blinking mask because I am one scary mother. When I take a ride on the Ghost Train at Blackpool Pleasure Beach, it's the ghosts that scream, not me! And another thing. - It would soon be Christmas!

Sex on Fire

(November 2014)

"November Rain", shivery mornings, drab overcast days and pitch-black-by-5pm evenings were to be faced once more. How I yearned for my old life in the tiny village of Gnommalard in southern Laos. This really was a place where the muddy side streets had no name. It was well off the beaten track, with a small ramshackle market selling fresh fruit and vegetables and a couple of hardware shops flogging shoddy Chinese 'bits and bobs' that would fall to bits within a week.

In the warm tropical evenings, I would sit comfortably in a homemade wooden chair outside the local bar - a tumbledown tin shack. I felt as 'snug as a bug in a rug' clad in my t-shirt and shorts, as the balmy equatorial breezes warmed my arms and legs and tantalised my nostrils with aromas of the nearby wild jungle. I was at one with the universe as I sipped an ice-cold Beer Lao under the Milky Way, while the crickets chirped loudly in the adjacent rice field. Bliss; I really had found what I was looking for. Yet now it was time to freeze my balls off once more as the harsh Blackpool winter was fast approaching. I was not only fighting the unforgiving UK weather; I was battling my unforgiving mind!

Ian sent a distressing text revealing that he was becoming weaker by the minute and needed to support his head with his hand to stop it flopping down. His speech was slurred. Now shaving and washing were becoming formidable tasks. He felt down in the dumps. Imagine a simple everyday job that we take for granted, such as washing your face, suddenly becoming a troublesome struggle. I fully related to his desperate situation because I too had experienced the sudden shock and despair of my life falling apart. He was still determined to complete the term at college. Just like me, he refused to give in.

Not only did he have to cope with his chronic and rapidly deteriorating health; he also had an angry Lao wife to boot. Been there, done that and worn my broken "Achy-Breaky Heart" on my t-shirt sleeve. His furious 'other half' was on the warpath. She was screaming outside his apartment demanding to be let in. She wanted money too. He knew beyond any shadow of a doubt that she had pinched his bank card but of course she would never admit to it. That would result in a loss of face, which was a massive no-no in that part of the world. Ian's ailing body stood firm by refusing to allow her entry into his flat. He didn't

273

hand over any cash either.

***

I remembered, remembered the 5th of November and treated the kids to a giant box of fireworks. For those of you from foreign lands, the 5th of November is an annual event celebrating the capture of Guy Fawkes, who in 1605 was caught red-handed with a cache of explosives in a cellar beneath the Houses of Parliament. The Gunpowder Plot was a scheme formulated by a group of Roman Catholics to assassinate the Protestant King James 1, because of his refusal to grant greater tolerance to their religion. The conspirators were betrayed and their plan to blow up the monarch and his powerful sidekicks was thwarted.

Guy Fawkes, dressed in cloak, hat, boots and spurs was discovered along with 36 barrels of gunpowder. He was arrested and taken away for interrogation. His fellow conspirators fled, and the lucky ones died fighting while the others met a gruesome execution. They were dragged on wooden panels through the crowded streets of London, then hanged. Then subsequently, cut down and while still conscious, castrated, disembowelled and finally quartered. Ouch! That is almost as bad as the chemo-radiotherapy nightmare!

It has been reported that Fawkes jumped from the gallows, broke his neck and died, thus avoiding the grisly finale of being slammed onto the quartering block, prior to having his dangly bits chopped off, his guts ripped out and his body cut into four. The lucky bugger.

Since that day way back in 1605, Bonfire Night, Fireworks Night or Guy Fawkes Night has been celebrated in Britain every fifth of November. Fires with an effigy of Guy Fawkes sitting atop them are set ablaze to commemorate the failure of the Gunpowder Plot. Spectators circling the raging inferno stand back in fear and respect at the ferocity of the wild beast's angry power. Red, yellow and orange tongues of flame leap up in orgasmic waves to lick the dark heavens. Their flickering reflections dance hypnotically on the eyeballs of the mesmerised crowd. Sparks twinkle like stars as they jitter above the rooftops. Plumes of grey smoke spiral upwards before vanishing into the "Black Night."

Children gaze in wonder as the pyrotechnics of fireworks paint the dark sky with kaleidoscopic floral masterpieces. These fire-flowers give birth to a chorus of 'oohs' and 'aahs' as the onlookers sing out in delight. Bangs, booms, whistles and screams are all part of this flower-power show. Friendly chatter and children's laughter echo in the murky air. The malevolent crackling, spluttering and spitting of the bonfire in the background completes the psychedelic symphony of Guy Fawkes Night to perfection.

The fragrant smell of burning wood and whiffs of sulphur from the gunpowder smoke evoke a hazy memory of a distant time that you struggle to recall. You force a vision of yourself witnessing some strange witching hour ritual in a medieval village. Could this be a past life recollection or is it just your imagination?

Your skin glows a molten golden colour as the fire warms your front while the icy fingers of winter chill your back. Holding the hot potato that has been carefully retrieved from the blaze, you cautiously take the first bite, always wary of getting a burnt gob. For afters, the traditional sticky treacle toffee and parkin cake. This cake made with oatmeal, molasses and ginger originates from the counties of Lancashire and Yorkshire in Northern England. No fireworks night would be complete without a slice of parkin.

Bonfire Night tantalisingly stimulates our senses; all six of them! November the fifth is indeed a night to remember.

Fireworks night in health-and-safety-conscious 2014 couldn't hold a candle to the Fireworks nights of my childhood. In 2014 you had the option of either mingling with the crowd at a regulated bonfire party to observe a supervised pyrotechnic display or buying a box of fireworks for a mini-event with your family back home. Personal bonfires were a rarity rather than the norm.

Yet, in my early-teens of the late 60s it was a full-on throbbing sensual orgy of heat, light and sound. Virtually every house on the council estate where I grew up had a whopper of a blaze burning lustily in the back garden. Powerful phallic rockets shot up into the wide-open heavens with cries of "Oh my god", as the climatic explosion covered the black satin sky. There were pretty catherine wheels screaming ecstatically from their bondage on old wooden posts. And don't get me started about the banging that lasted all night long.

OK dear reader; stop your moaning and groaning. If you have come this far on the journey with me then you must already have it in your head that my unzipped mind has slipped in another screwy paragraph. So, all apologies again. Time to get back down to business.

On the days leading up to the fifth we would dawdle outside pubs and shops with a homemade Guy Fawkes reeling off, "A penny for the Guy, please," to the passing shoppers and drunks. The Guy was made of old clothes stuffed with newspapers and finalised with a grotesque mask. When we didn't have a Guy, we would improvise with one of us sitting motionless wearing the mask. Joe Public wasn't fooled but usually saw the funny side and handed over some spare change.

The money was spent on fireworks and our weapon of choice was the banger. It was a small red tube stuffed with gunpowder which made an almighty deafening bang. We blatantly ignored the warning of 'do not hold' printed on this noisy firework as we hurled them at rival gangs in explosive street battles. Racing after our target, screaming abuse with our faces twisted in rage. Getting closer and closer with hand held high as the tiny red monster spat bright orange sparks. Then boom.

Each one of us had the short sharp shock of holding onto the explosive for one split-second too long branded onto our minds. Standing shaking in shock, with ringing ears as we stared open-mouthed and frog-eyed at our throbbing black-powdered hand. Of course, we played the brave soldier, thus keeping our street cred by laughing it off before screaming obscenities at our chums, who were inevitably rolling on the floor laughing their effing heads off. Alas, these powerful red demons were banned in 1998 on the grounds of misuse and noise pollution by some loud-mouthed spoilsports in suits.

The big night was pure bedlam with an unremitting cacophony of explosions and whirrs in the dense foggy atmosphere. Balls of fire shot from Roman Candles would screech past your head, rip-raps landing at your feet had you leaping for dear life and bangers would shatter your eardrums as they exploded right in front of your astonished eyes. This foolhardy bombardment came from the nearby parties, which were *Obscured by Clouds* of bonfire and gunpowder smoke. We needed no encouragement to hurl our own barrage of deafening fiery projectiles back. We were bouncing as we tasted the fear and excitement while the adrenalin ran riot around our brave young bodies. It was lunacy. It was war.

It was also known as 'Mischief Night' for a very good reason. Spiteful neighbours who had refused to return the football that had been accidentally kicked into their garden were the first to have their wooden front gate stolen and tossed on a fire. Nosy Parkers, bad-tempered busy-bodies and pathetic snobs who sneered down their toffee-noses as they pretended to be Lord Muck in their dingy terraced houses on a shithole council estate, were next in line to be gateless.

As a much older and I like to think, much wiser person, I now get the picture that those insane deadly days will remain where they belong; in the past. And in all honesty that is a good thing, because thousands were burnt and injured during that mad evening when all hell was let loose after Pandora's box of dangerous fireworks had been opened.

And they will never return for another reason; the world has changed beyond recognition. In my youth there were no computer games, so we had to create our own adventures. Playing football in the street, climbing trees, hide and seek in the local woods and skirmishes with other neighbourhood gangs were part and parcel of growing up. However, today's youth are programmed like robots in front of an Xbox, PlayStation or computer, which have ready-made artificial adventures. They hardly ever venture out into the real world and in my opinion that is not a good thing.

I led the kids into our tiny backyard for a tame, short-lived firework display. Eugene and Jo painted swirling patterns in the darkness with the sparklers. The volcanoes, screamers, catherine wheels and rockets were extinguished in a flash. The children promptly stepped back indoors, returning to the unreal world of Minecraft and Alien Warfare. I sat in the very real kitchen like a discarded spent firework, feeling used and worthless. I longed for the good old days when I sparkled like a shining star. Alfie my faithful best friend, wasn't the slightest bit troubled by the noisy commotion outside as he slouched indifferently on the chair next to me.

***

Another upsetting message from Ian accosted me the following morning. He had returned home after teaching and was aghast to discover that his girl had stolen his motorbike and computer. His Aussie flatmate had caved in to the hysterical hullabaloo she had been creating outside the door and timidly let her in. Ian was furious with his weak-kneed friend as well as his thieving other half.

In a rage he had seized all her clothes and commemorated the capture of Guy Fawkes one day late. He confessed to feeling triumphant as he gleefully witnessed her glad-rags going up in flames. Once he had cooled down, he made a spur-of-the-moment resolution to fly to Uganda at the end of term. He would visit his Japanese wife and two teenage kids, who were living in Kampala, the capital city. Once there he would decide what to do next with his atrophied body and his quickly disappearing life. Heartbreaking!

Ian's spontaneous act of revenge galvanised me into dashing upstairs and yanking my wife's clothes from the two wardrobes before flinging them onto the bedroom carpet. Jeans, coats, boots, shoes, tops, jackets, dresses and skirts. Each item had only been worn once or twice. I had spoilt her rotten. Sadly, I wasn't tasting avenged satisfaction like Ian; I just shuddered before crumbling inside. My hands trembled as I placed each item into a black plastic bin bag along with a tiny sliver from my shredded heart.

I gazed at each item as I painstakingly folded it. I floated back to a day of happiness and smiles, feeling that warm tingling sensation that you only taste when you are deeply in love. I glowed as I watched her beautiful face light up and smile, as she tried on her new light-blue skin-tight jeans for the very first time. I was so happy then because I didn't yet know that she hated me and wanted me to die. I was in heaven believing that she was smiling because she loved me. I had no idea that she was smiling because she was imagining her secret new boyfriend unzipping them before making love to her. My hands trembled, I struggled to breathe and my eyes almost spilt tears as my soul screamed in misery, as if slashed once again by a razor-sharp steely knife. This was a torment I was unprepared for. I still wasn't ready to face the truth.

It was torture; death by a thousand cuts as I pushed on with the anguish of condemning her garments to the bin bag. The next sharp slash was viewing the mind movie of my 'one and only' posing for seductive selfies in her brand-new gear before uploading them to her Facebook page. She was hungry for likes and flattering comments from her admirers. Of course, they were oblivious to the fact that she had a terminally ill husband. Even worse was that her husband had been mercilessly blocked from viewing the images of his wife wearing the new outfits he had bought. You just couldn't make it up, could you? Her narcissistic hunger needed feeding and nothing on earth was going to spoil her egotistical feast. Having a husband was just an awkward inconvenience.

I screamed as the blade sliced once more. I relived the moment when she towered over my broken body. Cut. She was dressed to the nines in her brand-new clothes as she screamed, "Ghost-face, hurry up and die." Cut, cut. She danced out of the house laughing her head off as she hurried to meet her new boyfriend in a hotel room for an afternoon of sex. Cut, cut, cut. She returned later that evening mocking my piteous bag of bones as she taunted me with tales of how good the sex had been with her new bloke. Cut, cut, cut, cut and one more fucking cut.

Now, if I had been an unfaithful, violent or abusive hubby then the trouble and strife (wife) could have had mitigating reasons for spooning me a gob full of my own medicine. But for the death and life of me I hadn't. I had been a loyal loving partner who had granted her every wish. A house, a baby, helping her parents, holidays overseas and more shopping and new clothes than she could ever have dreamed of. Her final wish for me to hurry up and die would be the first one denied. For crying out loud; my children needed me.

I felt dizzy and nauseous as the memories of that nightmare kept cutting deep. I carefully placed the bags into the car and dropped them off at the Easterleigh Animal Sanctuary charity shop. I had contemplated burning the bloody lot in a futile attempt to hit back at my wicked old flame. I realised that I would have been pissing in the wind because she wouldn't have given a toss. After all, she already had the house, the land and everything else I had flipping worked for. Donating my abusive partner's vast collection of garments to help abused animals seemed like a fitting end to the painful saga. Love and compassion is always the answer. Hate and anger just poisons the mind. Like selling the wedding ring in Bangkok, it was another painful step forward in accepting that the past was dead and buried.

I returned home still distraught, only to come across a pair of scanty panties underneath the bed. I did not lovingly place them beneath my pillow but tossed them into the rubbish bin outside. After all, I didn't want the stinking smell of treason to haunt my dreams each night, did I?

Now don't go grabbing the wrong end of the stick and assume that all Lao girls are cheats and thieves. Nothing could be further from the truth. I absolutely adore the Lao people. They are the friendliest, kindest, gentlest, most beautiful people I have ever encountered. I love them with all my heart and miss their beautiful, genuine smiles. Many of my friends have faithful Lao wives and have lived in harmony for years. The problems Ian and I suffered were the exception rather than the rule.

I was feeling "Down in the Sewer" the following day. I felt like shit; all alone and unloved. My life and dreams had just been flushed away down the shitter. I made the snap decision to nip across the road to the pub in the hope of finding a bit of adult company. As I was standing at the bar ordering a half-pint of real ale a middle-aged man to the right of me hollered, "I wouldn't speak to you if you had terminal cancer, you fat bastard."

I was startled. Surely, he couldn't have been gobbing off at me?

How the heck could I be described as a fat bastard after the big C had left me looking like a matchstick man? Without warning a jovial obese chap to the left of me roared with laughter as his blubbery beer-belly wobbled like jelly. He took a large swig of lager before retaliating with, "Fuck off." Good gracious me. A case of, buffoons to the left of me, comics to the right. And I was stuck in the blooming middle.

I grabbed my glass of ale and sat in solitary confinement at a table near the door. The cancer wisecrack hadn't offended me. In fact, I couldn't stop chuckling at the irony. In recent times I had occasionally overheard typical seventies comments such as: mong, window-licker and spaz. It didn't distress me, but I was concerned in case someone with a mentally or physically disabled child had overheard too. They would have been deeply hurt. Consequently, we must be mindful as to what we send out into the universe because, more often than not, it has a nasty habit of coming back to bite us on the arse.

Many years ago, in Bangkok, I had a slapstick couple of minutes walking down a road in the most ridiculous manner imaginable. I wasn't mocking the physically impaired but just mimicking a John Cleese silly-walk from the *Monty Python's Flying Circus* television series. My Thai girlfriend wasn't impressed and didn't find it amusing, giving me a right bollocking for taking the piss out of the disabled. Obviously, she had never seen the programme in that part of the world. Lost in translation once again. Anyway, lo and behold, that very evening I crashed my motorbike which resulted in me having to walk like a silly-billy for the next two months. Instant karma strikes again.

The beer stung like ant bites as I took tiny painful sips. The radiotherapy had kiboshed any aspirations of living life as a beer-monster and that was a good thing. I was destined to be a herbal tea fiend from then on, it seemed

I sat with my shadow watching happy couples holding hands as they smiled and gazed adoringly into each other's eyes. Their laughter, their jokes and their love was all around. The sweet smells of perfume mingled with the smell of beer which hung in the air. I recall sitting with my wife in a pub in Laos such a long, long time ago. I was so proud, so happy and so in love. And now she was sitting with her new man and she was so proud, so happy and so in love. Cut, cut. Janet was correct. Once you are over fifty and single in the UK you are invisible.

At that moment I regretted my decision to step outside and join the human race. Going to the pub had left me feeling even lonelier. Better to be a hermit at home in my kitchen. Nobody noticed as I stood up, left the pub and walked the 50 steps home.

A few bags of coffee were sold online. That was good but not really making a dent in the bank loan and certainly not covering the interest. I was far too ill to be giving out samples and selling to cafes and restaurants. Another fine mess, Syd.

On 18th November Jo joined the local Beaver Scouts and came home with a bird feeder. It was full of nuts and seeds. We took it into the back yard and hung it up. I was so happy that they had taught him to care about the local wildlife.

During the final few days of the month I was sweating then shivering with a full-on fever. My neck was swollen, and I was bringing up shedloads of yellow phlegm. The inside of my mouth and tongue were covered in painful sores. It was just like days after the chemo. I struggled with the housework and cooking and the school runs were just a daze. I was starting to panic in case the cancer had returned. Luckily, I was as right as "November Rain" on the final day of the month. Phew, that was a close shave.

Ian informed me that he had finally booked his flight to Kampala, Uganda to visit his wife and kids. His Japanese missus was employed by an NGO out in deepest darkest Africa. He was now flogging his furniture before his mid-December departure.

I dreamt that I was sitting on a plane flying across the sky to anywhere away from here. Would that make any difference though? Was I running away from Blackpool or was I running away from myself?

Starman

(December 2014)

The biting cold numbed my face and turned my fingers into clumsy ice pops as I scraped the frozen car windscreen in readiness for the school run. The bitter wind brutally lashed my shivering body as my lips turned blue and my teeth chattered like a pneumatic drill. I noticed my frosty breath and childishly likened it to cigarette smoke. "I Don't Want to Grow Up." December was here again, and I felt chilled to the bone; all 206 of them as bone number 207 had wisely disappeared. "Good job I am not on a blind date," I smirked.

Spending roughly half my life being kissed by glorious sunshine under never-ending clear blue skies made the cruel cold bite even deeper. After tasting life in shirt and shorts in paradise, the thought of another dark freezing winter in a big coat and thick pullovers made me want to vomit. And cry too. The tropical sunshine had made me shine, but now I was doomed to be dark and gloomy, just like all the other miserable cold grey sods here in the land of ice, snow, rain and cloud. I flipping loathed winter in bloody Blackpool.

On the 4th I wrapped up and plodded to the nearby school to attend Jo's nativity play. And lo and behold Jo was the star of the show; in fact, he was dressed as a star, shining brightly in my idolising eyeballs. He stood there on stage trying to hide at the back behind the other performers, frequently glancing over to check that his old man was doing a bit of stargazing. Jo didn't have a speaking part and just reluctantly mumbled some of the carols when the whole group sang. There were no aspirations of stardom in his mind; he just stayed in the background willingly letting the other kids take centre stage.

At the finale I joined the other doting mums and dads taking snapshots of their little sunshines. For once I didn't feel any self-pity at being the lone single dad; I had a twinkle in my eye as I sparkled with pride at having lovingly raised my little sun all alone. He was my favourite star in the whole universe.

On the 11th, Jo was the birthday boy for the sixth time. How the years had flown by, but on reflection the last three had dragged, like a sadist's knife. I floated back to that magical day at a private hospital in Thailand, when I held my newly born baby boy for the very first time. The love, the wonder and the tears of joy from that beautiful moment are lovingly stored deep within my big red heart. The recollection of his first birthday in the tiny village of Gnommalad in Southern Laos, when he had more chocolate cake on his face than in his mouth evoked a chuckle.

Finally, I remembered a wild celebration of running, cheering and dancing, but fortunately, not doing myself an injury by sensibly opting out of performing an acrobatic backflip. No, I hadn't just scored the last-minute winning goal in a world cup final; this was something far more important. My son had just uttered his very first words and those words were 'dada'. My clever little lad must have had an eerie premonition that his old man would be the only one looking after him in the very near future.

The party in the living room was a riot of laughter, happiness and spicy whiffs of South Asia as we scoffed an Indian feast of curry, samosas and onion bhajis. Eugene, yours truly, and our rescue mutt Alfie were the only guests. No need for a doggie bag as my faithful hound eagerly wolfed down the leftovers. We belted out "Happy Birthday to You" … prior to Jo proudly blowing out the candles with just one birthday blast of air. It suddenly struck me that this was Jo's first birthday without his mother. She had left us one and a half years ago but had made a brief visit last December. Speaking of the devil; the phone rang, and she demanded to talk with Jo. He wasn't very enthusiastic, but I insisted that he had a quick word. She wished him a happy birthday and promised to post him a laptop as a present, which of course never arrived. What a surprise!

She did have an unexpected gift for me though; an unwelcome foul-mouthed earful of abuse and yet another threat to use her rich boyfriend's dosh to take Jo away. I knew that this was just a bluff and that she was joyfully 'sticking the knife in' to mess with my mind. I informed Pauline, my family support worker of her provocation and was advised never to allow her into the house and to phone the police if she ever turned up unannounced. And Pauline wasn't pleased that I had granted Jo's mother the opportunity to speak with him. He was very young, and his mum's rare phone calls could do more damage than good, was the gist of her reasoning.

The subsequent knife-wound of painful news from the wicked one arrived a few days later. She cackled, "I don't need you to agree to a divorce because my lawyer has informed me that the marriage can be annulled because you haven't been sending me any support money." Was she calling my bluff again? I was flabbergasted and if what she had stated was true then the law really was a buffalo. In Laos a buffalo is an idiom

283

for stupid. Be careful though because if you are ever naïve or foolish enough to call a Lao person a buffalo, you'd better get ready for a violent confrontation. It is a massive insult and the offended person is guaranteed to lose the plot and go completely berserk because you have made him or her lose face big-time. Not recommended, unless you are prepared to spend a large chunk of time on a diet of hospital or prison food.

Shockingly, some legal jargon blabs that I must support a wife who has cheated and lied and send her money while she is lying on her back for every Tom, Dick and Harry, otherwise she will be granted a divorce. Something smelt very fishy to me. And it wasn't her scanty panties because I had thrown them away, remember. The odds-on favourite to this mind-boggling conundrum was that her rich fella had handed over *A Fistful of Dollars* under the table.

My dream of paying off the loan and taking the kids for a holiday in the sun had just gone up in a puff of wicked witchy-poo smoke. It was nothing more than a pipedream because she had never had any intention of returning what she had stolen. I'd better start saving up for a pot to piss in. I sat there like the proverbial buffalo. Now, if I really had been a stupid buffalo then I would have flown back to Laos and burnt the thieving cow alive before blowing my brains out. However, I cleverly elected to play the role of a wise old owl by allowing karma to take care of her while I took care of my kids. The following day the she-devil sent me this message: "Hurry Up and Die". Some things never change, do they?

***

On the 14th I attended the inaugural 'Blackpool and Fylde Vegans' meet-up at a café in the town centre. 'Toast' was the in-place for the in-crowd to be noticed as they casually sipped a latte, a tropical fruit smoothie or nibbled one of the Mediterranean dishes up for grabs. It was all shiny and clean with walls the colour of newly peeled apples as tantalising aromas of freshly brewed coffee tickled your sense of smell. This forward-thinking eatery had the insight to provide a vegan menu after realising that veganism was not just a passing fad but was a rapidly growing movement which was here to stay. It was either the first or one of the first places in town to have a vegan menu and I was ready to give it a two-thumbs up.

I grinned like a schoolboy as I sat with my fellow "Meat is Murder" mates. There were just eight of us but from little acorns mighty oaks grow. These included Roddy, a fortyish blonde haired punk whose claim to fame was being one of the first people to organise vegan festivals in the UK. Dennis was a fit young-looking bloke in his sixties who owned an interesting second-hand shop. Then we had Sarah, a middle-aged goth covered in inks and her twenty-something lad who would become a very close friend of mine. In fact, Dan the Man as I called him, helped me much more than you could possibly imagine but that comes in part two of this jaw-dropping tale.

I ordered a tasty roasted vegetable vegan wrap but only managed to eat half of it because of my radiotherapy-damaged throat. Shit happens hey! We all nattered away about our vegan lifestyles and a good time was had. I was glad that I had made the effort to crawl out from under my stone to show my ugly mush.

My busy northern monkey mind was doing my head in as it continued grabbing branch after branch and each branch was a trivial thought. To put a stop to this 'round-the-clock' monkey business I persevered with my daily meditation. I sharpened my mind by focusing on the breath entering and leaving my nostrils. At times I managed to gain control and by not following the frivolous thoughts, tasted the peace and bliss of living in the "Nothing Else Matters" dimension. I was making steady progress along the middle path, but knew it was a long journey to reach the promised land of Nirvana. These fleeting glimpses of true reality inspired me to plod on in my effort to flee the unreal world of mind-created madness.

I was still chatting and flirting with several vegan girls online. It was a great escape from my lonely kitchen life, but I realised in my broken heart of hearts that I would never bump into any of these plant-based angels in the flesh; my crushed body and mind were unworthy. Thank goodness I could let my non-existent hair down at the weekend meetings with Miss Bombshell. The banter just ebbed and flowed with my supportive caring bosom buddy.

On the 16th Jo attended his Beaver Scouts Christmas Party at the nearby Squirrel Pub and it was heart-warming watching him mixing and having fun with kids his own age. He needs more than just his decrepit old fella, doesn't he?

Throughout the concluding week of term Ian had been highly emotional at the thought of leaving Laos. He had miraculously managed to complete his teaching and had flogged all his meagre possessions too. Even treating himself to a new computer, to replace the one stolen by his

Lao missus. On the 17th when he got on the flight, he forwarded a text saying, "I have made a massive mistake." I fully understood where he was coming from. I always felt gutted when leaving paradise, because in my mind paradise was home. Although, I admit I was in too much pain and shock to feel anything the last time.

I gently replied to Ian, "No you haven't mate. It is imperative that you visit your kids and bear in mind that you can always fly back to Laos."

On the 18th Ian forwarded me a message notifying me that he had arrived in Kampala, the capital of Uganda. He continued, "My wife and kids are friendly, but the kids spend most of their time playing computer games."

"Tell me about it," I laughed.

More worryingly, he disclosed that he had lost 25kg in five months! I recall dropping 45kg in six months but have somehow managed to put 12kg back on.

Dead and Buried

(December 2014)

The 18th was also the day of another endoscopy to see if there was any sign of the big C. I swaggered out of Victoria Hospital once again with a massive Manc smirk on my mug after being informed that there was no sign of the bastard cancer. One more unexpected Christmas to celebrate, unless the Wicked Witch had an 'out of character' change of heart and sent me the money for the house she had stolen. In that unlikely event I would more than likely die of shock before Rudolph had finished his carrot and Santa had slurped the almond milk.

It seemed that I was in with a shout of escaping almost certain death by the skin of my radiotherapy-damaged teeth after all. In fact, I have had two other close encounters with death. Let me reveal all the spine-tingling details about these other two meetings with my scythe-carrying skeletal mate.

In my mid-teens I became a 'mad for it' potholer and weekends were enjoyed splashing about in the bone-chilling icy waters underground. A year later my enthusiasm for crawling around in muddy subterranean tubes disappeared because my 'mad for it' libido meant that adventures of another kind were all my one-track mind could focus on. I bet you are surprised that 'the devil in me' didn't scribble 'holes of another kind' and in all honesty so am I, ha-ha-ha. I initially considered using 'holes' as you can well imagine but decided to be a Simon Templar for once and change it to 'adventures.'

In my early twenties my lust for "Going Underground" and jamming myself in narrow passages returned with a vengeance, so I established my own potholing club – the Chorlton Cavemen. Our leader was Denis, a skilful experienced caver who was ideal for the role because he was only about four and a half feet tall. Kevin, a close friend, was a black belt karate expert and fitness fanatic. There was Mike, an amazing musician, who could play any song you named on the guitar and finally, me, who you know far too much about already. This handful of lunatics tackled several of the most dangerous caving challenges the UK had to offer. Super-severe grade five trips involving hour after hour of soul-crushing tight squeezes, eternal long wet crawls and descents into deep dark chasms.

Picture yourself lying flat on your back, chilled to the bone in freezing cold water in a very tight tube. Don't open your eyes though, because they are under water along with your mouth. The only part of your body above the water is your nose, which is scraping along the rock in the tiny bit of airspace available. Your helmet is off and being dragged along because the tube is far too cramped for helmet and head together. You understand that you are about three hours away from the surface and in the event of an accident, a rescue so deep in this system of narrow twisting waterlogged passages would be almost impossible. You try to banish from your mind the knowledge that if it rains on the surface, then many parts of this cave system including this very tube will quickly flood to the roof. However, it is always in the background, repeatedly projecting a mind movie of a terrifying finale of being trapped and drowning to death.You are shivering but know that any sudden movement will create a wave, causing your tiny airspace to disappear, resulting in a nose-full of icy water entering your lungs. You must be calm, focused and stay right in the moment as you negotiate this petrifying obstacle; panic and you are fucked. You continue moving inch by inch until you exit the tube into a slightly larger space, feeling ever so grateful for the luxury of four inches of airspace.

You fight on for another hour over boulders, navigating more tight wet crawls and tubes, down deep dark abysses until you eventually reach your destination; the end of the cave. You are overjoyed at having ticked another super-severe pothole off the list before realising that you now have the formidable four-hour task of overcoming all the intimidating squeezes and tight wet crawls once more. Of course, returning to the surface is far more strenuous because now you are fighting gravity and it will be a herculean effort to stop yourself sliding back down near-vertical muddy tubes. Eventually you spot daylight as you near the entrance. Your body is shattered as it struggles to take one step after another, but your mind is already racing back to the car; where you are eager to get changed for a piss-up in the local pub.

Once the booze starts to flow, the day's adventure is discussed with nonchalant laugher. "It was a piece of piss, an effing doddle," laughs one of the team.

"I could do it stark bollock naked with my hands tied behind my back," quips another. With boozy Dutch courage, discussion of the possibility of an illegal adventure down the notorious Mossdale Caverns begins. Access to this cave has not been granted since 1967, when six young men drowned after it flooded to the roof. Occasionally a group of mad rebels sneak onto Fountains Fell in Yorkshire to pirate (sneak into) this infamous system, but they are few and far between. And for very a good reason, because it is an eight-hour slog of mainly crawls, which flood to the roof if it rains on the surface. Therefore, if the heavens open while you are down the cave then you will have a nightmare farewell to life on planet Earth. Everyone agrees in the drunken haze that next week's adventure is Mossdale. However, you know it will never happen because that is just one mad crawl beyond, even for a group of nutters like us. This is how I spent most of my weekends and I blooming loved it.

Time to stop waxing lyrical about caving and get down to the nitty gritty and spit out the account of my first near-death experience. The Chorlton Cavemen travelled to the Mendip Hills in south-west England to explore Swildon's Hole. This undertaking consisted of freediving several submerged passages called sumps and a few shorter, partially or fully filled tubes of water known as ducks. It is intimidating and quite scary when you focus on a fixed-rope disappearing into the murky water of a submerged passage. It takes balls to go against your survival instinct and dive headfirst into the jet-black unknown.

We entered the system and after overcoming half a mile of underground passages with a descent of around 400 feet we arrived at a small chamber and our first major challenge; sump one. We stood in apprehension as we stared in fear at the way forward; a rope disappearing into a submerged tunnel. We shivered while plucking up the courage to test ourselves against this frightful obstacle.

Denis the bloody Menace shouted, "After me lads." He lay flat upon his stomach in the chilly water and took hold of the rope. We watched him vanish into the darkness. The last thing we saw were the bottoms of his wellington boots being swallowed up by the murky liquid. A short while later the rope moved five times, letting us know that he had emerged at the other end of the water-filled tunnel and that he was safely breathing in large lungsful of oxygen. It was also the signal that it was now my turn to pass this unnerving hazard.

With my heart in my mouth I reluctantly stepped towards my darkest nightmare. The sharp sound of my boots crunching on the small wet stones echoed in the subterranean chamber. My senses were fully focused and on high alert. The malevolent laughter of trickling water from a distant dark corner and the disturbing drip-drip-drip right next to my head were loud enough to wake the dead. A cold breeze kissed my right cheek and was that fear I could smell? I lay on my belly feeling each sharp stone pressing into my skin as my lamplight reflected off the murky water onto my frightened eyeballs. Then I gripped the rope tightly. I stared one last time into the inky blackness, took a deep breath and pulled my face into the unknown.

The bitter cold mugged me, stealing all my body heat. *For God's sake never let go of the rope, otherwise you are fucked,* I warned myself. I pulled and pulled repeatedly, banging the top of my helmet on the roof of the underwater tube, praying for the miraculous moment it popped-out at the other side. I was right there in the present moment, pulling and pulling, banging and banging and kicking like a madman until my head suddenly surfaced, whereupon I spotted Denis laughing his little head off as he gave me the two thumbs up. With immense relief I filled my lungs with wonderful life-giving oxygen.

A wicked smirk spread across my frozen face as I tugged the rope, letting the next poor sod know it was now his turn for a taste of hell. The adventure progressed nicely as we overcame further climbs, scrambles, descents and submerged passages with our usual gung-ho 'bring it on' attitude. After all, we were an elite group of experienced super-fit cavers; nothing could possibly go wrong. Or so I thought.

We arrived at an awkward duck. A tight tube with limited airspace. The option was to either lie on your back and slowly edge backwards with your nose against the roof or on your stomach with your face underwater and scramble through to the other end. Denis went first on his stomach, face in the water and quickly overcame this perilous obstacle.

My gut feeling advised, "Go through on your back, always keeping your nose above water," but my insane sense of humour laughed "Do it the hard way Syd." I lay on my stomach at the entrance to this rocky narrow tube of water. I could see Denis' lamp flickering about eight feet away. Sharp intake of breath, then with my face underwater I pulled like crazy to quickly exit this awkward tube. About half way I became stuck. My face was pressed against the stony floor with my helmet stuck fast to the roof. I pulled at rocks, kicked my legs but my body didn't budge. I was stuck with my face fully underwater and starting to panic.

Without warning, a sensation of pure ecstasy and peace filled my whole being. Thoughts and fears of drowning were replaced by a floaty feeling of perfect euphoria. I had the uncanny perception that I had been here before and was returning home. I yearned to remain forever in this timeless zone but that was not meant to be, because I was abruptly back in the land of the living, gasping for air. I was free at the other side, taking deep lungsful of air, looking wide-eyed at Denis. My flesh and bones must have been battling for dear life while I was blissing out in paradise. "Are you ok Syd?" asked a worried-looking Denis.

"Never felt better, mate," I said, smiling.

I shouted through to Mike, informing him that it would be far safer to come through on his back. He agreed but halfway he panicked and gashed the side of his head on a rock as he scrambled for safety and life-giving air. The trip went without further incident and that evening we were all laughing in the pub, drinking pints of Mendip Madness; the very potent local scrumpy cider. Even Mike, with a deep cut and angry purple bruise, was having a good time, strumming his guitar while we all had a right old sloshed-up singsong.

I never described my magical near-death experience and the rapture I felt to anyone. It seemed personal and like it had to be a secret never told. This otherworldly experience was meant only for the dead and not for the living. I mused that either it was the physical body releasing happy chemicals to make death more bearable, or perhaps I had just been permitted a secret glimpse of life after death. A little voice inside me whispered that it was the latter.

The Chorlton Cavemen disbanded shortly after this trip. In fact, Mike after getting a gashed face, was the first to see the insanity of our madcap bravado and never ventured underground again. The final Chorlton Cavemen adventure, undertaken by Denis, Kevin and me, was to Hammer Pot in Yorkshire. It was so named because bits of rock had to be bashed out with a lump hammer to allow a thin man to squeeze through. We struggled through the entrance, a series of unbelievably tight passages, gaining just a few inches every few minutes. No time for claustrophobia here.

After 20 minutes Kevin threw in the towel for the very first time. He said, "Fuck this, it is just getting tighter and tighter." He managed to find a bit of space to turn around and sensibly headed back to the surface. That was his caving days over.

Like a bloody idiot I followed Denis on the arduous struggle to the far reaches of this punishing underground network. There were amazing deep descents, large chambers and a fast-flowing stream at the bottom, but it was a ghastly nightmare escaping the tight tunnels leading to the entrance on the way back. I was like a contortionist twisting and bending in the tiniest of tubes and extremely relieved to eventually stand back on the surface. I was covered in mud, bruises, scrapes and sweat but presented my usual cocky 'it was nothing to write home about' grin as I inhaled deeply on a cancer stick. However, I knew deep down that my caving days were now dead and buried. What about Denis? I have not heard 'head or tail' of him but it wouldn't surprise me if he were happily crawling along some underground tunnel at this very moment.

***

Have you ever seen a dead person? Well I have and without further ado, let me supply the astonishing tale regarding my second smooch with the angel of death. It occurred in the mid-nineties when I was doing a spot of work at a sugar factory in Khampheang Phet in Northern Thailand. This city is famous for its historical park and small oval-shaped bananas.

On the day in question, I had a ticket for the front seat on the early morning express bus to Bangkok. Each weekend I would embark on the five-hour journey to the capital city to visit Eric Jay, my two-year-old son. Even though his mother and I had separated, my strong paternal instinct and deep love for my first-born meant that giving this weekly journey a miss was a non-starter.

I couldn't relax in the front seat to the left of the driver; something just didn't feel quite right. A strange sensation inside kept prodding me to move away from this spot. Was it my sub-consciousness or was it a supernatural message from my guardian angel? I will never know. The tropical storm was chucking itself against the windscreen as a cheery Thai pop song played on the radio. My inner-being continued screaming, "Get out of this seat."

I was keeping everything crossed that the bus would not fill up, so I could obey my gut-reaction and get the hell out of this seat. I was on a "Knife-Edge" counting the soaked-to-the-skin passengers stepping onto the bus. It was raining snakes and lizards here in the land of smiles. The hostess got on next, spotlessly dressed in her smart bus-company uniform. A royal blue jacket, skirt and hat, crisp white blouse and highly polished black shoes. She had been ushered to the bus by a colleague holding a brolly, so besides a few wet splashes on her shoes she was relatively dry. I would estimate that she was about 25 years old. Her shiny shoulder-length hair matched her demeanour, which sparkled with happiness. I managed to catch her eye and asked if I could possibly change my seat. She gave me a beautiful warm smile, studied her notes and led me to a place on the right, half-way down the bus. I thanked her, and she laughed, "You are welcome." I was able to relax my God-given arse in my new seat now that the alarm bells in my brain had stopped ringing.

The half-empty bus pulled away in the heavy rain. A middle-aged man was now sitting in the very seat that had given me bad vibrations, I considered warning him but of course I didn't. What could I say? Your seat is dangerous? Your seat is haunted? He would have thought the foreigner was off his blinking head.

The pretty hostess continued smiling and laughing as she handed out bottles of drinking water and face wipes to the passengers. I attempted to fathom the reason for her happiness. Had she recently fallen head over heels in love, so she was walking on cloud nine, wearing rose-coloured specs? Could she be dreaming about her young son or daughter's birthday party later that evening? Or was it the dinner she would be sharing with her devoted parents tomorrow? This young lady radiated with the joys of life and it was infectious. I felt happy too and was pleased that I had contemplated another person's life. Most of the time we only focus on me, me, me, imagining that the universe revolves only around our precious selves. We rarely wish to know anything about another person unless they are of benefit to us; usually sexually, financially or to boost our ego in some way. I find that so sad.

The rain was belting down as we sped along the highway towards the City of Angels. I perused the sports pages of yesterday's *Bangkok Post* before yawning. I was feeling the effects of last night's beer. We were only about 45 minutes into the journey when I eased back into my seat and closed my drowsy eyes. Pictures of a pizza with my boy that I had planned for later that day, played in my mind before I fell asleep. I was unexpectedly jolted from my cat-nap by frantic shouting and screaming, coming from the front of the bus. I instantly jumped up in alarm and gripped the back of the seat in front of me tightly. There was an almighty bang as we hit a truck, then everything went into slow-motion as the bus left the road. I thought to myself, *This is the day that I die.*

Still in slow motion, we bounced down a slope and came to a halt in a waterlogged field. I looked out of the window and was stunned to witness the bus driver running away in slow motion. It was like an action replay from a televised football match. However, his face was not lit up in pride after scoring a goal; it was white with shock as he looked back in horror at the carnage he had caused. It was surreal, just like an edge-of-your-seat scene from an old black and white Hitchcock film.

My focus returned to inside the bus, which was filled with hysterical screams and desperate cries for help from the front. I checked myself over and was gobsmacked to find that I was injury-free, as was a young lad who was sitting nearby. We just gazed at each other in astonishment before shrugging our shoulders and nervously smiling. I had lost a shoe but nevertheless managed to open the emergency door at the back and step out into the field. I walked in the rain to the front of the bus and noticed the young hostess lying on her back crying, *"Jep, jep, jep."* (I am in pain.) It was obvious that she had flown through the windscreen.

A shiver ran down my spine when I spotted that the front left-hand side of the bus was completely destroyed. This must have been the spot that impacted with the truck. Shit, that was where I was supposed to be sitting, I shuddered. An old man who was tightly holding a baby was pacing up and down frantically crying, "He isn't breathing," but refused to release the child to anyone.

In the chaos, I sprinted up the slope to the highway and frantically waved down a pick-up truck. With the driver and the young lad, we managed to get about eight injured people in the back including the hostess and the man with the baby. The driver put his foot down and continuously beeped the horn until we arrived at the nearest hospital five minutes later. I jumped out and placed an injured woman on a trolley bed and quickly wheeled her into the hospital. Once the doctors and nurses saw the seriousness of the situation, they informed me that this was just a small village hospital and that they didn't have the facilities to deal with it. We would have to drive another 15 kilometres to the main hospital. We carefully placed the injured woman back in the pick-up and raced down the highway.

The doctors and nurses were there at the ready. The smaller hospital must have phoned them. The injured were speedily transferred into the hospital. I stayed with the hostess, who was still breathing but in a lot of pain. After being mesmerised by her *Joie de vivre* plus my reflection on the possible reasons for her high-spirited attitude, I felt a deep connection to this girl. And not to forget, she was the angel who led me away from the death seat. I really wanted a happy ending for this lady. I sat outside the room where the doctor and nurses were treating her. I could hear her continuous low groan of *"Jep jep jep."* I clenched my fists tightly and whispered, "Come on girl, you can do it." Then suddenly, there was steely cold silence.

My heart sank as I stood up and walked straight into the tiny cream room and asked the doctor about the hostess. He remembered that I had accompanied her when she arrived and gently replied, "I'm very sorry, she is dead." He pointed to a body on a bed about a metre to my left. I had never seen a dead body before. As soon as I looked, I knew that it wasn't her. The sparkling energy, the laughter, the dreams, the smiles, the love and the joy I had witnessed just a couple of hours earlier weren't there. On the hospital bed was a slab of lifeless meat and it wasn't her. She had left already. My inner being had one last word with me that day. I was told that the physical body is nothing more than a suit and that the real being is the invisible energy which lives eternally; moving on after the physical body has died.

I thanked the doctor and slowly left his room to sit outside alone. I softly sobbed as I recalled the three words, she had spoken to me, "You are welcome." And those words had saved my life here on planet Earth. In fact, I am weeping now as I write. Visiting the past can be very painful can't it?

From my recollections, out of the 16 passengers seven died, including the hostess and the small baby, and seven were badly injured. Just the young lad and I were injury-free. I was interviewed by a TV reporter. He asked me if I had any amulets, which most Thais wear around their necks for good luck. I replied, "No, all I have is a bit of wood on a piece of string that I got from Phu Kradueng National Park." I pulled it from under my shirt and everyone gazed in wonder at my lucky bit of wood.

The sugar factory manager collected me and gave me a lift to Bangkok. I was in deep shock of course. I hugged my son and took him out for a pizza. As I lay in bed that night I reflected on the day's events. Firstly, I thought about the happy hostess and how her hopes and dreams were snatched away by a stupid driving error. Her partner, children, parents, grandparents, friends and relatives would all now be crying and suffering terrible grief, which would last for weeks, months or even years. Then, the little baby who had hardly started his life. He would never go to school, learn to ride a bike, fall in love or have children of his own. His mum and dad would be distraught. My heart went out to them all.

And what of me? Moving my seat had saved my life but had killed another. If I hadn't moved, the middle-aged man couldn't have sat there and may have chosen a place further down the bus. At first, I had a pang of guilt but then realised that the bus only had 16 passengers and that he was free to sit in any section of the bus. It was his fate to elect for a seat at the front. That was his decision, not mine.

I was still confused as to why I had such a strong feeling to change my seat. I had sat in the front seat of buses many times before. Why did I get the heebie-jeebies this time? I don't know and probably never will. One thing I do know is that life is fleeting and very fragile. All it takes is one fatal error or being in the wrong place at the wrong time and it is over. I suppose the answer is to live with love, compassion and kindness and try to experience as much as possible of this magical world without harming others. The only certainty is that you will die one day, so make the most of it while you still can.

Back at my office I was offered serious money for my lucky piece of wood, but I refused to sell it. The shock of that incident affected me greatly and I avoided travelling by bus whenever possible, and the times I had no alternative I would be a bag of nerves staring out of the front window. It took me over a year to feel safe on a bus again and of course I never sat at the front.

***

It was Christmas Eve 2014 and I wrapped up presents for the kids. Each of them got a pile of gifts. Eugene's main gift was a Canon DSLR and Jo's was a Game Boy he had been asking for. Alfie got some pressies too. After all, he was part of the family. On Christmas day the kids opened their gifts and we had a meal together. Life carried on. Kids playing games, taking the dog for a walk, doing housework. I was struggling to cope but always put on a brave face for my children.

On Boxing Day Ian informed me that his wife didn't want anything to do with him. She scolded, "You walked out on me in 2004 so don't involve me in anything now."

He admitted, "Harsh, but I deserve it I suppose."

On New Year's Eve Ian sent me a text letting me know that he was off out with $100 and that he was heading to the raunchiest place in town. I warned him to be careful, but he said, "It is very safe in Kampala. Everyone is partying, and the music is playing."

I felt so depressed and alone yet again. No one to hold and no one to love. Yes, of course I had my children and I loved them with all my heart. I hated my life and it was only the love for my children that kept me in the land of the living. They needed me. Why had I fought so hard for such a shite-cold lonely life? It was as if I was Sisyphus doomed to repeat the 'day in day out' mind-numbing tasks repeatedly. Any time I seemed to make progress my world would come tumbling down and I would have to start at rock bottom once more. Life was a living hell.

I told Ian to have a good time and went upstairs wishing I was "Dead and Buried."

Dry Your Eyes

(January 1st, 2015)

All was not so quiet on "New Year's Day" as the rockets exploded in an ear-splitting kaleidoscopic crescendo outside my bedroom window, welcoming in 2015. Sadly, there would be no cocks cockily cock-a-doodle-doo-ing in the overcast outskirts of Blackpool at daybreak. Woe is me, coz I wouldn't be washing the chicken's face at the crack of dawn either, because I was now a pitiful "Lonely Man"… my "Dream Lover" had left me almost a year ago and was now far away in the arms of another.

I dragged the grimy duvet over my head in a feeble endeavour to escape the celebrations and sobbed into my hands, hot salty tears dripping between my trembling fingers onto the ruffled unwashed bedsheet. The echoes of the rhythmic thrusts and lustful cries of passion in this very bed the night before she left, last January, stabbed deeply as they emphasised my singleness. And those erotic reflections of lovemaking were painful knife wounds to my soul as I struggled to accept that my wife had betrayed me.

I was trapped in a hopeless depression without a dream in my heart. I felt like giving up the ghost but couldn't, because my kids had no one else except their broken old man. And what a bloody failure he was. He had lost 'everything but the flipping kitchen sink' and just lived a gloomy sorrowful existence as he wished upon a "Twinkle Twinkle Little Star" to return to the good old days before the cancer. My worst nightmare had become a reality; I was now a "Solitary Man" with no name just living from hand to gob in Blackpool; you can call me Skint Eastwood!

I drifted back to my blissful life before the cancer, picturing myself standing hand-in-hand with my beautiful wife under a dazzling fruit tree in our tropical garden. The sun warmed my tanned flesh and my two kids warmed my heart as I observed them playing happily beneath the trees. My dreamy eyes focused on a line of bright orange fire ants making their way along a nearby branch before I spotted an enormous purple butterfly resting on a lime green leaf of an adjacent wild plant. Later that day I would drive my loved ones for a mouth-watering feast at a romantic outdoor restaurant on the banks of the mighty Mekong River. We would laugh and chat together as another fabulous sunset in paradise captivated the mesmerised diners.

Then under a velvety night sky with a thousand stars we would amble as one through the enchanting night market. The brilliant colours of a hundred lanterns were reflected on the inky blackness of the river and on my kids' excited faces too as they rummaged for a new toy. My wife sparkled with pleasure as she selected a bohemian black and white wrap-around tribal frock. I stood still and glowed with pure joy and deep love. I squeezed my partner's hand and gazed into her gorgeous eyes, realising that I had found what I was looking for; the perfect place and the perfect partner. I was living the dream and tingled with optimism because the future looked very shiny, happy and bright.

I lay back on my bed and pondered what might have been if I hadn't gotten cancer. Would I still be living the dream, or would some other cruel twist of fate have smashed my life into tiny little pieces? I will never know the answer to that hypothetical question, but I did know one thing…the higher the high, the lower the low.

In a flash I was stood trembling in terror inside a tiny white room at Blackpool's Victoria Hospital after being thumped in the face by the tragic news that I was a terminal cancer patient with just six months to live. In that one single moment my life crashed to the ground like a playing card disaster. And like Wild Bill Hickok I had been dealt the 'dead man's hand' and shot down in my prime. I screamed inside, not in fear of the cancer but with the heartbreak of knowing that I would soon be parted from the woman I lived for. I had clenched my fists in sorrowful fury because it was plain to see that the pleasure of watching my beautiful children grow up had been cruelly snatched away. I had endured the madness of the chemo, the agony of the radiotherapy and like a desperate crackpot had searched for the elusive magic-bullet to grant me more precious time in the land of the living. I had changed my diet, my lifestyle, my drinking water, taken herbs, minerals, vitamins, supplements and forced my dying body to exercise.

And unbelievably I was still breathing in and out two and a half years later. But what the hell for? To live a lonely soul-destroying life all alone? It just didn't seem fair. After battling like a lionhearted warrior and kicking the Grim Reaper's arse, surely, such a miraculous victory merited the reward of love and comfort rather than lying here as a defeated abandoned man, spitting out pieces of my broken life.

Then in a moment of bitter pain I fixated on the woman I loved so deeply, always believing that she had felt the same way about me.

The horror at discovering that her "Heart of gold" was in fact a heart of shit had knocked me spark out, leaving me broken on the floor, facing a double death from cancer and heartbreak. Searching for a droplet of compassion from my wife while I was battling the big C was like looking for weapons of mass destruction in Iraq; there was nothing there! I was on the brink of death and my heartbreaker didn't give a shite. The sooner the better as far as she was concerned. And the BBC tears she cried when she begged me to fly her back to the UK so she could take care of me was just fake news. Her sweet promise that she had no one else but me when in fact she had been 'at it' with a Hungarian bloke had crippled me inside.

And what about the time I watched her walk away in the busy airport as the crowded loneliness crushed my mind. Meeting her was the happiest moment in my life but, she was just a beautiful disaster that ripped my heart, dreams and soul to shreds. I had often wished that I had snuffed it prior to discovering that my perfect angel was in fact, a perfect demon. At least then I could have gone to the grave happy at having tasted true love with my faithful soul mate, rather than dying of a bleeding heart before my bag of bones was laid to rest.

I closed my eyes and felt fuzzy and warm as I visualised a noose around my burnt neck, knowing that escape was possible. Next, I was diving off Beachy Head with a massive kiss into the air because I was now free. I shivered as I pulled the duvet around my bony body and froze with sadness in my large double bed. I softly said my prayers, "Please God let me drop dead in my sleep. I am shit; I don't deserve life. I am a good for nothing failure."

More fireworks exploded, creating psychedelic rainbows in the night sky before my soul fragmented in a brilliant white supernova, painting a flawless white masterpiece in my damaged mind. I sat up in astonishment, gazing wide-eyed into the dazzling darkness - and saw the light. Saul had been blinded on the road to Damascus, but I had just been given second sight on the road to desolation. I had been so busy squirming in hell playing the wretched victim that I had failed to see the "Stairway to Heaven" which was right before my eyeballs.

It was a blinking miracle that I hadn't kicked the bucket already. For crying out loud, I should have been a rotting corpse feeding the creepy-crawlies, yet here I was alive, with tears in my eyes on a bit of rock flying through cosmic space. For heaven's sake, I had fought like a lunatic for my life. I had taken everything conventional medicine could fling at my dying body and had researched like an insane boffin for any so-called "Hocus Pocus" cure that I could get my skeletal hands on. I had been burnt, poisoned and curled up on the floor screaming in agony yet I had fought like a punch-drunk boxer to achieve the impossible. Surely, I didn't go through all that just to lie flat-out in bed with a death wish?

And back to my partner who I had trusted and loved with all my heart. The shocking truth that she detested me and had never loved me smashed my world to smithereens. The evil hatred on her twisted face as she screamed, "Hurry up and die, Ghost-face," gave me nightmares. The delight in her dancing eyes as she spitefully laughed in my aghast gaunt face while describing her sexual adventures with her new healthy lover, sliced my broken mind to bits. She had stolen everything I had worked for and had left me without a pot to piss in. Yet I had clung onto my sanity by the skin of my yellow teeth as my heart, soul and pride were tortured daily. I had survived the most horrific and inhumane abuse any man could take. Did I endure that abominable treatment just to continue living in the past feeling sorry for myself?

And even though I had been a very sick, death warmed-up corpse, I had devoted myself to my children. Their well-being was paramount. Single-handedly, I had cooked their meals, washed their clothes, driven them to school, fitted them out with smart new clobber, given them meals in cafes, afternoons at the cinema and days out in the countryside. And I had kept in contact with my two kids overseas, promising to see them again. Did I dedicate myself to my offspring just to lie here as a pathetic loser dreaming of doing myself in?

My grim bedroom transformed into a bright boudoir of hope. I had been crucifying myself with painful thoughts and wallowing in self-pity but now I was sparkling with optimism. It was time to grab this second opportunity of life with both hands. It was time to be reborn. I whispered to myself, "Dry Your Eyes, Mate." I wiped away my tears on my old t-shirt sleeve and slowly walked over to the bedroom window. An orange and blue fire flower exploded in the black sky, causing me to smirk as I realised it was in celebration of my rebirth. Then a massive grin erupted across my dead handsome face as I declared, "I am the Resurrection."

I was bubbling with enthusiasm as I eagerly began planning my *Second Coming*. Man alive, the walking dead had suddenly transformed into a born-again dazzling "Ray of Light". I was the "Master of the Universe" as I created my own reality because the place I lived in was my very own mind. I chuckled at the piles of unwashed clothes, cups, books and countless other odds and sods scattered about the floor of my unkempt bedroom, understanding that this squalid lifestyle was not for the brand-new me.

It was time for a bleak midwinter spring-clean before splashing the cash on some new bedsheets, a duvet, an arty duvet cover and three pillows, to revamp this shithole into a divine crash-pad to rest my enlightened head. Not forgetting a vase of flowers and a couple of scented candles because with my new-found self-belief the space between these four walls would soon become the in-place for nights of loving naughtiness. I licked my lips at the very thought.

Come to think about it, the rest of my bedraggled 'two-up two-down' needed a damn good spit and polish to fit in with my new shiny mindset. Uplifting pictures and posters too. And what about me? I had spent the last two years tramping about like a scruffy hillbilly, wearing the same dirty old clothes day after day. Well let's face it, no femme fatale would be gagging to enter my romantic boudoir to give me a spit and polish if I looked like a dirty old tramp now, would she? That would be sorted by grabbing some new glad rags in the winter sales. And another thing, it was about time I joined the Fatboy Slim (gym) and put a bit of muscle on my skeleton.

But the most important change would be to love and respect myself. No longer would I hide under my stone feeling ugly and unworthy, because it was now time to hold my head high in the sky and fly like Superman with superpowers because after all, this superhero had stared death in the face and had lived to tell the tale.

***

Even though I was buzzing with "Good Vibrations", I wasn't a "Dancing Fool" oblivious to the fact that I was still fighting the bastard cancer. It was crucial to continue with my raw vegan diet, herbs and supplements. I was not out of the brown and nasty just yet, so no junk food or processed shite would pass through my sugarless lips. I didn't want to create an unhealthy environment in my system to give the cancer the green light to run amok, did I?

And after suffering the most dreadful pain, the fear of death and appalling abuse, my compassionate eyes were now wide open to the plight of the poor animals on planet Earth. Look into the eyes of an animal and what do you see? If you see yourself then you have seen the truth because they are "Made of Stars" just like you. They have a central nervous system and feel pain, experience fear, have feelings and emotions and want to be happy, healthy and free just like you. It is a crying shame that so many people cannot see this. They will watch a tear-jerking movie such as '*Babe*' and weep tears of joy for the cute little pig, yet when they get home, they fill their big fat cakeholes with a bacon butty. When will they wake-up and realise that you can't love animals and eat them?

Therefore, my new sparkling life would take my love for A*ll Creatures Great and Small* to the next level. I would be a voice for the voiceless and oppose all forms of animal abuse. I would speak out for tigers, elephants, dogs, cats and the poor dolphins trapped in concrete tanks. I would oppose circuses with animals, the disgustingly cruel foie gras, dog-fighting, bull-fighting, badger culling, grouse shooting and the posh twats who dress up and ride around the countryside chasing a poor fox. Now most of you will more than likely agree with me up to this point, but I haven't finished yet. I would also speak up for the frightened squealing pig who is about to be slaughtered, the baby lamb who was murdered for an Easter scoff and the poor cow who cried for days after her calf had been taken away because some people still believed that drinking another species' milk as adults was normal. My mojo had returned. I was a liberator with a "Rebel Yell" as I cried "No more, no more, no more".

***

I recalled the time when I was at my wit's end, screaming in the unbearable world of madness and despair after my life had fallen apart. I was a sickly mess on the floor, just like a retched-up splodge of vomit. I was dying of cancer, had lost the whole shebang and even the woman I loved despised me. Only the love for my children kept my suicidal thoughts from becoming a razor-sharp reality.

I was trapped in a nightmare and didn't know which way to turn. My only option was to journey to the centre of my mind. And what a terrifying trip that was as punishing mental pictures tortured me all the hours under the sun and the moon. In this bitter school of pain, I learnt enlightening lessons in universal wisdom. My initial insight was that nothing was permanent. Nowt lasted forever. If the woman I loved hadn't ditched me, the relationship would have still ended when one of us snuffed it. And with the large age difference and the big C doing its damnedest to finish me off, it would more than likely have been me… unless I murdered the cheating cow first.

Attachment causes suffering was the next spiritual revelation because when you love something or someone you suffer when you lose it, and you also suffer while you still have it because you are afraid of losing it. And lose it you will because everything is transient. And as I have pointed out many times, the only true reality is the present moment, because the past and the future are just figments of your imagination; they don't exist.

A large stride along the sacred middle path was the realisation that I was not who I thought I was. I wasn't my mind… I was the being living beneath my mind. I would often sit back and watch as thoughts entered and left my mind. I quickly understood that my mind was a sick bastard because it continuously bombarded me with painful regrets and future fears.

So, the resurrected Psycho Syd would continue floating along the middle path towards enlightenment, with deep meditation and spiritual awareness. I would live in true reality by being the master of my mind rather than suffering in a distressing dreamworld like the poor unhappy people who were controlled by their thoughts. It was time to spread loving kindness by greeting everyone I met with a friendly smile as well as being there for anyone who needed a shoulder to cry on. If you are feeling sad, lonely, depressed or afraid, then "Sit Down" next to me because as an empath I will listen, share your sorrow and provide comfort. I snuggled under the duvet and felt at one with "Mother Universe". I knew that if I dived deep into my soul, I would grow up to be a wise old man.

Loving and taking care of my kids would still be my primary focus and so far, so good as they were happy and healthy, therefore I gave myself a well-deserved pat on the back. And my best mate Alfie, who had always been there to listen to my sorrow, would continue being spoilt to death with treats, cuddles and lots of walkies. And not forgetting my walkies with the wonderful Miss Bombshell who I would meet once a week for a cuppa in a village café, a cheerful chat and some fresh countryside air.

On a more serious note, I must get my shit together and start flogging all the coffee that I had foolishly bought in a moment of madness. I would lose money for sure but at least I hadn't lost my life. And it was vital that I stood side-by-side with poor Ian as he walked along the "Boulevard of Broken Dreams" I would be with him every bit of the way and help all I can because I had walked that road and fully understood the horror of each painful step. I was all alone and it almost killed me so I would be there for Ian 24 hours a day.

And as I continued to fight the cancer and regain my health it would be imperative to have a dream in my heart. The inspirational dream was to relocate to an island in Thailand with my kids and Alfie to make a brand-new life. The target was to be living in the land of smiles by 2020, because paradise was my home.

What about love and lust? Would I ever taste romance again? Bloody hell, would I ever make love again? Well, you can bet your arse that continuing to trudge about with a face like sour milk, feeling ugly and unworthy, would make the fairer sex run a country mile. However, with my new self-belief, my Manc charm, crazy sense of humour, flirty cheek and cocky pizzazz, I may well be in with a seductive scream of attracting a compatible playmate. If a femme fatale refused to snog my ghoulish gaunt mug then she wouldn't be the one for me, would she? But if she kissed my monster heart then she may well be the baby to "Light my Fire". Anyway, I must stop banging on forever about my future life between the sheets and live as a happy single bloke in the here and now. "Life's What You Make It".

And finally, it was time to pick a raw nerve and consider the Wicked Witch of the East. For my sanity, I would have to let go of my anger and bitterness towards my ex-partner, because I was only hurting myself. It had absolutely no effect on her because she would be oblivious to my angst and anger as she lived blissfully in her new life. I was a forgotten man who was poisoning himself daily with blind hatred towards someone who didn't give a rat's arse whether he lived or died. It was time to face the truth…I would never be with her again.

And would I have been happier if she had returned once more to scream at me in a psychotic fury because I still hadn't kicked the bucket? Would I have coped with more of her infidelity as she laughed in my face while describing her latest sexual encounter? No thanks, I couldn't live through that nightmare again. I should thank my lucky milky ways that she was a long way away. And when all is said and done, she didn't belong to me. She wasn't my slave, was she? She was free to love and hate whoever she liked. She had wanted to leave and begin a new life away from me and that was her choice.

So, my beautiful disaster, you should live your dreams and enjoy happiness while you still can because life is a funny old game and who knows what painful tragedy is around the next corner. Enjoy the good times while you can. I have heard that time is a great healer; and I sincerely hope that one day in the future I will be able to think about her without feeling hurt and be able to forgive her completely.

I lay back on my bed with newfound belief. I felt like the dog's bollocks. It was all in the mind and I had changed my mind which had changed my life. The world looked very different today; it was wonderful being alive. My soul danced with joy as I pictured myself standing in the light at the end of a long dark tunnel. I put my hands together once more and prayed to God, thanking him because I realised that heaven was on Earth. My psychedelic eyes sparkled with dreams as my happy Mancunian gob announced, "Syd, you must shine on like a crazy diamond."

And it's time to let the pussy cat out of the bag and let you know that I had a date later that New Year's Day. I was meeting a lovely vegan lady I had been flirting with on a spiritual dating site. With my new euphoric attitude, I was buzzing at the prospect; in fact, I was mad for it. However, this time there would be a couple of cheeky vegan condoms stashed in my ball-hugging blue jeans pocket because as Finbarr Saunders would say… the only way is up.

The future is bright; the future is Psycho.

Epilogue

Is This the End?

Is this the end? Well, my fellow voyager, no it isn't, in fact, far from it because we are only halfway there. And what do you think of it so far? Hopefully not rubbish. When I began scribbling this tale the plan was to have the complete trip in one book, but I soon realised I would have to split it into two; just like my "Achy Breaky Heart". As you know from experience, the first half of the trip, "Foxtrot Uniform Charlie Kilo" was a heart-stopping dark journey of pain and wretchedness, but I am glad to inform you that the second half, "I am the Resurrection" will be an uplifting page-turning adventure. You will be chuffed to hear that it will yet again be scrawled in my unique colourful style with strange wordplay, gobsmacking anecdotes and of course dollops of naughty but nice humour.

And let me give you a big high five my intrepid mate, for your courageous "Never Say Die" spirit during *The Perfect Storm*. The mountainous waves and the gale-force winds screaming under the angry black clouds on our journey were not for the lily-livered, were they? Yet you stood firm as Poseidon in his rage slammed his gigantic watery fists against our struggling battered vessel. His younger brother Zeus was no better, wickedly splitting the sky with jagged forks of white-hot lightning, followed by terrifying ear-shattering booms of wild thunder. We both looked to the sky and cursed that one-eyed bastard the Cyclops for handing the king of the Greek gods his weapon of choice: the thunderbolt. You were right beside me as we boldly stood as one, facing the fury of this savage turbulent tempest. Heavens above, it looked a dead certainty that we were doomed, soon to be a tasty snack for the fishes at the bottom of the sea, yet we heroically fought for our lives and miraculously survived. So, a massive ta very much for standing by me in my hour of need.

And just look at the reward for your bravery. Not a shiny medal but an extended, well-deserved time-out to chill on this gorgeous tropical island in the sun where our weather-beaten sailing ship has just dropped anchor. We could be here all summer, as we get our galleon shipshape for the final leg of this wondrous odyssey. Well, it could be a much worse place, like back in rainy Blackpool, couldn't it?

So, make the most of it and walk barefoot along the idyllic white sandy beaches while observing the fabulous seabirds. However, there will be no Honolulu "Peaches" wearing grass skirts with seductive 'come and get me eyes', to ogle at on these beaches, because our "Island in the Sun" is uninhabited. Why not go inland and shower under magical waterfalls, bathe in hot springs, explore magnificent caverns, walk through steamy jungles and climb the highest mountain for breathtaking views of paradise. Drink from the revitalising mineral-rich freshwater streams, feast on bananas, coconuts and all the other nutritious tropical fruits and take photographs of the abundant wild creatures living freely here.

You are fully aware that this is a trip of compassion and no sentient being will be killed and eaten as we travel towards the truth. Just be at one with the spiders, lizards, birds of paradise, wild pigs, snakes and psychedelic fishes in the sea and smile, because Nirvana here we come. Live blissfully on this dreamy island as you recuperate in paradise. Then before you know it you will be jumping aboard the good ship Psycho for the second episode of this fantastic voyage.

You are bound to have countless things on your mind. Will Psycho Syd beat the big C and get the all-clear? And what about his friend Ian? Will he miraculously defeat his terminal illness, or will the bastard Grim Reaper lead him by the hand to the other side? Will the Wicked Witch of the East suddenly mutate into the Good Witch of the North and return some of the money that she has effectively stolen? Will pigs fly? Will Syd manage to flog the coffee? Will his kids grow up happy and do well at school? Will Alfie still be loving life with the Psycho Syd tribe? Will Syd ever fall in love again? And finally, will Psycho Syd end up living ecstatically as an enlightened spiritual being or will he be living orgasmicaly as a well up for it, ladies' man. Well don't worry because you will find out during the subsequent part of the journey but in the meantime, sunbathe on the beach and turn "Golden Brown." This is a happy place where there is no time to frown. Enjoy it while you can.

I must stress that everything in this book is true. I couldn't make all that shit up, could I? I know it is true and you know it is true but if any smart-arse would like to challenge me then go for it, but the only outcome would be the doubting Thomas looking like a clown with vegan egg on his face while swallowing a big slice of humble pie. I am up for taking any lie detector test that you are willing to pay for. If it is proven that I am telling porky pies then I will cover the costs, leaving you with a victorious, 'I told you so' smirk on your mush. This only includes the major points of course so don't be a pedantic pleb by pointing out something like 'you wrote that you ate chips and beans when in fact you had chips and peas. Sad that I had to point that out but there are a lot of sad shitty arseholes in the world as you know. Anyway, I doubt that anyone is mug enough to take me on coz it is as plain as the hooter on your face that I don't do lies.

Now another thing I need to clarify is that I did not scribble this tale in a pathetic revengeful attempt to paint my missus blacker than black. My only motive for publishing this book was to flee a glum existence on benefits. I knew that I was clutching at straws, but I had a dream in my heart that maybe Lady Luck would smile on me and make it a success, to give me and my kids a better life. I knew the odds were stacked against me, but I could see no other way. And believe me, it has been almost four years of sorrow, despair and regret visiting those dark days.

Initially, I was bitter and angry and in shock at being ditched in my hour of need by the woman I worshipped and trusted. Who wouldn't be? However, over time as I grew spiritually my heart began to soften with compassion and understanding. I merely wrote my account of the events that took place. My emotions, my feelings, my fears, my pain were written straight from my shredded heart. These events did occur, and this book describes them from my point of view. However, if my wife was to give her version of the story it would be very different, wouldn't it? Remember, there are always two sides to every story.

Maybe her version would be something like this? I was born in a very poor family in Laos. One day a friend of mine introduced me to an older Englishman who was fluent in the Lao language. I saw this as my only opportunity to escape poverty. (A bit like my dream of writing this book lol.) Therefore, I decided to marry him and have a baby which would ensure I would be able to live in comfort for the rest of my days. I did my best for him and took care of his young son from a previous marriage too. However, the truth is that I never really loved him. Even so I enjoyed the comfortable lifestyle, holidays overseas, new clothes and it was amazing when he bought a house, ensuring I would always have something of value. When he was diagnosed with cancer, I was excited to travel to the UK and really did feel sorry for my husband. At this time, it was unfortunate because I now felt trapped and began to hate him. I needed to get away. I was contacted on Facebook by attractive males much closer to my age and hated being a married to my old husband. In my terrible frustration I said some terrible things to him and to my son too, in my desperation to be free. Eventually I got free but had to pay the heavy price of losing my son. So, as you can see life hasn't been easy for me either, has it?

That is just a guess of course because I have absolutely no idea what is in her skull. Therefore, I ask you to see things from her side too and feel compassion because it obviously wasn't a stroll in the park for her, was it Everyone has their own tale to tell and everyone has their own thoughts and feelings. You must walk in their shoes to see things from their perspective. I have less anger towards her now but still feel hurt by her betrayal. Of course, my mind often wanders to the past, recalling romantic days with my perfect partner in my perfect place, yet now I feel both happy and sad, there isn't the painful stab of gut-wrenching heartache I had a year back.

After walking in the Wicked Witch's shoes, a startling realisation slapped me in the face. She was my perfect partner, yet I wasn't her perfect partner, was I? And her discontent at being married to a man purely for economic reasons and not romantic love created an angry thunderstorm in her mind, invoking a tornado of abuse towards the cause of her misery; poor old me. But when you think about it, poor young her too. She was dreaming of escaping her imperfect partner to find true love while I was dreaming of staying together with my perfect partner. We were both suffering. Love isn't for the faint-hearted is it?

I recalled a story I had heard many moons ago. It was about two ex-prisoners of war who meet again after many years. The first one asked, "Have you forgiven your captors?" The second man answered, "No, never." The first man replied, "Well, you are still in prison then, aren't you?" Upon pondering this old story, I saw the truth, opened my cell door and walked out. As I forgave the Wicked Witch my inner pain left my soul. The chains to the past were snapped and I smiled like a wise old man as an overwhelming weight was lifted off my heart.

It was time to move on. Now, forgiveness is not weak, in fact, it takes courage to forgive those that have hurt us. However, we must understand what and why the harm, pain and wrongdoing occurred and take steps to ensure that we never permit the same things to happen to us again. For such a long time I had been strangled by horror, confusion, grief, pain and rage, unable to flee my self-imprisonment. The wisdom of this revelation is that when you let go of your anger, resentment and bitterness you stop harming yourself. By forgiving and allowing your maltreater to go free you also free yourself.

Anyway, my fellow crew member, that is my final spiritual message, so go forth and enjoy your stay after overcoming the harrowing part of the trip. I am already writing "I Am the Resurrection" and believe me there will be as many crazy twists and turns as you discovered in the first book. You will love it, and this will be the uplifting part of the voyage that we all deserve.

Love, Compassion and Peace to all Sentient Beings

Psycho Syd

Dance to the Music

You don't have to be a "Rock and Roll" star to see that this story is littered with musical references. Psychedelic and Psycho Syd's love of music clearly vibrates on each page. I hope you enjoyed all the bands and song titles you encountered on the journey and that they made you smile as you took a trip along a tuneful memory Lane.

I have been careful not to steal song lyrics for two reasons. Firstly, I feel that it is better for me to write the content from my very own crazy mind and secondly song lyrics are copyright. The thought of scribbling this heartbreaking tale in a desperate effort to escape benefits only to be sued would be too much to bear. However, if anyone feels that a certain phrase I have written is a bit close to a song they own the rights for then please let me know and of course I will edit it out. It would have been an unintentional error on my part and as anyone who has read the story would know any two or three words in the tale would have absolutely no bearing on the popularity of the book.

Hopefully, that covers my God-given Manc arse and stops any greedy heartless bugger trying to smash the dream of a better life for me, my kids and my dog..

Here is a list the songs used for chapter headings and the bands they belong to. Have a listen if you get a moment

My Name is Psycho .... Goldblade

I Hope You Die .... The Bloodhound Gang

Living in the Past .... Jethro Tull

Sugar Sugar .... The Archies

There She Goes .... The La's

Fifteen Minutes of Fame .... Sheep on Drugs

Ever Fallen in Love .... The Buzzcocks

Welcome to Paradise .... Green Day

Run .... Snow Patrol

Psycho Killer .... Talking Heads

Jump .... Van Halen

Highway to Hell .... AC/DC

Beat It	Michael Jackson
The Prettiest Star	David Bowie
Welcome to the Machine	Pink Floyd
Burn	Deep Purple
Too Sick to Pray	Alabama 3
Wish You Were Here	Pink Floyd
Epitaph	King Crimson
Living on the Ceiling	Blancmange
Secret agent Man	Devo
Where is my Mind?	The Pixies
Gobbing on Life	The Albertos
Sound of Silence	Simon and Garfunkle
Danger Zone	Kenny Loggins
Fox on the Run	The Sweet
Chirpy Chirpy Cheep Cheep	Middle of the Road
The Leaving of Liverpool	The Dubliners
Lucky Man	The Verve
Break on Through	The Doors
I Believe in Father Christmas	Greg Lake
Goodbye Kiss	Kasabian
I Had Too Much to Dream Last Night .	The Electric Prunes
Dizzy	The Wonder Stuff
River Deep, Mountain High	Ike and Tina Turner
If I Had a Hammer	Peter, Paul and Mary
Wake me up When September Ends....	Green Day
Apeman	The Kinks
You're Unbelievable	EMF
Sex on Fire	Kings of Leon
Starman	David Bowie
Dead and Buried	Alien Sex Fiend
Dry Your Eyes	The Streets
Is This the End?	Creed

A Massive Ta Very Much
To These Wonderful People

So many people were part of my journey and gave me a helping hand.

Firstly, my brother Jeff and his wife Ann who were always there for me. They helped my mum in her hour of need too.

And my old school pal Janet and her sister Jackie supported me.

Miss Bombshell who kept me sane.

Friends overseas including Bob, John, Vaughan, Peter, Tony and Jean-Luc. Heather Doyle who helped to proofread and Jon my editor.

Julie Cotterill and Jojo Bison-Dyke had some input too.

Keith Hoare of Ragged Cover Publishing who took me under his wing and helped make this book a reality.

Antonietta was an angel who appeared at just the right time.

Sandy the dizzy blonde and Anne Marie Nugent too.

Dan the man was a hero who did so much for me.

All the teachers and staff at Bispham Endowed Primary School who supported me and my kids during the dark days.

And Chris Curtis and The Swallows Head and Neck Cancer Support Group and Melanie Gamble at Together Against Cancer. I spent many an afternoon with the amazing Cleveleys Writers.

Not forgetting Peter Jefferson of Visionistic Photography who snapped the image of my ugly mug on the cover.

And my son Eugene for designing the cover.

My other three kids, Panvilas, Francesca and Jo who were there. And Alfie my faithful rescue staffy who never left my side.

The amazing Ken of Blake Mill artisan shirts who supplied me with so many fabulous shirts to wear at my events

All the hospital staff who looked after me during the nightmare including Jo Ashton, Mr. Nigam, Mr Kasmi and a Czech Oncoligist whose name I forget.

Craig at Purple Custard and John Flanagan for his advice.

I will no doubt have forgotten to include some people who should be here but will ensure they are mentioned in part two once my foggy mind remembers. All apologies

Also, all the other wonderful people who stood by me.

I love you all. xx

315

Lightning Source UK Ltd.
Milton Keynes UK
UKHW010210061122
411729UK00001B/33